ESSENTIAL DECISION MAKING AND CLINICAL JUDGEMENT FOR NURSES

Commissioning Editors: Steven Black, Mairi McCubbin
Development Editor: Sally Davies
Project Manager: Christine Johnston
Design Direction: George Ajayi
Illustration Manager: Merlyn Harvey
Illustrator: Chartwell

ESSENTIAL DECISION MAKING AND CLINICAL JUDGEMENT FOR NURSES

EDITED BY

Carl Thompson BSc(Hons) PhD RN
Senior Lecturer, Department of Health Sciences, University of York, York, UK

Dawn Dowding BSc(Hons) PhD RGN
Senior Lecturer in Clinical Decision Making, Department of Health Sciences,
The Hull York Medical School, University of York, York, UK

Foreword by
Anne Marie Rafferty CBE BSc MPhil DPhil(Oxon) RGN DN FRCN
Professor of Nursing Policy and Dean of the Florence Nightingale School of
Nursing and Midwifery, King's College London, London, UK

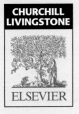

CHURCHILL
LIVINGSTONE

ELSEVIER

EDINBURGH LONDON NEW YORK OXFORD PHILADELPHIA ST LOUIS SYDNEY TORONTO 2009

CHURCHILL
LIVINGSTONE
ELSEVIER

First published 2009, © Elsevier Limited. All rights reserved.

No part of this publication may be reproduced or transmitted in any form or by any means, electronic or mechanical, including photocopying, recording, or any information storage and retrieval system, without permission in writing from the publisher. Permissions may be sought directly from Elsevier's Rights Department: phone: (+1) 215 239 3804 (US) or (+44) 1865 843830 (UK); fax: (+44) 1865 853333; e-mail: www.healthpermissions@elsevier.com. You may also complete your request online via the Elsevier website at http://www.elsevier.com/permissions.

ISBN 978-0-443-06727-3

British Library Cataloguing in Publication Data
A catalogue record for this book is available from the British Library

Library of Congress Cataloging in Publication Data
A catalog record for this book is available from the Library of Congress

Notice
Neither the Publisher nor the Editors assume any responsibility for any loss or injury and/or damage to persons or property arising out of or related to any use of the material contained in this book. It is the responsibility of the treating practitioner, relying on independent expertise and knowledge of the patient, to determine the best treatment and method of application for the patient.

The Publisher

your source for books, journals and multimedia in the health sciences

www.elsevierhealth.com

Working together to grow
libraries in developing countries

www.elsevier.com | www.bookaid.org | www.sabre.org

ELSEVIER   BOOK AID
            International   Sabre Foundation

The publisher's policy is to use paper manufactured from sustainable forests

Printed in China

CONTENTS

CONTENTS

CONTRIBUTORS

Martin Bland MSc PhD DIC ARCS FSS HonMRCR
Professor of Health Statistics, Department of Health Sciences,
University of York, York, UK

Dawn Dowding BSc(Hons) PhD RGN
Senior Lecturer in Clinical Decision Making, Department of Health
Sciences, The Hull York Medical School, University of York, York, UK

Jo C. Dumville MSc PhD
Research Fellow, Department of Health Sciences, University of York,
York, UK

Vikki Entwistle MA MSc PhD
Associate Director, Social Dimensions of Health Institute, Reader,
Professor of Values in Health Care, University of Dundee, Dundee, UK

Marta Soares MSc
Research Fellow, Department of Health Sciences, University of York,
York, UK

Carl Thompson BA(Hons) PhD RN
Senior Lecturer, Department of Health Sciences, University of York,
York, UK

Ian S. Watt BSc MB ChB MPH FFPH
Professor of Primary Care, The Hull York Medical School,
University of York, York, UK

FOREWORD

It is rare to find a volume which captures the challenge of clinical decision making in such a sensitive and sophisticated manner but this book pulls it off with flamboyance and flair. It also manages to sidestep the classic pitfalls of the genre where the omniscient author dispenses wisdom from afar, often in a patronising tone. The expert 'voice' in this case recognises that it is uncertainty and contingency that often pose the greatest challenge to decision making in clinical care. Moreover it addresses the topsy-turvy world of the busy clinician as much as the academic, managerial and patient communities, all of whom have an important stake in the outcomes of clinical care.

This book offers a fresh and open approach to clinical reasoning and support systems using a range of disciplinary perspectives to tell its story. It argues that it is principle and pragmatism that make up the cocktail of clinical acumen and recognises that we do not live in a perfect world: trade offs have to be made. Over time we have evolved rules and tools to help us cope with the variation that patients bring with them to the clinic. Heuristics, the cognitive short cuts we take in arriving at decisions, fast and frugal reasoning, satisficing and what we do to reach a given level of satisfaction are techniques we use to systematise our thinking. While some of these processes benefit from the insights of cognitive psychology, economics, statistics and assessments of risk, all impinge on the process. As this volume demonstrates there is a serious science to the art of clinical reasoning. The great strength of this volume is that it offers insights into concepts and principles that underpin some of these processes. Peering into the black box of decision making helps to unpack the pattern recognition, the puzzles we solve, the strategies we deploy to do so. This transparency helps to teach the skills and to examine how we as nurses stack up as clinicians. We need to do more of it. How else can we advance the art and science of nursing? We need to be prepared to benchmark ourselves against others and pull up performance where it falls short. We cannot do that without the confidence to question and that confidence comes from sound and rigorous clinical reasoning. We owe it to the profession, we owe it to our colleagues and fellow clinicians, and most of all we owe it to the public we serve. This book is most definitely a tonic that deserves to be taken in large doses.

London, 2009   Anne Marie Rafferty

PREFACE

Few nurses can have avoided the exhortation to become 'evidence-based' decision makers in the past decade. In theory, this sounds like a simple enough statement. In practice, however, decision-making ability is not something that we all share in equal amounts. Making choices requires the right skills and knowledge and a means of combining these correctly.

In this book we describe some of the skills and knowledge that nurses require to enable them to make decisions that consist of more than just good quality (but oh-so-variable) guesswork and professional intuition. We also try and go beyond simply presenting this information by illustrating ways of actually using the skills and knowledge to reach choices.

The book is aimed at the full range of nurses and other healthcare professionals from a variety of professional areas and at varying levels of expertise: from the first-year student nurse to the most experienced nurse consultant or specialist. In 2002, we edited a book with a similar title, *Clinical Decision Making and Judgement in Nursing* (Thompson and Dowding, 2002). Since then, many people have used the book and contacted us with their experiences, both good and bad. We have listened and tried to learn from the good ones and address the less positive in this text – an exercise that itself is a microcosm of the learning that must accompany good decision making! There are more exercises, more practical examples, more interactive components and a whole new set of chapters in areas that thus far have not been part of a text such as this for nurses.

The book remains an intentionally multidisciplinary endeavour built around a nursing focus, with input from a statistician, economists, a social scientist, and a GP. We have both benefited from being exposed to research methods taught by epidemiologists, health economics taught by economists, and psychology from psychologists. We think that nursing (and nurses) benefit from being exposed to those with the most relevant knowledge to help us solve the problems we all face. Sometimes, this knowledge doesn't come from nurses.

We hope that this book opens your eyes to the practice, research and educational possibilities that the field of decision making and judgement offers nursing. Please do not skip over the practical exercises. They are meant to be fun as well as instructional. Likewise, although few people like mathematics please don't avoid the theoretical or 'number-rich' chapters. Who knows, you might find – as we did – that once someone puts probability in context it is actually understandable *and* helps improve your choices.

We cannot promise that all the choices we made in the writing and production of this book were good ones. Let us know of the ones that you think can be improved; we promise we will at least listen. We hope that you will do the same with the ideas in Essential Clinical Decision Making and Judgement for Nurses.

York, 2008

Carl Thompson
Dawn Dowding

ACKNOWLEDGEMENTS

I would like to thank Issy, Lily, Spillers and all at the University of York (staff and students) who together constitute some of my better decisions. They also happen to be on the receiving end of my less-than-optimal ones, and yet remain tolerant of my need to learn.

Carl Thompson

I would like to thank John and Iddy for their constant support and understanding during the production of this book. Thanks should also go to my parents, Fay Dowding, friends and colleagues (past and present), who have been a constant source of guidance and advice for decisions taken, good and bad! Finally, thank you to all the students I have had the privilege of teaching and supervising to date. Their experiences and questions are the basis of many of the examples used in this book.

Dawn Dowding

Introduction

Carl Thompson and Dawn Dowding

There is nothing new about nurses and midwives using their clinical judgement, wisdom and foresight to make good quality choices. Mary Seacole used her knowledge and systematic observations in the 1850s to relieve the impact of cholera in Jamaica. Similarly, Florence Nightingale (often called a pioneer of clinical epidemiology) used systematic observation and recording of data to fight for improved conditions and resources in Scutari. Technology has improved, roles have changed, patients' expectations have developed, and knowledge (actually, information) has grown exponentially. At the heart of the healthcare endeavour, however, are professionals judging the value of perceptual and clinical information and making choices that provide more benefit to patients than harm.

The problem with delivering healthcare is that it is uncertain. Our choices have to be made (and they do have to be made) in the full knowledge that not everyone with certain symptoms will have a disease or be in a given health state, not everyone we provide with the most 'evidence-based' intervention will improve, and not everyone will feel the same about their future health and healthcare. Uncertainty is the only certainty in health. The problem for nurses, and the profession of nursing, is that we have traditionally taught nurses for certainty, as opposed to the uncertainty they will encounter as clinicians. They learn 'facts' about the causes of health states, what happens as a result of our interventions, and what happens to patients over the course of time. Once these facts are acquired we rely on 'reflection', a smattering of continuing professional development (usually consisting of more 'facts'), unsystematic observation and 'knowing' based on our own experience to marshal them(Thompson et al 2001, 2004). Most nurses, however, do not need to know more facts about diabetes, heart disease, anxiety and depression, or venous leg ulceration. Instead, they need to be able to make better use of the knowledge that they already have in the context of the uncertain world in which they make choices with patients. Knowing that type 1 diabetes is caused by the pancreas not producing enough insulin is important but probably doesn't help when a primary-care nurse practitioner is faced with a 20-year-old patient complaining of 'being thirsty all the time', 'peeing loads', 'feeling knackered', and 'having lost loads of weight'. What the nurse needs in this situation is a different kind of knowledge: given this constellation of signs what should I be thinking about? And – just as importantly – what should I be doing?

This book is about this different kind of knowledge and the way in which we can use it as nurses. It is a book that deals with the processes and outcomes of judgement and decision making in nursing. It is unashamedly *not* a 'how to' textbook of protocols or a 'cook book' of actions for given sets of circumstances (alternative texts that fulfil this task). Equally, although we are by nature 'evidence-based' clinicians and teachers, this is not a text on evidence-based practice and the science of critical appraisal; again, there are many such texts on the market that deal with this as a topic in its own right.

This book takes a deliberately multidisciplinary perspective on nursing decisions. The science of decision making and judgement is not the province of any one academic discipline. Psychologists, economists, statisticians, nurses, doctors, philosophers, and sometimes talented combinations of most of these (Eddy 1990), all contribute to our understanding of how we reach judgements and exercise choice. Any text that seeks to understand judgement and decision making needs to embrace the perspectives that each of these disciplines brings. That said, we have tried, where possible to draw on examples of relevance to most nurses.

Some of our examples are derived from roles that represent the outer boundaries of the profession, especially when dealing with the diagnostic, prognostic, and interventional choices that nurses face. This is intentional; roles such as nurse consultants, nurse practitioners and some of the specialist roles that have developed specifically around judgement and decision making (such as triage and critical-care outreach nurses), are a rich source of examples of clinicians grappling (by and large successfully) with uncertainty in a very visible way. However, just because decisions are relatively visible in these areas does not mean that 'ordinary' staff nurses in non-acute areas face any less of a judgement and decision challenge in their daily work. Nursing is, above all, about communication, and a key part of that communication is around the judgement that accompanies being presented with physical and verbal 'signs' (or cues) as to the underlying state of the patient: the wavering voice of an anxious patient, the clammy and pale skin of a patient whose haemodynamic status is compromised, the characteristic smell and look of a patient whose faeces contains fresh blood. From the day they enter practice, nurses must become adept at recognising not just the presence of such cues but the *value* of them for their judgements and choices.

WHAT ARE JUDGEMENTS AND DECISIONS?

It is probably helpful right at the beginning of this book to clarify what we mean when we talk about judgements and decisions. The nursing literature uses a number of terms to describe the same phenomena: clinical decision making (Field 1987), clinical judgement (Benner & Tanner 1987, Itano 1989), clinical inference (Hammond et al 1966), clinical reasoning (Grobe et al 1991) and diagnostic reasoning (Radwin 1990). However, in this book we consider them as two separate entities, which entail different types of thought process. Depending on the topic we are discussing, this distinction varies in its importance. However, and particularly when we are concerned with either trying to *describe* how nurses reach their judgements and decisions, or provide ways of *improving* those judgements and decisions, it is important to recognise exactly what it is we are describing or improving.

THE NATURE OF JUDGEMENT

In everyday life, we make judgements on people constantly (Weiss et al 2006): 'How attractive is that person?' 'Is this person being aggressive?' 'Is this person paying attention?' When these judgements are carried out in healthcare settings by professionals, they become 'clinical judgements'. Weiss et al (2006) suggest that these judgements should be considered as 'opinions' about other people. In healthcare, such opinions include health status and functional ability, or they may include predictions of future behaviour. Dowie (1993) provides us with a useful definition of judgement as, 'an assessment between alternatives'. The process of making a judgement involves the integration of information about a person (in nursing this could be information such as their vital sign readings, how they look, their medical condition, or their behaviour) to reach an evaluation or assessment of their state or condition (Crow et al 1995, Maule 2001).

Nursing practice is characterised by making judgements. Studies that have examined the focus of nursing practice suggest that nurses spend a lot of their time identifying clinical deterioration, assessing the patient's current and previous condition, and predicting future events (Cioffi 1998, 2000a, 2000b, Lamond et al 1996). In a study examining how nurses in acute medical and surgical wards carry out patient assessment, Lamond et al (1996) identified four different types of judgements made by nurses. A typology of judgements taken from this work, together with the evidence from studies by Cioffi (2000a, 2000b, 1998) is provided in Table 1.1.

Distinguishing between types of judgement might, at first glance, be difficult. The excerpt in Box 1.1 is data from a recent study carried out by the authors when they were examining how heart-failure specialist nurses make decisions during patient consultations. We have highlighted where the nurse reports different types of judgement. Also, note that most of the judgements the nurse makes are based on information collected about, or from, the patient.

CLINICAL DECISIONS

In contrast to clinical judgements, clinical decisions have been defined as, 'a *choice* between alternatives' (Dowie 1993). Like all choices, clinical decisions produce some kind of outcome, i.e. an action: to do (or not do) something. Decisions in healthcare are usually made under conditions of uncertainty: we do not know (with certainty) what will happen because of our decision

Table 1.1   Types of judgement

Type of judgement	Definition	Example
Causal judgement (diagnosis)	A statement expressing a state or condition based on the presence of attributes that are used to explain a problem	Nurse diagnoses the cause of a patient's incontinence (based on information collected during a full assessment)
Descriptive judgement	A statement expressing a state or condition based on the presence of attributes that had been observed directly or obtained from another source	Nurse judges that the patient is 'stable' (based on information collected during an assessment)
Evaluative judgement	A statement expressing a qualitative difference in a state or condition based on the presence of attributes that had been observed directly or obtained from another source	Nurse judges that the patient's condition has 'deteriorated' (based on information collected about the patient at this point in time, compared with a previous occasion)
Predictive judgement	A statement expressing a belief in the likely course of a patient's state or condition, based on presence of attributes that had been observed directly or obtained from another source	Nurse judges that the patient will have problems postoperatively (based on information collected about the patient preoperatively)

Adapted from Lamond et al (1996) and Cioffi (1998).

Box 1.1   An example of clinical judgements in practice

Although he's generally unwell (*descriptive judgement*), he wasn't dramatically worse than he had been (*evaluative judgement*), ... we started to through things like blood pressure, blood pressure OK (*descriptive judgement*), did his heart rate and it was 30, so it was, 'Oops' and obviously you're stopped in your tracks because there's something not quite right here (*descriptive judgement*) and went back over things, what's happened, what drugs was he on and we actually hadn't altered any of his medication. So we had to try and work it back and there wasn't anything obvious but obviously there had been some kind of acute event or some acute change (*causal judgement*), so we had to organise an ECG. No – in fact we didn't – we discussed it with the consultant and because of his age and he was so slow we actually admitted him (*decision*) and it turned out that he was in complete heart block, possibly related to his beta-blockers or an ischaemic event because he was a diabetic (*causal judgement/diagnosis*).

---

or action. In clinical decision making, the process involves the weighing up of the potential costs and benefits associated with each option you are considering, before deciding on a course of action (Baron 2000).

Nurses make a variety of different types of decision in clinical practice (a typology of the decisions nurses make is given in Chapter 2, p. 15). Decisions normally follow judgements, for instance in the example given in Box 1.1, the nurse has made a number of judgements: the patient is 'unwell', that his problem has 'probably' been caused by a 'new' event. On the basis of these judgements (as well as in discussion with the consultant) the nurse decides that the best course of action (i.e. the decision) is to admit the patient to hospital.

Judgements and decisions are closely related, and both elements can contribute to the appropriateness of a nurse's eventual actions. For instance, a nurse might make an accurate judgement based on the information they process about the patient (e.g. 'this patient is in extreme pain') but then go on to choose an inappropriate action (e.g. 'I will give her a heat pad'). Alternatively, a nurse might make a poor judgement (e.g. 'the patient's pain is due to indigestion', when in fact it is cardiac pain) but make a good decision on the basis of the poor judgement (e.g. 'I will give him indigestion medication'). What we strive for in clinical practice is a situation where, on the basis of an accurate evaluation of the patient's condition, the nurse takes appropriate action. How we can achieve this aim is the focus of much of the rest of this book.

WHY NURSES NEED TO KNOW ABOUT DECISION MAKING

Nurses' work is shaped by the organisational, professional, and regulatory frameworks within which they must operate. For nurses in many developed health systems, the past decade has seen a focus on clinical governance, regulation linked to professional competence, and patient safety. This focus, due in part to a recognition of the limitations (as well as strengths) of unaided and autonomous decision making by professionals, represents both a challenge and an opportunity for nurses. The challenge is to continue to develop nursing in ways that provide enough freedom to practise and to exercise judgement with the minimum of interference in the relationship between the patient and the nurse. The opportunity is to rethink the ways in which we train, develop, and self-regulate the profession; as well as the ways in which we establish and market our contribution to enhanced patient outcomes. Research by Scott et al (1999) has highlighted the contribution (on a population level) of skilled nursing care to patient outcomes. Although this is a valuable piece of work, the puzzle for the profession is to establish *why* some nurses produce better outcomes than others. We believe that one of the distinguishing factors that marks out exceptional nurses is their skill in judgement and decision making. There are many such nurses in existence – some feature in the seminal work of Patricia Benner (1984). We need – somehow – to describe and transfer (to other nurses) some of their decision-making skills; this book is designed to encourage the profession to engage in this debate.

THE STRUCTURE OF THE BOOK

To equip the reader with the tools needed to engage in the debate regarding the role of nurses in healthcare decision making, we have designed the book around six key themes.

1. Introducing and describing uncertainty

Chapters 2 and 3 are designed to introduce the concept of uncertainty to the reader. Uncertainty will be nothing new to most nurses. What we strive to do in these first two chapters is to provide some ways of *thinking* about and *talking* about uncertainty that may be new to many nurses. The rationale for placing uncertainty at the core of the book is because it is at the core of judgements and decisions, particularly when they go wrong. Uncertainty is not necessarily a negative force in healthcare; without some uncertainty in the future, there can be no hope. And it is hope that feeds the human condition. However, to stop uncertainty denigrating the choices of nurses and patients, it must be managed. Like all forms of management, without a grounding in the basics of the object, person or phenomenon that you seek to influence, you will invariably fail. Chapters 2 and 3 aim to ensure that you have this grounding.

2. Theories of judgement and decision making

'Theory' has something of a bad reputation for many nurses. The separation of theory from practice is something that many students (and teachers) have bemoaned and struggled with for many years. However, theory is not all bad. It connects concepts that might otherwise remain disconnected, abstract, and irrelevant. It weaves a coherent explanation around otherwise hard-to-unpick events, phenomena, and experiences. In short, theory helps us understand. Chapter 4 touches on both *how* nurses engage with information in the context of clinical decision making and *how they could* engage with the masses of information that exist on paper and in cyberspace. Chapter 5 explores the means by which we make our judgement-calls and choices. If we are to influence choices, we need to understand the role of the 'raw ingredients' required: cognition, information, memory, context. When we locate what really matters for nurses' decision making, we can begin to refine and improve the processes involved and the outcomes generated. Chapter 6 asks a fundamental question that many nurses ask us in our teaching sessions: 'What are good decisions?' In our day-to-day lives, we all need standards, criteria, and benchmarks against which to compare ourselves. Sometimes these are moral, sometimes logical; sometimes they are social in that they come from those around us. Chapter 6 discusses the complexities of trying to identify how we can evaluate the quality of our judgement and decision making.

3. When decision making goes wrong

Any nurse practising for an appreciable length of time will encounter errors and mistakes at the sharp end of clinical practice. After all, if 1 in 10 patients experience an adverse event while in hospital (Sari et al 2007) then it stands to reason that at least some nurses will encounter the same events. Just as good outcomes generated by receiving healthcare can be laid (at least in part) to the decisions made by nurses and doctors, the flip side is that the bad outcomes and iatrogenic harms that befall (too) many patients can also often be traced back to judgements and choices by professionals. Chapter 7 highlights the causative factors that lie behind many of these mistakes. Often, simply being aware of these factors is enough to prevent some common and entirely predictable flaws in our reasoning around decision making. Chapter 8 goes beyond this individual awareness strategy (valuable though it is) and asks 'What can we do at the organisational level to promote more good decisions than bad?'. It shows how relatively small changes to the 'way we do things round here' can have profound effects on systems, the people who work in them, and the patients who hope to benefit from them.

4. Assisting nurses' decision making

At the core of evidence-based approaches to decision making is the axiom, 'match the research evidence you bring to your reasoning to the kind of uncertainty you are faced with'. Just as the 'rules' of randomisation and blinding in a clinical trial can lead to unbiased, reliable, and valid results when examining 'what works', so there are rules for different kinds of reasoning given the uncertainty you are faced with. Thinking about a diagnostic problem requires different ingredients and processes for handling the probabilities involved, than for thinking about the future (prognosis), and for deciding whether choice A is more likely to be effective than choice B. Chapters 9, 10, and 11 look at the three main challenges facing the nurse decision maker: (1) how to classify objects based on incomplete information (diagnosis); (2) how to think about the future when all you have is the here and now and research derived from other peoples' futures (prognosis); and (3) how to balance the likelihood of outcomes occurring with how patients feel about the desirability of those outcomes (decision analysis). Having equipped the reader with some of the tools needed for handling probabilities from research and patient values, Chapter 12 provides a basic toolkit for getting to grips with the final piece of the evidence-based jigsaw: economic resources. Jo Dumville and Marta Soares steer us through making sense of economic analyses of the trade-off between the costs and benefits of healthcare.

5. Communicating with patients

Just as a huge proportion of nursing revolves around communication, so decision making (especially informed and shared decision making) also relies on communication. In Chapter 13, Vikki Entwistle and Ian Watt discuss how we can effectively involve patients in decision making about their care. In Chapter 14, we specifically look at ways in which complex ideas of risk, harm, and benefits can be communicated to patients. Decision making is rarely a solo activity and these two chapters are designed to ensure that both nurses and patients can take part in the dialogue that needs to happen before we can truly say that we have listened to what the patient wants.

6. Teaching

A large part of our lives for the past 10 years has involved teaching decision-making and judgement skills and knowledge to others. We use Chapter 15 to pass on some of the techniques that have served us well. When we produced our first book on clinical decision making and judgement in 2002 (Thompson & Dowding 2002) we neglected the needs of those tasked with preparing the next generation of nurse decision makers; we hope that Chapter 15 and the exercises included in it go someway to rectifying this.

Getting nurses to acknowledge and then use the necessary skills, tools, and knowledge to manage uncertainty in their reasoning and clinical decisions is a complicated business. We have tried to take the theoretical and research literature on clinical decision making and translate it into a form that, at the very least, serves to introduce the topics and skills that we think are of most use to nurses and nurse teachers. Policy makers the world over are busy constructing defensive layers to protect patients from the unavoidable errors that sometimes occur when professionals make choices. The uncomfortable reality for most patients (and, we suspect, for most policy makers) is that often the only effective barrier between the potential harms that accompany healthcare delivery are the communication, judgement, and decision skills of the professional making the choices with patients. This book is intended to strengthen this defence and ensure that nurses make better decisions.

Of course, as we will see, a proportion of errors will always creep into any complex professional task. With this in mind, we would like to confess right here – at the beginning – that any mistakes are entirely our fault. If you do spot any errors, please write to us and we promise to try and learn from them and do better next time.

REFERENCES

Baron J 2000 Thinking and deciding, 3rd edn. Cambridge University Press, Cambridge

Benner P 1984 From novice to expert: excellence and power in clinical nursing practice. Addison Wesley, Menlo Park, CA

Benner P, Tanner C 1987 How expert nurses use intuition. American Journal of Nursing 87(1):23–31

Cioffi J 1998 Decision making by emergency nurses in triage assessments. Accident and Emergency Nursing 6:184–191

Cioffi J 2000a Nurses' experiences of making decisions to call emergency assistance to their patients. Journal of Advanced Nursing 32(1):108–114

Cioffi J 2000b Recognition of patients who require emergency assistance: a descriptive study. Heart and Lung 29(4): 262–268

Crow R, Chase J, Lamond D 1995 The cognitive component of nursing assessment: an analysis. Journal of Advanced Nursing 22:206–212

Dowie J 1993 Clinical decision analysis: background and introduction. In: Llewelyn H, Hopkins A (eds) Analysing how we reach clinical decisions. Royal College of Physicians of London, London, p 7–26

Eddy D 1990 Clinical decision making: from theory to practice: the challenge. Journal of American Medical Association 263: 287–290

Field P A 1987 The impact of nursing theory on the clinical decision-making process. Journal of Advanced Nursing 12:563–571

Grobe S J, Drew J A, Fonteyn M E 1991 A descriptive analysis of experienced nurses' clinical reasoning during a planning task. Research in Nursing and Health 14:305–314

Hammond K R, Kelly K J, Castellan N J et al 1966 Clinical inference in nursing: use of information-seeking strategies by nurses. Nursing Research 15(4):330–336

Itano J K 1989 A comparison of the clinical judgment process in experienced registered nurses and student nurses. Journal of Nursing Education 28(3): 120–126

Lamond D, Crow R, Chase J 1996 Judgements and processes in care decisions in acute medical and surgical wards. Journal of Evaluation in Clinical Practice 2(3):211–216

Maule A J 2001 Studying judgement: some comments and suggestions for future research. Thinking and Reasoning 7(1):91–102

Radwin L E 1990 Research on diagnostic reasoning in nursing. Nursing Diagnosis 1(2):70–77

Sari A B A, Sheldon T A, Cracknell A et al 2007 Sensitivity of routine system for reporting patient safety incidents in an NHS hospital: retrospective patient case note review. British Medical Journal 334:79

Scott J G, Sochalski J, Aiken L 1999 Review of magnet hospital research: findings and implications for professional nursing practice. Journal of Nursing Administration 29(1):9–19

Thompson C, Dowding D 2002 Clinical decision making and judgement in nursing. Churchill Livingstone, Edinburgh

Thompson C, McCaughan D, Cullum N et al 2001 Research information in nurses' clinical decision making: what is useful? Journal of Advanced Nursing 36:376–388

Thompson C, Cullum N, McCaughan D, Sheldon T, Raynor P 2004 Nurses, information use, and clinical decision making – the real world potential for evidence-based decisions in nursing. Evidence-Based Nursing 7:68–72

Weiss D J, Shanteau J, Harries P 2006 People who judge people. Journal of Behavioral Decision Making 19:441–454

Uncertainty and nursing

Carl Thompson and Dawn Dowding

2

KEY ISSUES

- What is irreducible uncertainty and why does it matter?
- Clinical uncertainty is finite even if patients all differ
- Kinds of clinical uncertainty
- Sources of clinical uncertainty
- Some starting points for managing uncertainty in nursing

THE ONLY THING CERTAIN (IN NURSING) IS UNCERTAINTY

" We demand rigidly defined areas of doubt and uncertainty!
(Douglas Adams, *Hitchhiker's Guide to the Galaxy*) "

Nurses wishing to use their judgement and decision-making skills face a key challenge: each decision they make requires them to think about an uncertain future, in the present, using evidence that comes from a (more) certain past. As every healthcare professional knows, everyone is unique and no intervention ever leads with complete certainty to a given outcome. However, nurses still have to make decisions about what to do, given the uncertainty with which they are faced.

IRREDUCIBLE UNCERTAINTY

When you acknowledge the pervasive nature of uncertainty, it can sometimes feel as if healthcare is overwhelmingly characterised by the uncertain. You might feel that there is never enough information available to avoid feeling uncomfortable when faced with situations in which judgement is required or when faced with having to make clinical choices. If you have ever experienced these feelings then you will probably not need telling that uncertainty in healthcare is 'irreducible' (Eddy 1990). Irreducible uncertainty is uncertainty that cannot be reduced by *any* activity at the moment that action is required (Hammond 1996).

Despite the permanence of uncertainty in decision making, nurses (like all human beings) must learn to live with it. Uncertainty cannot be completely eliminated, and yet we all still face choices. At first glance, it might appear that uncertainty is something negative; something that detracts from our existence. This view of uncertainty would be wrong. Imagine a world in which, on reaching your 13th birthday, you would know with absolute certainty your future income levels, educational attainment, social class, the year and cause of your death. Having such knowledge might remove any incentives to work to improve the quality of your remaining life. It would impact on how you might view your role as parent, and even if you wanted to become a parent at all. It would affect who you married; it would impact on every aspect of who you are. Without uncertainty, as Hastie and Dawes remind us:

" ... there would be no hope, no ethics, and no freedom of choice. It is only because we do not know what the future holds for us that we can have hope. It is only because we do not know exactly the results of our choices that our choice can be free and pose a true ethical dilemma. (Hastie & Dawes 2001, p 328)"

Hope itself is a phenomenon that is central to how nurses shape their interactions with patients (Kylma & Vehvilainen-Julkunen 1997). By denying uncertainty, we fail to grasp the centrality of hope for patients.

Beginning to break down irreducible uncertainty: subjective and objective uncertainty

Not all things in life are uncertain; for example, it is certain that we will all die, we will all suffer ill health at some point, and we will always have to pay taxes! For these *classes* of event there is 100% certainty, and very little judgement is required regarding how likely they are. As a nurse, you will know that you must plan for patients dying eventually of something, as well as other certainties such as staff becoming sick. It is the planning that is required to cope with the uncertainty *within* these classes of certain events that demands so much of nurses. 'Is patient X likely to die in the next 12 hours?' or, 'how will we manage the ward if 5% of staff go sick with diarrhoea and vomiting due to the gastroenteritis that is spreading throughout the ward? What if it's 25% of staff?' These questions are examples of uncertainty that occur within a class of certain events (death and sickness: each of us will die and/or get sick at some point).

To break down irreducible uncertainty it is important to realise that two kinds of uncertainty are present in any clinical judgement or decision: subjective and objective uncertainty. Subjective uncertainty is a reference to the *strength of belief* present in the mind of the individual making a judgement. Objective uncertainty is the impact of chance on the system about which a judgement is to be made (Hammond 1996). To conceptualise the distinction, ask yourself as you read this sentence, 'what time is it?' (don't look at the clock!). Now have a look at the clock (or a couple of clocks to be even more accurate) and see what time it is. Your initial estimate of the time was a product of your subjective belief and the clock provides an objective assessment of the time. How accurate where you? The gap between the two assessments represents the gap between your subjective belief and some other form of objective 'truth' (or at least measure).

PATIENTS ARE INFINITELY DIFFERENT BUT UNCERTAINTY IS FINITE

The possible combinations of patients' genders, ages, presenting conditions, clinical signs, symptoms, social factors, co-morbidities, and expectations of the healthcare system are almost infinite. In the face of such overwhelming uncertainty, it is tempting to either deny it (and undertake practice in an ill-informed way) or to adopt the 'frightened bunny' approach and simply freeze and do nothing. With regard to decision making, however, it is important to recognise two things:

1. Information and objective uncertainty are probabilistically related (meaning that some information is more important for decision making than other information). For example, when faced with a child admitted to accident and emergency (A&E) from school, with photosensitivity, a rash on the torso, and a fever, the admission from school is only poorly related (if at all) to the likelihood that they have meningitis.
2. Core uncertainties associated with healthcare provision are a product of the kinds of question that nurses ask in practice. Although patients' details change (ages, gender, signs and symptoms), at the heart of each question are some core uncertainties: 'What is going on here?' 'What will happen if I do nothing?' 'What will happen if I do something?' 'Which of my "do something" options should I take?'

Consider the scenario in Box 2.1. How might you describe and classify the uncertainties that are present?

In the example, we do not know what is causing the girl's symptoms (diagnostic uncertainty); we do not know what will happen if we do nothing (prognostic uncertainty); if it is an infection, we do not know if referral, antibiotics, or 'test-and-wait' is most likely to clear up the infection fastest (treatment or intervention uncertainty).

Box 2.1   Clinical scenario

You are a nurse practitioner working in an NHS walk-in centre and a young mother brings her 6-year-old daughter in. She has been complaining about her 'tiddler' stinging and 'tummy ache'. The mum has brought in a jam-jar full of urine, which is cloudy and smells 'fishy'. You are not sure whether to refer her to the doctor (because she is a young patient), send off a urine culture and wait for the results before deciding what next, or send off a culture and at the same time go ahead and treat with antibiotics.

THE TYPES OF UNCERTAINTY IN NURSING

In a series of studies examining the potential for evidence-based nursing, one of us (CT) examined the kinds of decision that nurses make in practice. By examining the decisions that nurses make, we can learn something about the uncertainties that surround them (Table 2.1).

From this decision-led perspective, there are three main forms of uncertainty in healthcare: diagnostic, prognostic, and treatment or interventional. These three *primary uncertainties* are important because, as we progress through the book, you will learn the rules and skills required to make sense of and use the information required to address these uncertainties.

A decision-based approach to uncertainty in healthcare is not the only approach. Beresford (1991) examines uncertainty from a position that incorporates the information available to healthcare professionals, the nature of the decisions and broader relationships between healthcare professionals, patients, and families. Beresford (1991) puts forward three types of uncertainty: technical, personal, and conceptual.

Technical (or 'first-order') uncertainty occurs when insufficient information exists for adequate prognosis, diagnosis, or estimation of the effects of intervening. Technical uncertainty also arises because of the speed of growth in the knowledge for healthcare decision making. In nursing alone, 3384 pieces of qualitative research were published between 1982 and 2005, as well as 457 randomised controlled trials and 334 systematic reviews (Cullum et al 2008). Obviously, many, many more pieces of research can be accessed if the entire biomedical literature is searched (and don't forget that the social sciences such as psychology, sociology, and health services research can also feed nurses' knowledge needs). Moreover, these figures cover only a small sample of the possible research designs available – staying on top of the literature by casually 'grazing' a few regular journals is too tall an order for most mortals. Technical uncertainty also arises as a result of natural variability in understanding, cognition, and physical condition in patients (and nurses). Sometimes, technical uncertainty is a result of a lack of confidence in the models or schemas we use to explain what we see and do. For example, some models of nursing can, in our experience introduce *more* uncertainty into what we do (albeit unintentionally). Sometimes, these models induce a sense of cognitive dissonance or disconnect between our thoughts on what we should be doing (empowering or progressing towards self-actualisation) and what we are actually doing (feeding, bathing, or listening).

Table 2.1 Decision types, associated uncertainties, and examples of what they look like in practice

Decision type	Uncertainty	Example of how it looks in practice
Intervention: decision that involves choosing among interventions	Treatment	Choosing a mattress for a frail elderly man who has been admitted with an acute bowel obstruction
Targeting: a subcategory of intervention decisions, in the form of choosing which patient will benefit most from the intervention	Treatment	Deciding which patients should receive antiembolic stockings
Prevention: deciding which intervention is most likely to prevent occurrence of a particular health state or outcome	Treatment	Choosing which management strategy is likely to prevent recurrence of a healed leg ulcer
Timing: choosing the best time to deploy an intervention	Treatment	Choosing a time to begin asthma education for a newly diagnosed patient with asthma
Referral: deciding to whom a patient's diagnosis or management should be referred.	Treatment	Choosing that a patient's leg ulcer is arterial rather than venous and so merits medical rather than nursing management in the community
Communication: choosing how to communicate information to patients and relatives for maximum impact/understanding. Also, choosing what information to communicate	Treatment (how to communicate) Prognostic (what to communicate, i.e. what is likely to happen in the future)	Choosing how to approach cardiac rehabilitation with an elderly patient who has had a myocardial infarction, whose family lives nearby and are worrying about her chances of another heart attack
Service delivery, organisation and management: choosing how to configure service delivery or process	Treatment	Choosing how to organise handover so that communication is most effective
Assessment: deciding that an assessment is required and/or what mode of assessment to use	Diagnostic and/or treatment	Deciding to use the Edinburgh Postnatal Depression screening tool instead of an alternative instrument
Diagnosis: classifying signs and symptoms as a basis for a management or treatment strategy	Diagnostic	Deciding whether thrush or another cause is the reason for a woman's sore and cracked nipples
Information seeking: the choice to seek (or not) further information before making a further clinical decision	Prognostic (what is likely to happen with no intervention) or intervention (i.e. wait versus decide)	Deciding that a guideline for monitoring patients who have had their ACE inhibitor dosage adjusted might be of use but choosing not to use it before asking a colleague
Experiential, understanding or 'hermeneutic': how to interpret cues in the process of care	Diagnostic uncertainty (but is unlikely to be resolved using quantitative research knowledge)	Choosing how to reassure a patient who is worried about cardiac arrest after witnessing another patient arresting

Personal forms of uncertainty are rooted in the relationship between nurses and patients, for example, when a patient cannot express his or her preferences or wishes and the nurse is unable to solicit these. Becoming emotionally attached to patients can also generate uncertainty such that nurses might feel as if their decision-making ability is impaired or compromised because of their attachment. In a study of heart-failure specialist nurses (Thompson et al 2008), we found that many nurses felt that their end-of-life decision making with patients was made more complex because of a sense of responsibility to '*their*' patients.

Conceptual uncertainty arises when trying to apply general criteria or rules (such as clinical guidelines) to specific or individual patients. Making sense of past experiences for current patients is also a source of conceptual uncertainty. Hall (2002) highlights the general, existential, uncertainty that surrounds the idea of 'the future' in all decision making, and that does not disappear in healthcare. Conceptual and personal uncertainties are sometimes referred to as second-order or *meta* uncertainties; a reference to uncertainty about how uncertain one is.

When we consider uncertainty along these first- and second-order lines it is clear why some of the solutions traditionally employed by nurses to help reduce the uncertainties in their practice might not work. For example, simply 'reading the literature', making a 'ward file' of articles, or 'producing a protocol' introduces *more* information into the decision-making arena. Increased (better quality) information can reduce some of the technical uncertainties associated with decision-making but will not reduce personal or conceptual uncertainty.

UNCERTAINTY GENERATED BY DELIVERING HEALTHCARE

Any nurse who has worked in an area for more than a few weeks will realise the enormous variations in practice and outcomes that exist. In a seminal piece of work, David Eddy (1994) outlined the role of uncertainty in the delivery of healthcare and how it causes the variations that we experience.

Defining ill health and disease

When looking after a person who is obviously ill, it is often easy to establish the underlying disorders causing the illness and alleviate or cure them. However, most patients, aside from those already with a diagnosis, will have signs and symptoms that might – or crucially, might not – indicate an illness or health state that requires diagnosis, treatment, or alleviation; hence the uncertainty. 'Normal' or 'abnormal' signs and symptoms are often harder to spot than textbooks would have us believe. Often, diseases or health states are self-limiting and/or do only limited harm to the patient. Examples of such include hypertension in the elderly (most people over 70 have higher blood pressure than 'normal') and obesity (large sections of the population are 'overweight'). Definitions of disease vary. Diabetes is defined in practice by varying criteria. In fact, there are different criteria depending on whether a diagnosis of diabetes is required for individual or epidemiological reasons (Expert Committee on the Diagnosis and Classification of Diabetes Mellitus

1997). For many nursing conditions, there is no clear definition of a 'disease' to provide an unequivocal basis for action. Consider, for example, 'anxiety', 'stress', 'pain', or many other of the myriad of possible diagnostic categories into which nurses classify patients. Almost all of us will experience stress at some point; and not only do categories such as stress, anxiety, and pain interact but there are no well-defined thresholds above which we should always act.

Making a diagnosis

Even if we could agree that particular patterns of signs and symptoms were perfectly indicative of a given health state, it is unlikely that the uncertainty and variation would disappear. Nurses, like all clinicians, vary in their abilities to see signs, ask the right questions, and apply diagnostic criteria.

Aylott (2006) reports the variability in nurses' abilities to count the simple sign of respiratory rate in breaths per minute. Eddy (1994) uses the examples of doctors disagreeing over degree of cyanosis, X-ray findings, and chronological events when taking a medical history. There is no reason to suspect that nurses are any less likely to vary in their recording of a diagnosis. Studies that have looked at nurses and doctors in the same samples have found just as much variability. For example, Buntinx et al (1996) looked at the variability in wound care assessment and found variations in areas such as colour and presence of exudate.

Selecting a diagnostic procedure

There are two reasons why selecting the right approach to help establish a diagnosis causes uncertainty. First, for each diagnosis there are often multiple ways of 'testing' for the presence or absence of a condition. Think about a patient who comes into the A&E department with chest pain. The kinds of diagnostic test that you apply range from asking, 'Where is the pain?'or, 'How does the pain feel?' through to ordering blood tests and electrocardiograms (ECGs). Each test will be differently able to correctly suggest particular diagnoses (e.g. 'crushing' chest pain is more likely to suggest a cardiac cause then a 'sharp and intermittent' pain). More pragmatically, each test will have different pros and cons, such as the time required to conduct the test, or its financial cost. The second reason why choosing procedures causes uncertainty is that the diagnostic value of a test often differs depending on who is administering it. Anyone who has ever watched a novice student nurse applying a blood-pressure cuff and listening for a sound that is still unfamiliar will recognise that experience matters; different nurses will record different blood pressure readings on the same patient at the same time.

The outcome of a test will also depend on the person carrying out the test, the characteristics of the person receiving the test, and the context in which the test is carried out. Sticking with our blood pressure example, many nurses and doctors routinely do not follow guidelines on resting patients prior to measurement. For an illustration of why this matters, consider the variation in average readings in Table 2.2.

Table 2.2 Average change in blood pressure associated with 14 everyday activities

Activity	Change in blood pressure, mmHg*	
	Systolic	Diastolic
Attending a meeting	+20.2	+15.0
Working	+16.0	+13.0
Commuting	+14.0	+9.2
Walking	+12.0	+5.5
Dressing	+11.5	+9.7
Doing chores	+10.7	+6.7
Talking on the telephone	+9.5	+7.2
Eating	+8.8	+9.6
Talking	+6.7	+6.7
Doing desk work	+5.9	+5.3
Reading	+1.9	+2.2
Doing business (at home)	+1.6	+3.2
Watching television	+0.3	+1.1
Sleeping	−10.0	−7.6

*Changes are relative to blood pressure when relaxed.
Adapted from Campbell & McKay (1999).

Many nurses use a regular-sized blood-pressure cuff on patients with large arms; a practice that causes an average 6 mmHg overestimation. Estimates of manual sphygmomanometer accuracy suggest that 50% are 'out' by between 4 and 10 mmHg. Together, this natural variability means that errors of more than 10 mmHg are common. You might think that such 'small' errors do not matter, but a consistent (but systematic) overestimate of diastolic blood pressure of more than 5 mmHg would increase by 100% (or double if you prefer) the number of patients with hypertension in an average general practice (Campbell & McKay 1999). Consider what an erroneous diagnosis of hypertension would mean for key aspects of your life: increased life insurance, unnecessary treatment, reduced job opportunities, and changes to how you view yourself and your health status.

Looking at the outcomes of healthcare interventions

If it were possible to conduct limitless experiments involving all of the interventions that are considered by nurses, in all the contexts in which healthcare is delivered, and observe what happens to patients, then, in theory, many nursing uncertainties could be removed. This is not going to happen; although it should be noted that the efforts of the Cochrane and Campbell Collaborations (www.theCochraneLibrary.com; www.campbellcollaboration.org/) are making some headway. Leaving aside the difficulties in financing and organising such a venture, and the fact that nursing (and healthcare) knowledge is always evolving faster than we can evaluate it, there is another – far more fundamental – barrier to be overcome. The most fundamental difficulty is that people respond differently to the care they receive. Imagine two patients with an identical 'diagnosis' (e.g. a venous leg ulcer), they both receive the same compression therapy, non-adherent dressing, district nursing input, share a GP, are the same age and gender, have a similar medical history, and so on. One patient's ulcer heals in 5 months whereas the other's takes over a year. This variation illustrates the need for a language of clinical reasoning that is probabilistic: the chances of diagnostic test being positive when the disease is present (sensitivity), the probability that a wound will heal in 6 months, the chances that a negative test result means you do not have a urinary tract infection (the negative predictive value) and so on. Don't worry about some of these expressions (sensitivity, negative predictive value), we will meet them more fully in later chapters.

Researchers get around this natural variation by studying what happens to samples of people who represent the same kinds of patients likely to be involved in the decisions. This too is challenging; it means multiple nurses and recruiting multiple patients in many different geographical areas. The problem is compounded when what we would like to see happen (or not happen) as a result of our interventions is a relatively rare event. For example, imagine you are a practice nurse and a 37-year-old patient asks, 'How often do I need to get my cervical smear done? Ultimately, the way to conceptualise screening is as a form of intervention; so the core uncertainty becomes, 'Does this procedure actually prevent any cancers?' This, after all, is what the patient (and probably you) are worried about. In women between 20 and 39 years of age, the evidence suggests that 41% of new cancers are prevented with 3-year screening and 30% with a 5-year regimen (www.cancerscreening.nhs.uk/cervical/#effective). However, because of the relatively low frequency of cervical cancers in younger women and the small relative difference expected between 3- and 5-year screening, gathering this evidence requires the observation of hundreds of thousands of women – a serious undertaking.

Many nursing interventions have multiple outcomes, each of which might be more important to one patient than another. Take the example of nurse-led cognitive behavioural therapy (CBT) for treating depression in a young (35-year-old) married man. The CBT might have a positive effect on depression but will also affect our patient's experience of employment, his ability to enjoy family life and make love, his anxiety when carrying out daily activities or having contact with new people, even his financial well-being. It is not possible to measure all the outcomes on which the intervention will impact (even if we could, the list would be too long) and so choices about which outcomes matter most have to be made. Many nursing interventions are designed with long-term well-being in mind. The problem with long-term interventions is that their effects take a long time to emerge. Consider a health visitor who wants to know whether families who are in a Sure Start (www.surestart.gov.uk/) programme go on to bring up healthier and wealthier children. The health visitor will have to wait more than 20 years for enough children to grow up.

Finally, even when the evidence does exist, making sense of it and combining it with our own experience is problematic. 'Evidence' (in evidence-based nursing) can be a mix of randomised controlled trials, uncontrolled experiments, surveys, and clinical experience; all of which can provide contradictory answers. The upshot of this 'decisional uncertainty' is that we most often turn to unsystematic clinical experience as the primary source of 'evidence' for our choices (Thompson et al 2001, 2004) a strategy that leaves us open to all kinds of biases and mistakes (see Chapter 7).

Therefore with regard to the measurement of outcomes for clinical decision making:

1. The consequences of using a particular intervention for particular patients are always uncertain.
2. This uncertainty cannot be resolved in the short term (i.e. when you need it to be resolved!).
3. Any actions a nurse chooses to undertake in the face of such uncertainty cannot be right or wrong, only more or less likely to produce an outcome.

Preferences

Assume that for a given intervention we know what the outcome will be. Is it possible to say whether those outcomes are good or bad? No. Every nursing intervention produces multiple outcomes, some of which will be desirable (to the patient, the nurse, or both) and some of which will not. Choosing interventions involves trading off preferred outcomes against outcomes that are not desired but that cannot be avoided. There is a natural, in-built variability in the values that people exhibit. Consider patients trying to manage their type 2 diabetes: they must trade-off feeling better and long-term control of symptoms (increased thirst, polyuria, fatigue, frequent, or slow-healing infections, and erectile dysfunction) against having to measure the carbohydrate content of their meals and daily monitoring of blood sugar – possibly involving equipment that singles them out as 'a diabetic'.

Eddy (1994) uses the following thought experiment, which we have slightly adapted here, to illustrate variability in preferences:

" Pretend that you have just had a breast biopsy. You have already got your biopsy results and you know you do not have cancer. There is more information to be gained from further studies. However, after the biopsy, you have in the upper outer quadrant of your left breast a small 1-inch scar that is slightly indented from the removal of tissue – it is about the size of a pecan nut. I am a wizard and I can snap my fingers and make that scar disappear without a trace. I cannot erase the memory of your hospitalisation, any anxiety you had prior to my surgery, or any of the other events surrounding your biopsy, but if I snap my fingers, your scar will disappear. How much will you pay me to snap my fingers? "

People vary widely in their estimates to this question. They vary because women attach different valuations to the importance of having a small scar on their breast. For some, it will be of little importance (and they would pay little) whereas others would willingly pay far more because for them not having a scar on their breast is very important.

Putting it all together: synthesising information and reaching a decision

In the end, making a choice comes down to the ways in which we synthesise and 'make sense' of information. Information comes in the form of patient signs and symptoms, research, and experiential evidence of the effectiveness of the 'tests' that we use, the interventions that we deploy, and the possible impact on outcomes. Uncertainty surrounds each of these pieces of information. Time pressure and a possible lack of computing skills, hardware, and software mean that for many clinical decisions this synthesis must happen in the heads of nurses. Given the ranges of possible information values, and the underlying uncertainty around those values, it is challenging in the extreme to try to do this. It is no surprise, then, that nurses vary widely both in the decisions that they make and in the ways in which they use information. Some of this variation can be seen in the following example.

Figures 2.1 and 2.2 represent 48 critical care outreach nurses, each with between 5 and 7 years' experience in critical care and more than 10 years' experience as qualified nurses. Each nurse was faced with the familiar task of deciding whether to intervene in the case of a surgical ward patient at risk of a 'critical event'. Critical events include respiratory and cardiac arrest and strokes. Each nurse was presented with the *same* 50 scenarios with the *same* information presented in the *same* order. The information and the values used were drawn from *real* assessments of risk in a *real* hospital ward. Thus, we controlled for the information and the only bits of the experiment that altered were the nurses themselves and how they interpreted the information with which they were confronted.

First, let us examine the differences in the actual judgements reached by the nurses (remember, they were all given the same information): it is clear that there are considerable differences between nurses. Now, if we look at how they used just one piece of information (the patient's respiratory rate in Figure 2.2) we can see that there was considerable variation in the 'weight'

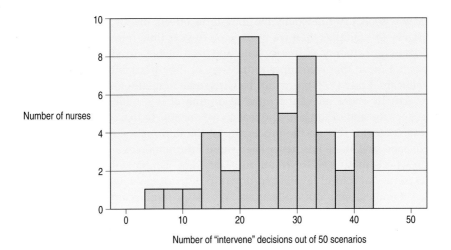

Figure 2.1 Histogram of number of critical care nurses' (*n* = 48) decisions to intervene in a sample of 50 'at risk' critical event scenarios.

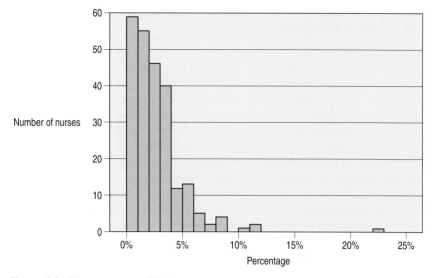

Figure 2.2 The percentage (%) that respiratory rate contributes to the decisions of 48 critical care nurses.

(or value) given to the information. Even though there is considerable uncertainty associated with this task, the limited information presented to nurses was able to predict around 70% of critical events (Subbe et al 2001).

WHAT CAN BE DONE WITH UNCERTAINTY?

At this point, it should be clear that there is no escaping clinical uncertainty. Many of the causes that lie behind how we experience uncertainty in practice are simply not within our control. For example, rare events in nursing will remain rare, and so base rates (see Chapter 9 on diagnosis) will remain low. Different patients will quite naturally vary in the preferences and values they have for the options that nurses suggest. Finally, if we decide that we need to understand the long-term effects of our interventions on patients and families then we need 5- or 10-year time frames.

Thus, uncertainty is inescapable and irreducible. Irreducible, however, does not mean that we cannot reduce *any* of the uncertainty that surrounds healthcare. Eddy (1994) provides us with some remedies for uncertainty that are actually more relevant for the beginning of this millennium than they were for the end of the last. The reason we are able to make this claim is that these strategies rely on the processing of the information available to us as clinicians, and there has never been more information available to the clinician who is motivated to seek it out. These are also remedies that lie within our control at a local level; even down to individual contacts with patients, their families, and our colleagues. We have five recommendations that nurses might like to consider incorporating into their practice as starting points for managing uncertainty:

1. *Admit uncertainty*: only if we acknowledge that uncertainty exists in our choices with and for patients and families (and colleagues) can we search

for ways to address the type and scale of the uncertainties that we face. This will be an uncomfortable task for some practitioners, but if we fail to do it then truly informed choices will never be a reality.

2. *Learn the language(s) of uncertainty*: many of the sources of uncertainty have well-established languages to describe and make sense of them. So for example, the language of statistics is the means by which we describe the collection and interpretation of evidence; the language of uncertainty itself is probability theory; and the problems of choosing between options in which outcomes are uncertain and values different is economics and decision theory. It is unrealistic to expect all nurses to be conversant in these languages, but we should certainly expect that those who produce the information sources to guide practice (protocols, guidelines, care pathways) should make use of the language (and underlying concepts) in the production process.

3. *Learn to look beyond the headlines*: even if you are a nurse who follows policies, you should always enquire (and question if necessary) the underlying logic and supporting evidence. Simply having a policy in place and implemented does not make it correct.

4. *Being clear about what is important*: when we design a policy that we expect nurses to adopt locally, then we should specify: (1) the clinical and economic outcomes that we considered when designing the policy; (2) our estimate of the impact locally of the likely impact on these outcomes if the policy were adopted; and (3) the basis for this estimate.

5. *Encourage our patients to play a role in stimulating professional acceptance of uncertainty*: when you tell a patient that a procedure will involve 'some discomfort' how might you respond if the patient asks you to rate it against a sensation that you have both experienced (e.g. a dental filling); when you tell a patient that 'some patients' find a procedure uncomfortable, how might you respond if asked, 'What proportion?'; when you suggest that a procedure is likely to be helpful, how might you respond if asked, 'With regard to what?' or, 'What is the likelihood of benefit?'

SUMMARY

Uncertainty is inescapable in healthcare, but without it there would be little hope associated with the choices we face; and hope is an important commodity in caring. Although patients vary in their characteristics, the outcomes they value, and their responses to our interventions, there are enough similarities between them to make healthcare a worthwhile enterprise. Alongside these patient-centred sources of uncertainty, the very act of delivering healthcare generates further uncertainty and variability. As nurses, we can all look at the same information and reach different conclusions, and we can all consider the same outcomes and hold different valuations.

Although the possible combinations of patient information, preferences and outcomes may appear infinite, at the heart of our judgements and choices are some finite *types* of choice: diagnostic, interventional, prognostic, and experiential. The good news is that for each of the possible types of uncertainty there is an appropriate set of information requirements and techniques for handling the information retrieved (more on this in later chapters). Making use of this information is sometimes counterintuitive; it involves learning new languages and skills, and ultimately requires the reader to expend some energy to acquire the necessary competences. In this book, we introduce you to these skills, languages, and points of focus – the motivation and effort are down to you.

EXERCISES

1. Write down ten decisions you made during your last shift or day's work.
2. What kinds of uncertainty are present in these choices?
3. What sort of information would you require to reduce these uncertainties?
4. Did you have this information available and if not why not? If you did, did you make the most of it?
5. What personal development opportunities can you identify to help you manage uncertainty (maybe critical appraisal or evidence searching opportunities).

RESOURCES

www.content.healthaffairs.org/cgi/reprint/3/2/74.pdf

This is a copy of Eddy's seminal exploration of medical ('healthcare' is a better expression) variations and the role of uncertainty. Every professional in healthcare should read this at least once.

Fox R C 1980 The evolution of medical uncertainty. Milbank Memorial Fund. Quarterly Health Society 58:1–49.

Another classic from another key author; again, essential reading for any one serious about understanding uncertainty.

REFERENCES

Aylott M 2006 Observing the sick child. Part 2A: respiratory assessment. Paediatric Nursing 18:38–44

Beresford P 1991 Uncertainty and the shaping of medical decisions. Hastings Centre Report 21:6–11

Buntinx F, Beckers H, De Keyser G et al 1996 Inter-observer variation in the assessment of skin ulceration. Journal of Wound Care 5:166–170

Campbell N R C, McKay D W 1999 Accurate blood pressure measurement: why does it matter? Canadian Medical Association Journal 161:277–278

Cullum N, Ciliska D, Marks S et al 2008 An introduction to evidence-based nursing. In: Cullum N, Ciliska D, Haynes B et al (eds) Evidence-based nursing. Blackwell, London, p 1–8

Eddy D 1990 Clinical decision making: from theory to practice: the challenge. Journal of American Medical Association 263:287–290

Eddy D 1994 Variations in physician practice: the role of uncertainty. Health affairs 3:74–89

Expert Committee on the Diagnosis and
Classification of Diabetes Mellitus 1997
Report of the expert committee on the
diagnosis and classification of Diabetes
Mellitus. Diabetes Care 20:1183–1197
Hall K H 2002 Reviewing intuitive decision
making and uncertainty: the implications
for medical education. Medical Education
36(3):216–224
Hammond K R 1996 Human judgment and
social policy. Oxford University Press,
Oxford
Hastie R, Dawes R M 2001 Rational choice
in an uncertain world. Sage, London
Kylma J, Vehvilainen-Julkunen K 1997
Hope in nursing research: a meta-
analysis of the ontological and
epistemological foundations of research
on hope. Journal of Advanced Nursing
25:364–371

Subbe C P, Kruger M, Rutherford P et al
2001 Validation of a modified early
warning score in medical admissions.
Quarterly Journal of Medicine 94:521–526
Thompson C, McCaughan D, Cullum N
et al 2001 Research information in nurses'
clinical decision making: what is useful?
Journal of Advanced Nursing 36:376–388
Thompson C, Spilsbury K, Dowding D et al
2008 Does whether a choice is perceived
as 'easy' or 'difficult' make a difference to
heart failure nurses' clinical judgements?
Journal of Clinical Nursing in press
Thompson C, Cullum N, McCaughan D
et al 2004 Nurses, information use, and
clinical decision-making – the real world
potential for evidence-based decisions in
nursing. Evidence-based Nursing 7:68–72

Uncertainty and nursing

Probability: the language of uncertainty

Carl Thompson and Martin Bland

3

CHAPTER CONTENTS

KEY ISSUES

- Why probability is useful to help deal with uncertainty
- Definitions of probability
- How to calculate probabilities

As discussed in Chapter 2, uncertainty is inherent within decision making in healthcare. Although we can use everyday English to express our uncertainty using terms such as 'likely' or 'rare', there is another far more specific language that we can use to discuss uncertainty: probability. Probability is a measure or representation of the uncertainty associated with our decision making, represented numerically.

NUMBERS, FEAR AND UNCERTAINTY

People don't like using numbers to think about the uncertainties we face. Our innate aversion to numbers can be seen in the ways in which we describe uncertainty itself. When nurses and doctors talk about the uncertainties in their practice, they use words to describe them. For example, most surgical nurses don't say there is a 1 in 10 (or 10%) chance of you not passing wind in the first 24 hours after gastric surgery, they say it is 'unlikely' that you will pass wind in the first 24 hours after your operation. Similarly, community nurses will rarely say, 'I think that if we put a compression bandage on that venous leg ulcer there is a 60% chance of it healing in 24 weeks'. People prefer to express their belief in a treatment working by saying that there is a 'good' chance that the leg will get better in the next 6 months. Although using 'qualitative' expressions of (un)certainty can be more comfortable for us as nurses, there are some downsides; not least the potential for introducing *more* rather than less uncertainty into a decision. When we ask individuals to quantify their degree of belief in response to a label such as 'rarely' or 'likely' they can vary enormously (Shaw & Dear 1990). This variability is a problem when we are trying to encourage *informed* decision making with our patients.

With over 10 years experience of teaching nurses about decision making and statistics, we know that that a fear of numbers is a very real perception amongst clinicians. Gerd Gigerenzer (2002) goes further than this and suggests that such fear amounts to a kind of societal 'innumeracy'. Innumeracy is a strong word, but if we take a moment to consider how it might look in our practice then we can see how Gigerenzer's use of the term becomes understandable. Paradoxically, it is not uncertainty that reveals our innumeracy but our misplaced belief in certainty; or the 'illusion' of certainty.

Consider the statement, 'Everyone in the A&E who comes in wanting pethidine uses other illegal drugs so we don't give them pethidine' (this is a real statement conveyed by a staff nurse in an A&E unit in which one of the authors – CT - worked). The nurse was clearly pretty certain of the correctness of her view, but why was the statement probably wrong? Let us look at the statement graphically (Figure 3.1). In this figure, we can see that many illegal drug users have indeed used pethidine, as the shaded section of the diagram shows. However, the same shaded portion covers only a small proportion of the population of pethidine users. When we view it this way we can see that such a statement (in the absence of any other evidence) is just plain wrong. Innumeracy presents itself in three main ways: ignorance, miscommunication, and clouded thinking (Gigerenzer 2002).

Ignorance of risk

This is a common form of innumeracy in healthcare. It occurs when individuals have no idea of the size of a relevant risk. This is not the same as our 'illusion of certainty' example above. When people are ignorant of risk they might be aware of uncertainties but fail to recognise the scale of them. An example is the (common) misconception among some nurses that an X-ray is a definitive test for a fracture; even X-rays yield positives and false negatives.

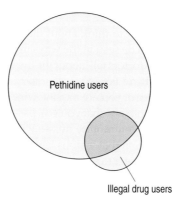

Figure 3.1 Most illegal drug users use pethidine but this does not mean that most pethidine users are illegal drug users.

Miscommunication of risk

At the root of this form of innumeracy is the inability to communicate known risks to others. Sometimes, thinking about risks differently can help us better understand and communicate them. For example, people often think that $p = 0.05$ on a research report means a 5% chance of the outcome being measured happening to them. Figure 3.1 is an example of how presenting a risk differently can help understanding (we discuss this further in Chapter 14). Similarly, each year we ask groups of nurses which is bigger, 0.05 or 0.01? A sizeable (usually around 20%) number of each group always get it wrong (the answer is 0.05). Once you express it as a percentage though (i.e. 5% or 1%), the task is made somewhat simpler, although – worryingly – some still get it wrong, and using percentages rather than integers or whole numbers is usually not a recipe for good communication of risk (Gigerenzer 2002).

Clouded thinking

This is one of the most common forms of innumeracy; it happens when a clinician knows the risks but is unable to draw useful conclusions from them. A classic example is that nurses know that 'base rates' (prevalence) of diseases differ in different settings (e.g. there are more people with diabetes in a medical ward than in the community) but do not know how to adjust the chances of a 'positive' diagnostic test, indicating the presence of disease, in the light of these differences. We can help avoid clouded thinking by using natural frequencies (such as 1 out of 5 patients) rather than proportions or percentages (e.g. 20% of patients). Other tools, such as decision trees, can also help in our attempts to reconceptualise problems (see Chapter 11).

One way of handling risk, and making thinking about uncertainty easier, in clinical decision making and judgement is by using a common language to describe it. The common language for describing uncertainty is probability. As with any language, there are definitions and rules to be learned if you are to use it effectively. This issue is really important and if you are serious about using some of the techniques outlined in the rest of the book (decision analysis, 2×2 tables and understanding diagnostic reasoning, for example) then you really should not skip this chapter. Make sure you understand it and try the exercises at the end of it until you are comfortable with them (and get the answers right!) before moving on.

DEFINITIONS OF PROBABILITY

There is no single definition of probability and the two definitions that most concern us in healthcare are: (1) the idea that probability is an expression of a subjective *degree of belief*; and (2) the notion that probability represents *frequencies* of a phenomenon in a sample of observations.

Probability as a degree of belief: Bayesian approaches

From this perspective, a probability reflects a subjective belief that an event or phenomenon will happen. You can see this in action in healthcare when, for example, you carry out a procedure that you have never done before with a patient and he or she asks you about some of the uncertainties around it (e.g. 'How likely is this dressing to heal my scar in the next 4 weeks?'). How do you answer if you have no previous experience to draw on? If you had to quantify your answer you would use a number to express how strongly you believed that the procedure would generate the outcome you wanted. If you answered, 'I'm pretty confident, I would say 80% likely', then you would be using probability as a measure of how strongly you believe it will work. We will come across the idea of probability as subjective belief and the notion of Bayesian probability in Chapter 9 when we look at diagnosis.

Frequentist probability

Far more common in healthcare, and particularly healthcare research, is the idea of probability as a reflection of the number of occurrences of a phenomenon within a sample of observations: the *relative frequency* of an event in a specified *reference* class. For example, the statement 4% (or 1 in 25) of men are likely to die from prostate cancer suggests that there is a relative frequency of 4 men dying of prostate cancer out of every 100 of the reference class (all men).

There are many ways of expressing probabilities but they are all measures of the uncertainty surrounding an event (see Table 3.1 for the most common).

PROBABILITY: THE RULES AND SOME SHORTHAND

Probabilities range from 0 to 1 (or 0% to 100%). A probability of 0 means there is no chance at all that you will see whatever it is that you are interested in and a probability of 1 (or 100%) means that it is certain that the

Table 3.1 Different ways of measuring probability

Term	Definition	Formula	Range
Probability measures that do not involve time			
Probability	The chance of an event	P	0–1
Proportion	The relative frequency of a state	P	0–1
Prevalence	The proportion of a group with a specific disease	P	0–1
Percentage	Probability expressed as a frequency per 100	$P \times 100$	0–100
Frequency	Probability expressed per sample (e.g. 1 per 10,000)	P	0–denominator
Odds	The ratio of the probability of an event to its complement	$P/(1 - P)$	0–infinity
Probability measures that involve time			
Incidence rate	The occurrence of new disease cases or events per unit of person-time	P/t	0–infinity
Incidence proportion	The proportion of people who develop a new disease or have an event during a specified time period	P	0–1
Risk	The probability that an individual develops a new disease or has an event during a specified period of time	P	0–1

P, probability of an event; t, time.

phenomenon you are interested in will occur. The easiest way to appreciate probability is to use the example of a die (not 'dice', which is the plural of a 'die'). We realise that using the 'abstract' example of a die means that its relevance to healthcare is not immediately obvious. Trust us, you need to grasp the key concepts, rules and calculations surrounding probability and a die is the easiest starting point. Once you grasp the key elements then we can make more use of healthcare decision problems. A die has six sides and so we expect that there is a 16.6% (or 1 [side] in 6 [possible sides]) chance that a particular one of the numbered sides will be face up. In practice, if we throw the die five times, the same number *might* come up four out of the five times. This does not mean that the probability is any less than 0.16; probability is a measure of the *relative* frequency of an event for a large number of events. So, if we throw the die five times and the number 4 shows face up on four occasions, we should not be too worried. However, if we threw it 200 times and it came up with the number four on 160 occasions, we might think that the die was not fair. If we threw it 2000 times and the number 4 was face up on 1600 occasions then you should definitely worry that the game you are playing is not going your way (unless you are betting on the number 4!). The proportion of outcomes to observations has not altered in any of these examples (it is 80% in each) but as the number of observations gets bigger, your assumptions alter; or at least we hope they do. When you appreciate this relationship between uncertainty and numbers of observations, the importance of large sample sizes in research studies that make claims about the 'significance' of their results should become clearer.

Probability of an event

When we talk about the probability of an event the notation used is P[event]. So, the probability of obtaining of 4 on our die is expressed as P[number 4 on a die].

Probability of something not happening

Sometimes we are interested in the probability of something not happening, as in the probability that a patient does not have a disease. Again, using our die example, there is a 5-out-of-6-throws (or 84%) chance that the die will show a number apart from four on its uppermost face. We can write this as $P[\bar{4}]$. The bar over the four means 'not'. One other important thing to remember about probabilities is that the chances of something happening and not happening must add up to 1. This makes sense. Consider a coin being flipped; if there is a 50% (0.5) chance that it lands heads up and that it doesn't land heads up, then there has to be a 50% (0.5) chance that it has landed tails up instead; 100% of all possibilities are covered. This is important in clinical practice because if, for example, there is a 5% chance that a person is diabetic then there must be a 95% chance that he or she is not. Such 'rules' are vital for rational and logical reasoning about problems. In Chapter 7, we will see that when we don't follow such rules we leave ourselves open to mistakes and errors.

The summation rule

The example of the coin toss is an example of the *summation rule* for probabilities. This rule says that all mutually exclusive outcomes must sum to 1. The rule applies whether there are just two possibilities or if there are more than two. Consider the example of establishing the probability that a patient post-myocardial infarction will comply with a cardiac rehabilitation programme consisting of dietary changes and psychological self-help. We need to consider diet alone, self-help alone, both, and neither. Thus, the possibilities can be expressed as:

$$P(\text{diet}) + P(\text{self-help}) + P(\text{both}) + P(\text{neither}) = 1$$

The usefulness of this rule becomes clear when one considers groups such as the elderly, who often have multiple conditions (comorbidities) all present simultaneously (e.g. diabetes, hypertension, and arthritis).

Odds and probabilities

Sometimes in decision making, and especially in research used in decision making, you will encounter the concept of odds (as has already been seen in Table 3.1). Odds are just another way of expressing uncertainty, but they have slightly different properties to probabilities. Probabilities, as we have seen, range from 0 (impossible) to 1 (certainty). Odds, however, range from 0 to infinity. Why? They have such a broad spread because they represent the ratio of the chance of something happening to the chance of something not happening. So, if we have a phenomenon with a 0.75 (75%) chance of happening and so a 0.25 (or 25%) chance of not happening then the odds of it happening are 0.75/0.25 or 3 (often written as 3:1 or 3 to 1). Odds mean that you will see three occurrences for every one where it is absent. Or, if you had four potential examples in which the phenomenon might be found, you would expect to see it three times. So, the odds are 3 to 1 but the probability is 1/4 or 0.25 (Box 3.1).

Box 3.1 Odds and horse racing

Not a clinical example this, but potentially useful nevertheless. Sharp-eyed readers might have noticed that the notion of odds is often applied to horse and dog racing. Sharp-eyed *and* sharp-witted readers will have gone further and recognised that a horse with odds of 4:1 does not win 25% of the time. The odds in racing are always *against* the horse winning (or the chances of the horse losing divided by the chances of the horse winning). To decide on the probability that a horse will win you need to convert the odds into probabilities, which is quite simple: our horse with 4 to 1 odds means that, out of 5 (4 + 1) horses/chances, our single horse has 1 chance of winning. So the probability of the horse winning is 1/5, 0.2, or 20%. This means that the probability of the horse not winning is 80% or 0.8.

Conditional probabilities

Sometimes we are interested only in certain outcomes in certain reference classes. For example, as a community nurse specialising in diabetes, I might want to know only the prevalence of venous leg ulcers in patients with type 2 diabetes (rather than all patients); or as a mental health nurse I might be interested in parasuicide attempts only in patients in forensic mental health settings (rather than all care settings). These kinds of probability are termed conditional: we have placed a condition on the possible chances. Namely, that they should come from type 2 diabetic or forensic populations. This probability can be written using the symbol '|':

$$P(\text{venous leg ulcers} \mid \text{type 2 diabetes})$$

This should be read as, 'What is the probability of a venous leg ulcer in a patient *given* that he or she has type 2 diabetes?'. We will come across the idea of conditional probabilities again in Chapter 9, because test results are often interpreted with reference to conditional probabilities. For example, the *sensitivity* of a diagnostic test is the probability of a positive test result *given* that the person has the disease we are interested in.

If the condition makes no difference to the probability then we say that the factors are 'independent'. For example, if being older makes no difference to the prevalence of venous leg ulcers then age and prevalence of venous leg ulcer are independent (so, clinically, you would not need to be more aware of the likelihood of an ulcer in an older patient than a younger patient). Actually, they are not independent $P(\text{ulcer} \mid \text{more than 70 years age}) > P(\text{ulcer} \mid \text{less than 70 years age})$; the prevalence in younger patients in the UK is 3 ulcers per 1000, rising to 20 ulcers per 1000 if you are older than 70. Plainly, 0.003 (3/1000) is not equal to 0.02 (20/1000) and so the two are not independent.

Combining information for single probabilities

Let us consider two outcomes of interest and lets call them A and B. We can ask three questions:

1. What is the probability of seeing A AND B?
2. What is the probability of seeing A OR B?
3. What is the probability of seeing A GIVEN B?

Remember, we can also estimate negative outcomes (e.g. what is the probability of not seeing A or B) by the summation rule and the fact that all alternatives must add to 1. So the probability of not seeing A OR B is 1 minus the probability of seeing A OR B.

If our possibilities are mutually exclusive (i.e. they cannot possibly occur together) then all we have to do to find out the probability of the events is add them together. For example, taking our die again, we can say that the probability of landing a 2 OR a 4 is 0.16 + 0.16 = 0.32 or 32%.

What about when we are interested in the chances of events that are not mutually exclusive; for example, suppose we are a practice nurse and interested in whether a patient is diabetic OR has hypertension. Figure 3.2 demonstrates that the two categories of patients with diabetes and hypertension overlap. In

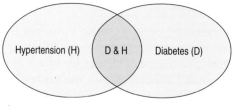

Figure 3.2 Possible relationships between diabetes and hypertension.

this case we need to sum the probabilities of having hypertension and diabetes but *subtract* the probability of having both. We would write this as:

$$P[\text{hypertension}] + P[\text{diabetes}] - P[\text{hypertension and diabetes}].$$

This is really just an extension of the summation rule because if the events [hypertension and diabetes] were independent then the 'overlap' P[hypertension and diabetes] will be 0.

Multiplying probabilities and handling multiple uncertainties

So far, we have been concerned with uncertainties about a single event but healthcare often involves multiple uncertainties. When one outcome does not affect the probability of the other occurring then it is easy: you simply multiply the two (or more) probabilities. For example, if you want to know the probability that a young mum-to-be planning a family will give birth to two boys (separately, not as twins) then the probability is simply $0.5 \times 0.5 = 0.25$ or 25% (assuming, of course, that there is a 50% chance of having a boy).

Far more realistic, though, is the scenario in which multiple, related uncertainties are present. If you think about the number of problems in healthcare that are related, the list soon becomes extensive (e.g. smokers and heart disease; alcohol abuse and memory loss; social class, educational level, and healthy eating). Let us use our example of the nurse concerned about the conditional probability that a patient is BOTH diabetic AND hypertensive. The probability we are interested in is the overlap in Figure 3.2. There are two ways of handling this: (1) using probability notation and simple maths; and (2) using tables.

Taking the simple mathematical route first, we can reconfigure our problem into two independent probabilities and just multiply as if they were unrelated. Thus, our question becomes P[hypertensive and diabetic] = P[diabetic] × P[hypertensive | diabetic] or even P[hypertensive and diabetic] = P[hypertensive] × P[diabetic | hypertensive] – it doesn't matter which way round they go in this instance.

The second way of getting the correct probability is by using the information from a 'contingency' table. Consider the relationship between body mass index (BMI) and depression in people with diabetes; that is, what is the probability of being overweight AND having depression if you have diabetes (being overweight and depressed are linked and thus not independent). Looking at data from a study of 3010 patients in the USA (Katon et al 2004), we can work out the appropriate probabilities (Table 3.2).

We can see that by organising the numbers in this way it is easier to make sense of the information present. For example, by looking at the 'depressed'

Table 3.2 Body mass index (BMI) and depression in diabetes			
	Depressed	*Not depressed*	*Total*
BMI > 30	216	1285	1501
BMI < 31	104	1364	1468
Total	320	2649	2969

P(depressed) = 0.10 or 10%; P(depressed | overweight) = 216/1501 = 0.14 or 14%;
P(depressed | not overweight) = 104/1468 = 0.07 or 7%.
Adapted from Katon et al (2004).

column we can see that 320 people out of the 2969 for whom data was available in the study were depressed; so the chances of being depressed are around 10% (320/2969). How does the table help us with learning more about the chances of depression if you are overweight? If we examine the row representing people with a body mass index (BMI) of more than 30 we can see that there are 1501 such individuals in our sample. If we examine the 'depressed' column we can see that there were 216 individuals with both depression and a BMI of more than 30. The probability, then, that a person is depressed *given* that he or she is overweight is therefore 216/1501 or 0.14 or 14%. This is clearly much higher than the probability of being depressed if you are not overweight; which is 104/1468 or 7%. So, the probability of being depressed if you are not overweight is half that of someone who is obese. Aside from concluding that being overweight increases your chances of being depressed, we can also be clear that depression and weight are dependent on each other. If they had been statistically independent of each other then the three probabilities would have been identical.

If we go back to our mathematical route to multiplying probabilities (now that we have them) we can write down the multiplication rule. For any two events A and B:

$$P(\text{A and B}) = P(\text{A} \mid \text{B}) \times (\text{B}) = P(\text{B} \mid \text{A}) \times (\text{A})$$

This, you will recall, is exactly what we did earlier in the chapter when we looked at the relationship between diabetes and hypertension.

It might appear as if it does not matter which way round we express the probabilities, e.g. $P(\text{B} \mid \text{A})$ is the same as $P(\text{A} \mid \text{B})$ This is not the case. Look at Table 3.3, which examines the relationship between hay fever and eczema at age 11 in the National Child Development Study (www.cls.ioe.ac.uk).

Table 3.3 Hay fever and eczema in 11-year-old children			
Eczema	Hay fever		Total
	Yes	*No*	
Yes	141	420	561
No	928	13525	14453
Total	1069	13945	15522

To understand that $P(A \mid B)$ and $P(B \mid A)$ are not the same, work out the probabilities that a child will have hay fever given that they have eczema – P(hay fever | eczema) – and then work out the probability that a child will have eczema given that they have hay fever – P(eczema | hay fever).

The probability that in this group a child with hay fever will also have eczema is P(eczema | hay fever) $= 141/1069 = 0.13$. This is clearly much less than the probability that a child with eczema will have hay fever: P(hay fever | eczema) $= 141/561 = 0.25$.

This might be obvious but in fact this confusion between conditional probabilities is common and has serious consequences. For example, forensic evidence (such as the DNA tests that you often hear about on the news, or Jerry Springer!) typically produces the probability that material found at a crime scene (DNA, clothing fibres, etc.) will match the suspect as closely as it does given that the material did *not come* from the suspect. This is P(evidence | suspect not at crime scene). It is not the same as P(suspect not at crime scene | evidence). Unfortunately, for the innocent, this is often how it is interpreted; an inversion known as the prosecutor's fallacy.

Another example of the prosecutor's fallacy can occur when two children in the same family die unexpectedly. This example of the fallacy had very real consequences for the Clarke family, in Cheshire in the UK, who lost two children to sudden infant death syndrome in 1999. In a now infamous piece of innumeracy, the expert witness to the court provided the chances of two children in the same (affluent, non-smoking) family both dying of cot death as 1 in 73 million. This figure of 1 in 73 million was derived from the Confidential Enquiry for Stillbirths and Deaths in Infancy (CESDI). The chances of a randomly chosen baby dying a cot death are 1 in 1303 if one examines CESDI data. If the child is from an affluent, non-smoking family, with a mother older than 26 years, the odds fall to around 1 in 8500. If it were possible to eliminate the known, and possibly shared, factors influencing cot death rates then the chances of two children from the same family suffering a cot death are 1/8500 squared or 1 chance in 73 million.

The problem with this estimate is that sibling cot deaths are not independent. In a thorough analysis of the data in CESDI, Ray Hill (2004) estimates that siblings of children who die of cot death are between 10 and 22 times more likely than average to die the same way. Using the figure of 1 in 1303 for the chance of a first cot death, we see that the chances of a second cot death in the same family are somewhere between 1 in 60 and 1 in 130. In the absence of enough data for more precision or to take familial factors into account, it seems reasonable to use a ballpark figure of 1 in 100.

Multiplying 1/1303 by 1/100 gives an estimate for the incidence of double cot death of around 1 in 130,000. As 650,000 children are born every year in England and Wales, we can expect around five families a year to suffer a second tragic loss. The 1 in 73 million figure quoted by Professor Meadows implied that double cot deaths were so rare that we could expect them to happen once in a century – clearly not so.

Yet another example of this confusion can be found in the measles mumps and rubella (MMR) public health scare of the late 1990s. During this crisis, the public was led to believe that the MMR triple vaccination was linked to an increased risk of autism in children. At the heart of the scare was a fundamental confusion in the minds of many parents (and healthcare professionals) that the probability of developing autism given that a child has had the MMR vaccine was the same as the probability of having had the MMR vaccine given that the child is autistic. The symptoms of autism develop slowly, thus many (indeed most) autistic children have the MMR vaccine before symptoms start to show. If, however, we took a random sample of all children and gave half the MMR vaccine and half no immunisation and followed them up to see if they developed autism, it is likely that the numbers of children developing autism in the two groups would be no different (Wilson et al 2003). Confusion over conditional probabilities is not just confined to the psychology lab; it matters in everyday healthcare practice.

In this chapter, we have endeavoured to introduce you to some of the basic concepts, definitions, rules, and notation associated with probability. If you have taken the time to engage with these ideas – although we are aware that P(engagement | numbers) is far lower than P(engagement | no numbers!) – then this will help you better understand and appreciate other chapters in the book.

EXERCISES

For teachers

Start by filling in the blank in the following statement with the probability expressions: 'certain', 'unlikely', 'frequent', 'probable', 'never', 'possible':

'One of the clinical nurse specialists in your hospital tells you that a particular symptom of chest infection is _____'.

1. For each of the probability expressions, ask your learners to write down the probability (from 0 to 1 or 0 to 100) that they think the expression represents.
2. Ask them to order the expressions from high to low.
3. Compare the answers between students.
4. Look at the paper by Kong et al 1986 (details in the Reference list). How do your group's answers compare?
5. What might explain these differences?

For learners

Exercise 1

A mother has an equal chance of giving birth to a boy or a girl:

1. If she gives birth to one child, what is the probability that it is a boy?
2. If she has twins what is the probability that they are both boys? (Assume that the sex of neither one can influence the sex of the other.)

Exercise 2

You are a nurse manager in charge of an outpatient clinic in a large NHS hospital. The Trust has promised its local population that 99% of its cancer patients will be seen in your clinic within 2 weeks. Of 1800 patients seen in a year, 15 were not seen in 2 weeks. Are the Trust's promises being met?

RESOURCES

The following website provides a *simple* introduction to probability, with self-assessment and interactive opportunities. It is a fantastic introduction to the building blocks of probability. Some readers might find it be too simple, but have a go before you decide!

www.bbc.co.uk/skillswise/numbers/handlingdata/probability/index.shtml

REFERENCES

Gigerenzer G 2002 Reckoning with risk: learning to live with uncertainty. Penguin, London

Hill R 2004 Multiple sudden infant deaths – coincidence or beyond coincidence? Paediatric and Perinatal Epidemiology 18:320–326

Katon W J L: In Russo, E H J et al 2004 Cardiac risk factors in patients with diabetes mellitus and major depression. Journal of General Internal Medicine 19:1192–1199

Kong A, Barnett G O, Mosteller F et al 1986 How medical professionals evaluate expressions of probability. New England Journal of Medicine 315:740–744

Shaw N J, Dear P R 1990 How do parents of babies interpret qualitative expressions of probability? Archives of Disease in Childhood 65:520–523

Wilson K, Mills E, Ross C et al 2003 Association of autistic spectrum disorder and the measles, mumps, and rubella vaccine: a systematic review of current epidemiological evidence. Archives of Pediatrics and Adolescent Medicine 157:628–634

Using information in decision making

Dawn Dowding and Carl Thompson

4

KEY ISSUES

- The issues surrounding information use in decision making
- The barriers to nurses' use of research information (as opposed to other forms of information) in their decision making
- How to use the PICO framework for structuring clinical questions and focusing your information searching
- Strategies for improving your ability to search for research based information to assist with decision making

INTRODUCTION

The process of making judgements and decisions involves the person making the judgement or decision *using* information. Think for a moment of a recent situation that you have been in, where you decided to *do* something – it could be related to a patient you have cared for (e.g. you gave some medication) or in relation to your own personal life (e.g. you have decided to move house). Those decisions or actions will have been based on your evaluation of items of information. For instance, when giving the patient medication, you might have (either consciously or subconsciously) taken into account factors such as the patient saying she is in pain, the patient looking as though she is in pain, when the patient last had pain medication, and the pain medication she is prescribed. In some instances, you might have had to look (or search) for the information you needed to make your decision. For instance, you might have examined the patient's prescription charts to find out when she last had pain relief and what that pain relief was.

How individuals use information, the information they use, and where that information comes from are key to successful decision making. From the perspective of evidence-based decision making, we want to know if nurses are using information from research evidence to inform their decisions, rather than relying on anecdote (which might result in poorer quality care). If anecdote and personal experience dominate, we need to know why, and how to try to assist nurses to make greater use of research information.

In this chapter, we look first at some of the research on how nurses use information in decision making, the sources of information that have been found to be used more frequently, how nurses identify that they have a need for information, and where they go to get it. We then examine the evidence on nurses' use of research information, in order to identify *why* nurses might not be using research as much as we would like to aid their decision making. In the final part of the chapter, we introduce a framework for helping with the structuring of uncertainty and information (known as the PICO) and give some tips on how to try to include information based on good research evidence into the decisions you take in the future.

NURSES' USE OF INFORMATION IN DECISION MAKING

One of the earliest studies examining how nurses make judgements and decisions was carried out by Hammond et al (1966) into the types of information that nurses used to inform their judgements. The study consisted of two stages; in the first stage, nurses were asked to record the judgements they made over a 24-hour period, together with the characteristics of those judgements (such as the information they used to inform them). The researchers concluded that they had found more varied decisions and more information cues used by nurses than they had originally anticipated (perhaps indicating that nursing was more complex than they had thought). Therefore, in the second stage of the study they examined the information used by nurses and the decisions they made when faced with a patient who was complaining of abdominal pain following abdominal surgery. They found that in response to the same 'decision task' nurses responded in 17 different ways (giving a patient PRN analgesia was the most common action) and used a total of 165 different information cues to inform their decisions. What the study indicated was the vast amount of information available, and used by, nurses to inform their decisions about practice.

More recent studies have examined the sources of information nurses use to inform their decision making in practice. A common picture occurs, in that nurses report using information gathered verbally from asking patients or other colleagues, observing the patient, or simply drawing on their own experience, rather than actively seeking evidence-based guidance via guidelines, protocols, or online resources (Lamond et al 1996, McCaughan et al 2005, McKnight 2006, Tannery et al 2007, Thompson et al 2001a). In particular, nurses value their own personal experience and information from 'human' sources – such as specialist nurses – over information from research reports (McCaughan et al 2005). Therefore, from an evidence-based decision-making viewpoint, it appears that, in practice, very few everyday decisions made by nurses are based explicitly on information obtained from reports of research.

The precise information on which nurses focus when making a judgement or decision has been less well examined. Offredy (2002) compared the information used by nurse practitioners and general practitioners (GPs) when making decisions based on patient scenarios. This study found that whereas nurses collected more information than GPs, GPs were more efficient in their ability to represent or describe the information they received. Being able to make an accurate judgement or decision about patient care is related to the ability to focus on the important or 'critical cues' in that situation (Offredy 2002). Therefore, developing ways of accurately identifying information that can help you with a judgement or decision is an important skill to develop.

NURSES' INFORMATION NEEDS

What is apparent from the research described in the previous section is that nurses do not appear to 'seek out' research-based information to inform their decision making. Moreover, research points to the problems some nurses have on focusing on the information that is *important* in order to make a decision effectively.

As we have seen, nurses make decisions in conditions of 'irreducible uncertainty'. One of the causes of this uncertainty is a lack of information on which to base your decision. As an example, imagine that you are a primary-care nurse visiting a woman with multiple sclerosis (MS) for the first time. You haven't looked after a person with MS before and cannot remember much about the condition from your initial nurse training. What would you do? In essence, you are *uncertain* about the situation and might have a number of *questions* that arise on the basis of it. Perhaps some of these questions occur to you before you even make your first visit, such as, 'What do I know about MS?' The answer might be, 'Not much', so perhaps you would learn more about the condition from sources such as textbooks, the internet, or just asking a more knowledgeable colleague. What you have identified is an *information need* expressed as a *clinical question* that you have addressed through *searching for* information.

Different information needs or clinical questions require different sources of information to answer them, which might be why nurses don't appear to use research-based information to inform their decision making. It could be that the types of information needs that nurses have are not amenable to the types of information provided by research evidence. Luker & Kenrick (1992) suggest four categories of clinical decisions, each of which requires different types of knowledge (Table 4.1). It could be that the majority of nurses' information needs result from clinical-support, social-support, and educational procedures types of clinical decisions. Luker & Kenrick (1992) suggest that these types of decisions need different types of knowledge to research; an argument that might partially explain why nurses seem so ill-disposed toward actively seeking research-based information.

Few studies examine the information needs of nurses. Cogdill (2003) used questionnaires and interviews with nurse practitioners immediately after patient consultations to examine their information needs. The study found most information needs were to do with drug and other therapies and diagnosis. In other words, nurses reported that they were often uncertain about

Table 4.1 Categories of clinical decision and their associated knowledge	
Decision category	*Type of knowledge*
Clinical-technical procedures	Research-based or scientific knowledge
Clinical-support procedures	Aspects of practice that can be described as 'general nursing care'. Require a knowledge and experience of nursing
Social-support procedures	Require common-sense knowledge and practical experience
Educational procedures	Concerned with teaching a patient or their carers

Adapted from Luker & Kenrick (1992).

issues such as what dosage of a drug they should give a patient, what the results of a diagnostic test meant, or whether or not a specific nursing intervention was effective. All of these types of question could (and should) be answered with reference to research evidence (more on this later). However, Cogdill (2003) found that nurse practitioners sought out information from physicians, colleagues other than a physician, drug reference manuals, or textbooks/protocol manuals. Like the studies examining nurses' information use in general, research-based evidence (accessed via print journals or electronically) was not likely to be used by nurses to answer their clinical questions and so reduce the uncertainty they encountered in the decision situation.

BARRIERS TO USING RESEARCH INFORMATION IN NURSING PRACTICE

The preference for non-research information begs the question, 'Why do nurses appear not to use information generated from research evidence to inform their practice?' Nurses certainly appear to have information needs or clinical questions that *could* be answered by research-based information but they choose not to (McCaughan et al 2005, Thompson et al 2001b).

A number of studies have addressed this non-use; normally by sending out questionnaires to nurses in a variety of settings asking them to identify both the barriers and facilitators to using research information in everyday clinical practice (e.g. Bryar et al 2003, Carrion et al 2004, Griffiths et al 2001, Parahoo 2000, Veeramah 2004). There is considerable commonality in the results of these studies; nurses feel that the setting or organisation where they work is often the most important barrier to them using research information in their daily clinical practice. Issues that have been identified include not having enough authority to change procedures or policies and not enough time to implement ideas or read research (Bryar et al 2003, Carrion et al 2004, Griffiths et al 2001, Pallen & Timmins 2002, Parahoo 2000, Veeramah 2004).

However, one of the limitations of the approaches taken by the above research is that it asks nurses about their use of research evidence in general, whereas what is important from an evidence-based decision-making viewpoint is how they use information from research to evidence their *individual clinical decisions*. In general, nurses might feel that they don't have enough authority to change practice based on a guideline, but in practice they may make decisions about individual patients that are based on some form of evidence. The exception to the approach taken by the majority of studies examining nurses' information use are the studies, reported by McCaughan et al (2002) and Thompson et al (2005), examining nurses' use of research information in the context of their clinical decision making. Thompson et al (2005) identified barriers reported by nurses in the context of their everyday clinical decisions. These included a lack of information-handling skills (such as using computers and understanding statistics) and a lack of time to carry out information seeking and appraisal of research. What this body of work tells us is that for nurses to use research evidence to inform their clinical decisions, they need to be able to find research evidence quickly, in a format that is easy to read or interpret and understand. Clinical nurse specialists provide this type of knowledge-translation function to nurses, which is why they were seen as such a valuable source of information to nurses in the McCaughan et al (2002) study.

FINDING RESEARCH EVIDENCE TO INFORM CLINICAL DECISION MAKING ABOUT INDIVIDUAL PATIENTS

The majority of decisions that nurses seem to make in practice are related to some form of intervention (Thompson et al 2000). Similarly, studies of nurses' information needs have identified that the majority of 'questions' nurses ask about the care they provide appear to be related to drug therapy, diagnosis or other types of nursing intervention (Cogdill 2003). Although these may be the most common types of question that arise in nurses' clinical practice, in reality nurses must grapple with other factors that induce uncertainty in their routine clinical practice. A typology of the most common types of question nurses face can be seen in Table 4.2. As well as questions about interventions or therapy (such as whether an intervention is effective or harmful), you might also want to know whether a specific diagnostic test is accurate (diagnosis), what might happen to a patient either with or without treatment (prognosis), how a patient feels about his or her illness (meaning), or how cost effective an intervention is (economics).

One of the ways in which you can reduce the uncertainty relating to the question you face is to search for information to help you make a decision. Ideally, this information should be based on good quality research evidence that is less likely to be subject to bias (a systematic deviation from the truth) than unsystematic clinical observations (DiCenso et al 2005).

To find research evidence, you will need to carry out some form of search of the existing research literature. We will assume that this search will be electronic (although most of the principles we cover can be adapted for hand searching), as this is the most efficient way to find information easily. It is also worth noting that what follows is a brief overview of the *principles* associated with effective searching for research information for decision making.

Table 4.2	**Common clinical questions**	
Question type	Definition	Example
Intervention	Examining the effect of an intervention on patient outcomes (either in terms of improving outcomes or avoiding harmful events)	Are nicotine patches effective in helping an individual stop smoking?
Harm (or causation)	Examining the effect of potentially harmful agents on patient outcomes (such as function, mortality and morbidity)	Does smoking tobacco cause lung cancer?
Prognosis	Estimating the future course of an individual's disease or condition	What is the life expectancy of an individual who is diagnosed with lung cancer?
Diagnosis (assessment)	Examining the ability of a diagnostic tool to distinguish between individuals with and individuals without a disease or condition?	How accurate is an X-ray at identifying individuals with lung cancer?
Meaning	Describing, exploring and explaining the phenomena of interest	How do individuals who have been diagnosed with lung cancer feel about their diagnosis?
Economics	Examining the economic efficiency of healthcare programs or interventions	What are the economic costs and benefits of using nicotine patches to help individuals stop smoking?

Adapted from Collins et al (2005).

The resources listed at the end of this chapter provide pointers to more detailed advice and guidance.

To search for evidence effectively, you need to consider the following issues:

1. Developing a *structured clinical question* you can use as the basis for your search.
2. Identifying what *type of research* study will give you the evidence you need.
3. Identifying *where* to search.

We cover each of these issues in turn, using the clinical example given in Box 4.1 to illustrate the processes you could go through.

Box 4.1   Clinical scenario

Mrs Jackson is a 69-year-old woman who has been referred to the community nursing services on discharge from hospital. She has a 5 cm × 5 cm venous leg ulcer on her left calf. The diagnosis of a venous ulcer was confirmed whilst she was in hospital. You are new to the community nursing team and are carrying out a first assessment visit to Mrs Jackson.

Developing a structured clinical question

To search electronic databases effectively, you need to be able to produce a search strategy that enables you to identify relevant research easily without also retrieving loads of irrelevant material. In our experience, one of the main problems that nurses have when trying to search for information is that their searches are unfocused. If we use the clinical example in Box 4.1, one of the clinical questions you might have is, 'What is the best treatment for Mrs Jackson's leg ulcer?' You could ask your clinical colleagues for advice; one might tell you that he would use a four-layer compression bandage; another colleague would use a two-layer bandage. Asking your colleagues has resulted in you remaining uncertain; you are still unsure what treatment might be best. One possible search you could use is to look for 'compression bandages' using the clinic's computer and PubMed connection. Doing this on one of the databases (Medline; how to do this is discussed later in the chapter), retrieves 128 titles and abstracts. You could look through all 128 to see if any of them could help you; a strategy that would probably be far too time consuming for most clinicians.

However, if you *structure* the question so that you focus in on the key issues you are interested in, you can identify *keywords* from the question you can use as the basis for your search. This is a far more effective approach. One framework often used to structure searches is known as PICO. PICO stands for:

Population: specification of the patient or client group that is the focus of your question. This could be defined according to age, sex, or the health problem.
Intervention/exposure: the intervention you are interested in knowing about.
Control/alternative intervention/exposure: you often need to compare the intervention you are interested in either to a control or other intervention (which might be normal practice).
Outcome: the outcome you are interested in for the patient or group of patients who are the focus of the question.

The clinical question generated from our scenario has been reformulated into the PICO framework in Table 4.3. We have also included the search terms we used to search the same database (Medline; Table 4.4).

Table 4.3	Clinical question in PICO format with search terms	
PICO element	*Question*	*Search Term*
Patient	Patient with venous leg ulcer	Leg ulcer
Intervention	4-layer compression bandaging	4-layer compression Compression
[Comparison]	2-layer compression bandaging	2-layer compression
Outcome	Ulcer healing	Healing

Table 4.4   Search used in Medline (1950 to February week 2 2008)

Search term used	Hits
Leg ulcer (MeSH subheading*) **OR** Leg Ulcer (free text search)	6283
Compression (free text search) **OR** Stockings, Compression (MeSH subheading*)	56,745
4-layer	229
2-layer	1029
Healing (free text search) **OR** Wound Healing (MeSH subheading*)	97,871
1 **AND** 2 **AND** 3 **AND** 4 **AND** 5	1

*In databases such as Medline and Cinahl, articles are indexed according to keywords, which are categorised into subheadings known as Medical SubHeadings (MeSH). A good search would encompass both the MeSH headings and use a free text search, as relevant articles might not be indexed using the keyword you have chosen.

We used 'Boolean' operators to combine the search terms to focus the search down. Boolean operators are a way of combining search terms to enable you to either broaden or focus your search in a structured way. A pictorial example of how the most common Boolean operators (AND/OR) work is provided by Figure 4.1. Normally, you combine those search terms describing the same element of the PICO (for instance 'randomised' and its American counterpart 'randomized') with the 'OR' Boolean operator. This retrieves titles using *either* term. You might then combine the different elements of your PICO (such as leg ulcers and compression bandaging) with the 'AND' Boolean operator. This would yield titles from the database that contain *both* the search terms.

By using this type of structured search in Medline we retrieved one journal article (Moffatt et al 2003). Using the PICO format to structure our question has produced a more focused search. However, you still need to

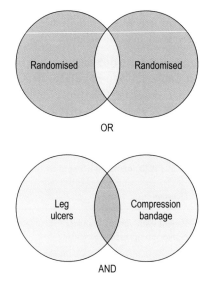

Figure 4.1   Boolean search operators.

evaluate (or appraise) the study to see if it provides reliable and valid evidence on which to base your decision (we don't cover critical appraisal in this book, but see the further reading at the end of the chapter for resources that do).

Identifying the type of study design you need to answer your question

If you are looking for research evidence to help you answer a specific clinical question, you also need to know what *type* of research study would provide you with the best evidence to do so. There are a number of different ways of carrying out research studies, each designed to answer different types of questions whilst avoiding different types of bias. You need to try to match your clinical question with the study design most likely to give you good-quality evidence to inform your decision. Table 4.5 provides an overview of the different types of study design for the different types of clinical question you might be faced with (Collins et al 2005). So, for instance, if you wanted to know the prognosis for a patient with a certain diagnosis, you would look for a cohort study. This study design follows patients up over a long period of time to try and identify what happens to them. You couldn't use a randomised controlled trial for this type of research question, normally because you either can't randomise patients to either have or not have an illness or it would not be ethical to do so (e.g. if you are interested in the effects of a possibly harmful substance like tobacco on an individual's health). Similarly, if you were interested in finding out how patients feel about having a specific treatment you would look for qualitative studies.

Returning to our example, our clinical question is concerned with 'intervention': we want to know the best treatment for a venous leg ulcer. The best study design to help answer this question is either a systematic review of the evidence or, if that isn't available, a randomised controlled trial. We could have restricted our search to these types of study if we had retrieved more than the one study. This would have limited our search further and ensured that the research retrieved was best suited to answering our clinical question. Refer to the examples of study designs at the end of this chapter (p. 50), where we have used the same scenario to illustrate the different study designs.

Table 4.5 Matching study designs with clinical questions	
Clinical question	*Study design*
Intervention	Systematic review of randomised controlled trials
	Randomised controlled trial
Harm (or causation)	Randomised controlled trial
	Observational study (cohort or case-control)
Prognosis	Observational study
Diagnosis (Assessment)	Diagnostic test study
Meaning	Qualitative study

Adapted from Collins et al (2005).

Identifying where to search

Thus far, we have given you a brief overview of the principles of searching for research evidence on databases such as Medline and Cinahl. These databases bring together the details of reports of research published in journals. This is a great approach if you have the time, knowledge, and confidence to read and understand journal articles. A far more efficient means of accessing research knowledge is to use information resources that do the critical reading and appraisal for you.

Haynes (2006) provides a model built around the '5Ss': systems, summaries, synopses, syntheses, and studies (Figure 4.2). At the top of this hierarchy are clinical decision-support systems. These give evidence-based guidance to a clinician and combine it with individual patient data (Haynes 2006) to provide tailored advice. Nursing has few such systems, and the evidence for their effectiveness in changing clinical practice and improving patient outcomes is limited (Randell et al 2007). Nevertheless, as a way of informing individual practice, they have a roll.

Moving down the hierarchy, the next source likely to yield useful information are summaries of evidence, such as evidence-based textbooks. Summaries integrate the best possible evidence from the lower 'layers' in the hierarchy such as systematic reviews, to provide an overview of the evidence for the management of a health problem (Haynes 2006). This is in contrast to systematic reviews and randomised trials, which often provide evidence about only one element of a management strategy. As can be seen from the hierarchy, if no summaries exist, the next best place to search for evidence is evidence-based journal abstracts, followed by systematic reviews, and then randomised controlled trials and other studies.

Let us use the 5S approach to informing the decisions surrounding the management of Mrs Jackson's venous leg ulcer. Starting at the top of the hierarchy, we would consult a decision-support system, but these do not exist in our case and so we look at the next best thing: an online evidence-based textbook. One such resource is Clinical Evidence (www.clinicalevidence.bmj.com/ceweb/index.jsp). Clinical Evidence provides an up-to-date

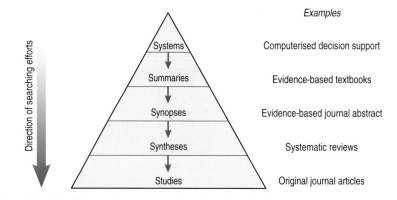

Figure 4.2 The 5S levels of organisation of evidence from health care research (adapted from Haynes 2006).

ESSENTIAL DECISION MAKING AND CLINICAL JUDGEMENT

overview of evidence-based systematic reviews to assist with the management of patient conditions. Accessing the wounds section (we did this in February 2008) highlights a summary of evidence for venous leg ulcers. This provides details of therapy likely to be beneficial, together with an indication of the quality of evidence for the recommendations. If we had accessed this source at the beginning of our search we would have seen that using *any* form of compression bandaging is beneficial for healing leg ulcers. In this case, it is uncertain whether using two or four layers is better; your clinical judgement, informed by a discussion with the patient, would still need to be employed in the final decision.

What if Clinical Evidence or some other summary had not helped us? The next level down on the hierarchy of information sources is synopses, examples of which are provided by the 'evidence-based' family of journals; one of which is *Evidence-based Nursing* (*EBN*; available online at www.ebn.bmj.com/). The 'evidence-based' journals review articles published in a wide range of medical and nursing journals, assessing them for the quality and validity of the research that has been published. The best studies are then selected and an abstract is produced, which provides the paired-down, essential details of a study. This is published alongside an assessment of its applicability to clinical practice in the form of a commentary. Searching EBN online for 'leg ulcer compression bandage' in the title retrieved 28 hits. One of the summaries retrieved was an overview and commentary on the systematic review of compression therapy (Fernell 1998). There is also a more recent commentary on a trial comparing four-layer bandages with one-layer bandages for compression therapy (Betts 2007). Both of these summaries are one page in length, with the commentary giving a useful overview on the clinical significance of the results of the original studies. Overall, as with the recommendations from clinical evidence, the results of these two studies suggest that compression therapy is better than no therapy; with the trial results suggesting that a four-layer system is better than just using a one-layer bandage.

Finally, if we were unable to find any relevant articles in a synopsis, we would then look for a synthesis of research evidence in a systematic review. The main resource for systematic reviews is the Cochrane library (www.thecochranelibrary.com), which publishes the results of good quality systematic reviews. A simple search on the term 'leg ulcer' in the Cochrane library database retrieves 34 reviews, of which one is directly relevant to our research question (Cullum et al 2001). The review concludes that using compression is better than no compression for healing leg ulcers, and that multilayer systems are better than single-layer systems.

When looking for research information, you are more likely to find relevant information that you can easily use to help you make decisions about patient care if you start at the top of the 5S hierarchy of information sources. Resources such as Clinical Evidence and Evidence-based Nursing have been developed to provide up-to-date information in quick and easy-to-read format. Using such resources has the potential to help nurses access research evidence they can use for their everyday decision making.

Using information in decision making

SUMMARY

This chapter has provided an overview of the issues surrounding how nurses use information to inform their decision making in clinical practice. Nurses face a number of challenges when making decisions in practice; not least, distinguishing that patient information which is important from the vast array of possibly less important information available to them. Being able to identify relevant information, and to distinguish it from less relevant information, is a key skill for good decision making, and one that probably comes only with experience.

One strategy that can be used to reduce uncertainty in a decision is to formulate a clinical question about patient care. Such questions might be related to the patient's treatment, to the diagnostic tests you are using, or to how the patient feels about his or her condition or experiences. Such questions can (and indeed, should) form the basis for searching for research evidence to help you access the experiences of far more patients than you could ever meet in your own practice.

The second half of this chapter provided an overview of the basic principles of using the above approach. If you wish to develop these skills further, we recommend that you access the resources listed at the end of the chapter and the further reading.

EXERCISES

Imagine that you are a community mental health nurse, who has been asked by a local GP to visit a 37-year-old man who lives alone, is recently unemployed, and has a history of alcohol misuse. The GP thinks that the man has 'moderate' depression and would value your opinion about treatment options, after you have discussed them with patient. The options the team are considering are cognitive behavioural therapy delivered primarily via the telephone or the traditional approach of drug-based therapy using selective serotonin reuptake inhibitors (SSRIs). You are uncertain which is most likely to work.

1. Formulate a clinical question based on the above scenario.
2. Where might you look for evidence giving the research you need that is most likely to be useful for answering your question?
3. Develop a search strategy that could be used for the source(s) you have chosen.
4. Run the search – was it useful or not? If not, what went wrong, and how might you improve it next time?

Examples of study designs

In the following examples, we have used the same scenario – the link between cigarette smoking and lung cancer – to illustrate the different study designs.

A randomised controlled trial (RCT)

In an RCT, patients are allocated randomly to either 'smoke cigarettes' or 'not smoke cigarettes' groups, and are followed up over time to see if they develop the outcome of interest (lung cancer). In this instance, because we think the intervention could be harmful, it would be unethical to randomise individuals, so we would need a different type of study design (Figure 4.3).

A cohort study (observational)
In a cohort study, you identify individuals who have been exposed to the intervention (in this case cigarette smoking) and compare them with individuals who have not been exposed (non-smokers) and follow them up over time to see if they develop the outcome of interest (Figure 4.4).

A case-control study (observational)
In a case-control study, you identify individuals who have the outcome of interest (in this case, individuals with lung cancer) and match them to controls who do not have the outcome. You then work backwards to see if they have been exposed to the intervention (in this case, you would identify how many in each group were cigarette smokers) (Figure 4.5).

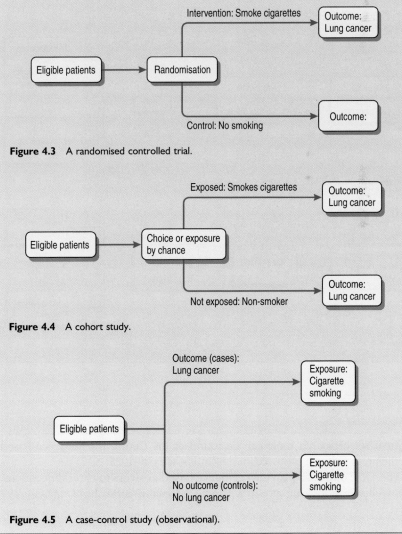

Figure 4.3 A randomised controlled trial.

Figure 4.4 A cohort study.

Figure 4.5 A case-control study (observational).

Continued

ESSENTIAL DECISION MAKING AND CLINICAL JUDGEMENT

EXERCISES—CONT'D

A study to determine prognosis

In prognostic studies, we are interested in identifying whether any variables modified the prognosis of an individual with a certain condition. Perhaps we are interested in whether eating five portions of fruit and vegetables a day modifies the chances of cigarette smokers developing lung cancer. We would identify patients with lung cancer, measure their fruit and vegetable intake over time and then monitor who does or does not develop the outcome of interest (Figure 4.6).

A study to determine the accuracy of a diagnostic test

When examining the performance of a diagnostic test, we want to compare the performance of the new text with some form of 'gold standard' test that is considered to be the diagnostic standard for a particular condition. As an example, say we have developed a new imaging test for the diagnosis of lung cancer and we want to establish how good it is. A lung biopsy is the 'gold standard' test, so this is what we would compare the new test to (Figure 4.7).

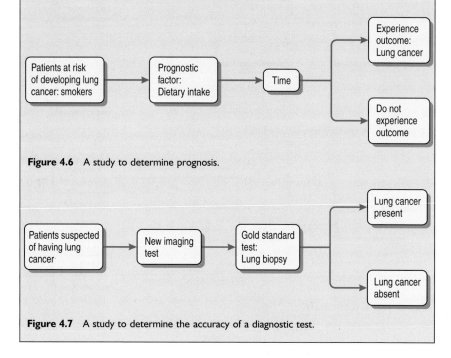

Figure 4.6 A study to determine prognosis.

Figure 4.7 A study to determine the accuracy of a diagnostic test.

RESOURCES

A great set of search tools can be found at the Centre for Evidence-Based Medicine at Oxford: www.cebm.net/index.aspx?o=1038

The TRIP database provides evidence-based answers to clinical questions. It is well worth looking at: www.tripdatabase.com/index.html

The Centre for Evidence-Based Medicine at Toronto has fantastic help, advice and tools sections for all of the stages of evidence-based practice: www.cebm.utoronto.ca/practise/formulate/

The journal *Evidence-based Nursing* has a useful search facility for synopses (an abstract and commentary from a nurse) of good quality research of relevance and importance for nurses: www.ebn.bmj.com

If you want to learn more about how to appraise research evidence, then the following text by Nicky Cullum and colleagues is an accessible guide for nurses: Cullum N, Ciliska D, Haynes R B et al 2008 Evidence-based nursing: an introduction. Blackwell, Oxford.

An excellent chapter by Trisha Greenhalgh, on how to search the literature, appears in the following book: Greenhalgh T 2006 How to read a paper, 3rd edn. Blackwell BMJ Books, Oxford.

REFERENCES

Betts J 2007 4-layer bandages were better than 1-layer bandages, and pentoxifylline may be better than placebo for venous leg ulcers. Evidence-Based Nursing 10:87

Bryar R M, Closs S J, Baum G et al 2003 The Yorkshire BARRIERS project: diagnostic analysis of barriers to research utilisation. International Journal of Nursing Studies 40:73–84

Carrion M, Woods P, Norman I 2004 Barriers to research utilisation among forensic mental health nurses. International Journal of Nursing Studies 41:613–619

Cogdill K W 2003 Information needs and information seeking in primary care: a study of nurse practitioners. Journal of the Medical Libraries Association 91:203–215

Collins S, Voth T, DiCenso A et al 2005 Finding the evidence. In: DiCenso A, Guyatt G, Ciliska D (eds) Evidence-based nursing: a guide to clinical practice. Mosby, St Louis, p 20–43

Cullum N, Nelson E A, Fletcher AW et al 2001 Compression for venous leg ulcers. Cochrane Database of Systematic Reviews, Issue 2, edn p. DOI: 10.1002/14651858.CD000265

DiCenso A, Ciliska D, Guyatt G 2005 Introduction to evidence-based nursing. In: DiCenso A, Guyatt G, Ciliska D (eds) Evidence-based nursing. a guide to clinical practice. Mosby, St Louis, p 3–19

Fernell J 1998 Review: compression treatment improves healing of venous leg ulcers. Evidence-Based Nursing 1:50

Griffiths J, Bryar R M, Closs S J et al 2001 Barriers to research implementation by community nurses. British Journal of Community Nursing 6:501–510

Hammond K R, Kelly K J, Schneider R J et al 1966 Clinical inference in nursing. Analyzing cognitive tasks representative of nursing problems. Nursing Research 15: 134–138

Haynes R 2006 Of studies, syntheses, synopses, summaries and systems: the '5S' evolution of information services for evidence-based healthcare decisions. Evidence-Based Medicine 11:162–164

Lamond D, Crow R, Chase J et al 1996 Information sources used in decision-making: considerations for simulation development. International Journal of Nursing Studies 33: 47–57

Luker K A, Kenrick M 1992 An exploratory study of the sources of influence on the clinical decisions of community nurses. Journal of Advanced Nursing 17:457–466

McCaughan D, Thompson C, Cullum N et al 2002 Acute care nurses' perceptions of barriers to using research information in clinical decision making. Journal of Advanced Nursing 39:46–60

McCaughan D, Thompson C, Cullum N et al 2005 Nurse practitioner and practice nurses' use of research information in decision making: findings from an exploratory study. Family Practice 22:490–497

McKnight M 2006 The information seeking of on-duty critical care nurses: evidence from participant observation and in-context interviews. Journal of the Medical Libraries Association 94:145–151

Moffatt C, McCullagh L, O'Connor T et al 2003 Randomized trial of four-layer and two-layer bandage systems in the management of chronic venous ulceration. Wound Repair and Regeneration 11:166–171

Offredy M 2002 Decision making in primary care: outcomes from a study using patient scenarios. Journal of Advanced Nursing 40:532–541

Pallen N, Timmins F 2002 Research-based practice: myth or reality? A review of the barriers affecting research utilisation in practice. Nurse Education in Practice 2:99–108

Parahoo K 2000 Barriers to, and facilitators of, research utilization among nurses in Northern Ireland. Journal of Advanced Nursing 31:89–98

Randell R, Mitchell N, Dowding D et al 2007 Effects of computerized decision-support systems on nursing performance and patient outcomes: a systematic review. Journal of Health Services Research and Policy 12:242–249

Tannery N H, Wessel C B, Epstein B A et al (2007) Hospital nurses' use of knowledge-based information resources. Nursing Outlook 55:15–19

Thompson C, McCaughan D, Cullum N et al 2000 Nurses' use of research information in clinical decision making: a descriptive and analytical study. University of York, York

Thompson C, McCaughan D, Cullum N et al 2001a Research information in nurses' clinical decision making: what is useful? Journal of Advanced Nursing 36:376–388

Thompson C, McCaughan D, Cullum N et al 2001b The accessibility of research-based knowledge for nurses in United Kingdom acute care settings. Journal of Advanced Nursing 36:11–22

Thompson C, McCaughan D, Cullum N et al 2005 Barriers to evidence-based practice in primary care nursing – why viewing decision making as context is helpful. Journal of Advanced Nursing 52:432–444

Veeramah V 2004 Utilization of research findings by graduate nurses and midwives. Journal of Advanced Nursing 47:183–191

Theoretical approaches

Carl Thompson and Dawn Dowding

KEY ISSUES

- What do we mean by a rational decision?
- The distinction between *normative* theories of how we should make decisions, *descriptive* theories of how we actually make decisions and the importance of *prescriptive* theories for helping us close the gap between the two
- How the characteristics of decisions influence how we make a choice between alternatives and use our professional judgement

INTRODUCTION

This chapter is about the theories that provide a foundation for our choices and judgements in clinical practice. Theory shapes our understanding. Theoretical models of phenomena we experience help us connect the dots between seemingly disparate facts about the world. Theory helps us describe experiences and helps us predict events yet to be encountered. Perhaps most importantly, theory allows us to test our ideas against our experiences. Through understanding relevant theories, comes knowledge. Knowledge provides understanding that provides a basis for our actions.

Although much of this book is concerned with the action part of 'actionable understanding', it is important to recognise that by understanding the theories of why we do what we do (and, just as importantly, why we fail to do what we should do) we can make more informed choices and possibly even better decisions.

Theory in nursing often gets a bad press; how many teachers have heard the clarion call of the disgruntled student, 'I hate theory, it's just not relevant'. We think that the theories we present in this chapter *are* relevant for nurses making decisions. Many of the practical techniques invoked in this book rely on these theoretical models of the way the world works. For example, Bayes' rule, which we discuss in Chapter 9 when we look at diagnosis, is a technique for ensuring that the theoretical rules of probability (specifically, conditional probabilities) are not broken when making a diagnosis. Before we try to distinguish between the various theories of decision making, we need a reference point or benchmark for comparison. One such reference point is rationality.

RATIONALITY

All decision making must deal with the selection of a preferred alternative using the facts and values associated with the choice. One standard to judge a decision by is whether it is a 'rational' decision. The *Oxford English Dictionary* defines rationality as:

> **1** based on or in accordance with reason or logic **2** able to think sensibly or logically **3** having the capacity to reason.

Although concise, these definitions do little to advance our understanding of *why* rationality is desirable when making decisions. To proceed, we need to break the concept of the rationality down a little further.

First, because decisions are a combination of our thinking *and* our actions, let us make the distinction between rational beliefs and rational actions. In slightly more academic language, we can term this distinction as one of 'epistemic rationality' (beliefs) versus 'instrumental rationality' (actions). Rational beliefs are rational in the sense that they are true (or most likely true) given the premises they are founded on. So, asking a nurse to describe their reasoning behind why they gave a patient analgesia reveals an entirely rational set of beliefs:

> *The patient has a headache and says this is the reason why he will not eat.*
> *I don't want the patient to have a headache (because then he will eat).*
> *If I give him some analgesia, the headache will most likely improve.*
> *So, I gave him some analgesia.*

The problem with this kind of abstract or *theoretical* reasoning is that it is just that: abstract. Our day-to-day reasoning is of a more *practical* kind and focuses not on the underlying logic of our reasoning, but on the selection of rational actions. Imagine a scenario in primary care in which you are faced with a patient with diabetes. The patient's theoretical reasoning enables her to infer that her lack of adherence to a balanced diet is hampering her efforts at controlling her blood sugar. However, the practical reasoning that accompanies choosing the best course of corrective action might mean she decides (entirely rationally) not to change her lifestyle. How can this be the case? How can it be rational for her to not change her lifestyle and so expose herself to greater potential harm? The patient is rational because our actions are a result not just of logical inference, but logical inference *given* our goals or values. In this case, the woman might value improved control of her blood sugar but she might place an even higher value on eating an unrestricted diet.

To be useful, rationality has to be of the instrumental kind: a rational action is one that is most likely to achieve the goals we set ourselves. Moreover, goals are a function of our beliefs, preferences and desires. Herbert Simon (1983) sums it up:

" Reason is wholly instrumental. It cannot tell us where to go; at best, it can tell us how to get there. It is a gun for hire that can be employed in the service of any goals we have, good or bad. (Simon 1983, p 7–8)"

On limited or 'bounded' rationality

Human beings, of course, are rarely purely rational. For a choice to be entirely rational, the decision maker would have to have answers to four basic questions (March 1994, p 2):

1. The question of *alternatives*: what actions are possible?
2. The question of *expectations*: what future consequences might follow from each alternative? How likely is each possible consequence, assuming that an alternative is chosen?
3. The question of *preferences*: how valuable (to the decision maker) are the consequences associated with each of the alternatives?
4. The question of the *decision rule*: how is a choice to be made among the alternatives in terms of the values of their consequences?

Getting complete answers to these questions is rarely possible. In reality, individuals have a number of limitations that together led to the (Nobel prize-winning) recognition that rationality is 'bounded' and constrained by these limitations:

" ... in an information-rich world, the wealth of information means a dearth of something else: a scarcity of whatever it is that information consumes. What information consumes is rather obvious: it consumes the attention of its recipients. Hence a wealth of information creates a poverty of attention and a need to allocate that attention efficiently among the overabundance of information sources that might consume it ... (Simon 1971 p 40–41)"

The limitations of human beings when it comes to instrumental rationality can be summarised as:

1. *Problems of attention*: as the above quote from Simon (1971) illustrates, time and the ability to focus one's attention on too many things at once means decision making is often about searching and attention rather than choice *per se*.
2. *Problems of memory*: individual and organisational memories are not like bank vaults in which memories are stored cumulatively and able to be withdrawn at will. Memories are constructs; our storage capacity is finite and recall is flawed.
3. *Problems of comprehension*: synthesising, summarising, and organising information to infer beyond what is simply experienced is difficult for humans. The relevance of information is often unnoticed; the connections between elements in a situation go unconnected. Coherent interpretations

of the decision problem and solutions are thus more difficult than they need to be.

4. *Problems of communication*: communicating information, particularly complex information, is difficult. The problem is compounded by specialisation (or the 'division of labour' in the language of sociology), as a differentiation of knowledge, competence, and language means that different groups make sense of decision problems differently.

Together, these limitations result in bounded rational decision makers engaging in two classic traits: (1) adaptive psychological behaviour; and (2) 'satisficing' (explained below). Adaptive behaviour takes a variety of forms including using cognitive shortcuts or heuristics (which we will explore in more detail in Chapter 7) such as stereotyping, typologising behaviour (e.g. people are classed as 'extravert' or 'introvert'), and attitude (e.g. people are 'liberal' or 'anti-professional') (March 1994 p 11). People pay attention to the core components of problems and ignore the peripheral elements. They use schemas, or socially developed scripts, to fill in missing information and discrepancies in understanding (the nurse's 'role in a typical primary care practice nurse-patient consultation' being one example) (Offredy 2002).

Satisficing is an important term and refers to the human tendency to make choices that are 'good enough' rather than optimal. Recall that a purely rational choice is the one that represents the most effective means to a specified goal. From this perspective, a rational decision maker is one who compares all the possible choices and chooses the one that best meets his or her goals. In economic terms, a rational choice is the option that *maximises* the outcome the decision maker is interested in (e.g. chances of healing, amount of health, maximum reduction in harm). Satisficing, however, involves choosing a decision that merely exceeds some kind of threshold or personal decision criterion.

We can see the difference between maximising and satisficing if we consider planning a new nurse-led service. A maximising decision would involve identifying and specifying, in advance, each service stakeholder's preferences for a variety of options and important goals and then choosing an approach to delivering the service that maximises those goals. Alternatively, a satisficing strategy would involve developing a range of options against a broad measure of 'average' value (such as greater 'patient choice') and then choosing the one that meets this broad goal (i.e. most likely to increase choice). Therefore, individuals can still be rational even when intellectual, cognitive, and environmental constraints mean that rationality itself is necessarily limited.

THEORIES OF JUDGEMENT AND DECISION MAKING

Ultimately, we all want to make good clinical decisions. The problem, which will be discussed further in Chapter 6, is how to define a 'good' choice. *Normative* theories help in this regard by steering us towards decisions as they would be made if we were *rational* decision makers. They offer a series of benchmarks against which we can compare our decisions and decision making and to try to gauge how far off the mark we are. When we discover that our decisions fall short of normative theories of decision making we try to discover and explain why. This explanatory function is where *descriptive* theories of judgement and decision making come in. With some idea of how we should make choices (normative theories) and some idea of how we actually make choices (via descriptive theories), the final task of decision improvers is to find ways that enmesh our real world decision making with normative approaches. This synthesis is the preserve of *prescriptive* approaches to decision making (which are discussed further in Chapters 9 and 11).

Normative theories of decision making: expected and subjective utility theory

As we have previously discussed, a 'rational' decision is a function of how likely an outcome is given a decision option and the value that the individual places on the outcome. Very few decisions in healthcare are a straight choice: most involve trade-offs. For example, if you have a venous leg ulcer and are offered compression bandaging, you must trade-off an improvement in your chances of the ulcer healing in 6 months against the discomfort and unsightly bandage of compression therapy. If you are an older mother and antenatal screening for Down syndrome is offered, you must trade-off the chance of identifying a baby with Down syndrome against having to live with the knowledge that you might give birth to a child with Down syndrome for the following 6 months of gestation (as well as how you might feel about mothering a child with Down syndrome once it is born). Such trade-offs revolve around how you feel about the potential outcomes of your choices. Utility is the means by which those feelings or 'valuations' are captured and represented in our decision making.

Trade-offs, outcomes, and decisional complexity

The concept of trade-offs is central to understanding why some decisions are more complex than others. Decision trade-offs can take three possible forms depending on the outcomes.

First, a decision can have just two possible outcomes. Examples include 'die or survive', 'cure or no cure', 'success or failure'. An example here is the patient who exhibits all the signs of someone having a cardiac arrest. You have a choice: do nothing or intervene. Doing nothing equates to almost certain death for the patient and intervening means at least a chance of survival. There is no need here to try to represent the trade-off by explicitly measuring preferences for outcomes; you simply choose the decision that is most likely to lead to the better outcome (survival).

The next level of complexity comes when a decision has a range of possible outcomes that can be measured on a single scale of 'least preferred' through to 'most preferred'. A common scale that forms the basis for this kind of choices is time – specifically, survival time. So, for example, consider a mental health nurse working with an adolescent engaged in self-destructive patterns of drinking and drug taking. The nurse is faced with having to choose which of a variety of effective management strategies to adopt. If the patient just wants to live for the longest possible time then a good decision is simply the one that is most likely to maximise their life expectancy. However, the decision might be more complex because of the patient's preference for 5 years of certain (but shortened) life rather than only a 50/50 chance of survival for 20 more years, should he or she change their behaviour.

The most complex kinds of choices are those in which there is more than a single dimension to be valued. Most commonly, these involve trade-offs between length of life and quality of life. A classic example for women is in the area of prophylactic mastectomy, in which women must choose to either undertake regular surveillance of their breast(s) or have them removed to decrease the risk of cancer. In this case, the woman must trade-off longer life expectancy with no breasts against a shorter life expectancy with breasts. A managerial, rather than clinical, example can be seen in a paper by Brennan & Anthony (2000), in which nurses were asked to value approaches to the management of nurses, such as continuity of care versus participation versus leadership.

Utility defined

One of the ways in which to examine how individuals feel about the outcomes of such complex decision trade-offs is utility. Utility is a numerical measure of the value that individuals or groups place on the different outcomes or consequences of a decision. Utility is also referred to as a health state preference. Whatever terminology is used, individuals are asked to provide an explicit valuation of how they feel about the different health states that may occur as the result of a decision taken about their health condition.

We will look at how to measure utilities in Chapter 11. However, at the theoretical level it is important to recognise that utility measures (as an evaluation of the value attached to a health state or health outcome) are different to quality-of-life measures. Quality-of-life measures (such as the EQ5D: www.euroqol.org/) focus on the characteristics of that health state. Utility can be thought of as an individual's emotional reaction to that health state and the quality of life it entails.

Expected and subjective expected utility theory

If we consider that a rational decision is a function of how likely an option is, given a decision option (its probability), and the value that an individual places on the outcome (utility), we can now consider how these two elements can be combined to make choices.

To understand why people make different choices despite being faced with the same information, we need to step outside the realm of clinical practice. Gambling provides an ideal environment in which to explore ideas of choice as they are often familiar, easily envisaged and well defined. Consider the following choice (gamble):

A. A 20% ($p = 0.20$) of winning £45, and an 80% ($p = 0.80$) chance of winning nothing.

B. A 25% ($p = 0.25$) of winning £30, and a 75% ($p = 0.75$) chance of winning nothing.

Which one would you choose? Actually, most people choose option A (Hastie & Dawes 2001). Do you know why? One explanation – although at this stage you might not have realised it yet – is that the *expected value* of option A is higher.

Expected value is the probability of winning multiplied by the value of the outcome (as distinct from the valuation we put on it). So option A's expected value is $0.2 \times £45 = £9$, whereas option B's expected value is only $0.25 \times £30 = £7.50$. If you chose option A, all well and good. However, how do we explain that at least some of you will have preferred option B?

In 1738, the mathematician Daniel Bernoulli said that, 'a gain of one thousand ducats is more significant to a pauper than to a rich man, though both gain the same amount'. In more modern language, this sentiment can be restated as, 'the value of money declines in line with the amount you win or already possess'. Returning to our examples A and B above, imagine a situation in which you are asked to make the choice on the Wednesday prior to a Friday payday; you might prefer the gamble with the higher chance of winning £30 to the one with the lower chance of winning £45. It all depends what the money will mean to you. We can see the effect of valuing outcomes even more dramatically if we look at the following gamble:

A. An 80% chance of winning £45 or a 20% chance of nothing.
B. A 100% chance of winning £30.

Which option do you prefer? Work out the expected value of both gambles (answers at the end of the chapter). Assuming you preferred option A in the first gamble and option B in the second – and most people do – what's wrong with your answer? In decision theoretic terms, you have violated the key principle of expected utility: that you will choose the option that gives you the largest expected value. Based on this simple starting point we can now expand our working approach to rational decision making with reference to six key principles (or axioms) (Box 5.1). Taken together, these constitute normative rules for a rational decision.

Thus far, we have encountered choices in which the probabilities are 'objective' and known. In nursing many of the probabilities we have to work with are unknown or can only be guessed. Savage (1954) took the idea of expected utility and recast it using 'subjective' probabilities (see also Chapter 3 and Chapter 9 for subjective probabilities in the form of Bayesian statistics and probability revision). Despite the subjective nature of the probabilities, rational choices are still a function of probabilities and the value that people place on the outcomes that might occur. We discuss how you can use the principles of subjective epected utility theory (SEUT) to help you make clinical decisions further in Chapter 11.

Although the axioms of Box 5.1 are remarkably robust at a societal level (Becker 1976), it is clear that the assumptions are violated at least some of the time by individuals. Descriptive theories of decision making can help us to understand why this might be the case.

Box 5.1   The six key axioms of a rational decision maker (one who seeks to maximise the expected value of their choices) (adapted from Plous 1993)

1. *Ordering*: rational decision makers will compare any two choices. Either they prefer one to the other, or if they don't they will be indifferent.
2. *Dominance*: rational decision makers will not choose decision options that are dominated by other decision options. Dominance can be weak or strong. If a decision is better than another decision in just a single respect then it is weakly dominant. If a decision is better than another decision in almost all respects it is strongly dominant. To appreciate the difference, a car (A) strongly dominates another car (B) if its colour is more agreeable to you, it gets more miles to the gallon, and it looks sexier (if having a 'sexy' car is your thing). It is only weakly dominant if the only difference between the two cars is that A does more miles to the gallon than B. There should be uncertainty at the point of decision making not 'dominance', otherwise the decision becomes a 'no brainer' and not a decision at all.
3. *Cancellation*: rational decision makers should base their decisions on those outcomes that differ between the options under consideration. Outcomes that are shared between the options will cancel each other out.
4. *Transitivity*: a rational decision maker who prefers outcome A to outcome B and outcome B to outcome C, should also prefer outcome A to outcome C.
5. *Continuity*: rational decision makers will prefer a gamble between the best and worst outcome to a definite intermediate outcome, as long as the probability of the good outcome is 'good enough'. So, rational decision makers will prefer a gamble between option A (£100 or bankruptcy) to a sure gain of £10; but only if the chances of bankruptcy are 0.0001 (i.e. the chances of £100 are greater than 99%).
6. *Invariance*: rational decision makers should not be affected by the order in which choices are presented. Sticking with our gambling examples; a rational person will not prefer a 'compound' gamble (a lottery with two phases each with a 50/50 chance) for a £100 win if both phases are 'wins' and a single phase lottery with a 25% chance of winning £100.

DESCRIPTIVE THEORIES OF DECISION MAKING

This section explores different approaches to describing *how* individuals reach judgements and decisions. It includes Information-processing theory, heuristics, fast and frugal thinking, social judgement theory (SJT), and cognitive continuum theory (CCT). All these approaches share an ability to describe how people reach a decision and use their judgement. In some circumstances (CCT, SJT, and fast and frugal thinking), they also have a normative dimension in that they offer us some rules to help improve our decision making in the real world. This real-world emphasis makes them distinct from truly normative theories such as expected utility and so for this reason we will say that they have a *prescriptive* element to them.

Information-processing theory

As has already been highlighted earlier in this chapter human rationality is 'bounded' by the limitations of our ability to process information. Newell

& Simon (1972) proposed that as a response to these limitations we have developed ways of thinking (processing information) that allow us to make judgements and decisions effectively. It is these assumptions regarding the limitations of human rationality that underpin most of the research on how nurses (and doctors) reason and is broadly known as an information-processing approach to reasoning.

Research into how doctors and nurses reason when making judgements and decisions has identified a number of different processes that are used to make judgements and decisions. These include hypothetico-deductive reasoning, the use of heuristics, and fast and frugal reasoning.

Hypothetico-deductive reasoning

A number of studies examining the reasoning of both doctors and nurses have suggested that individuals go through a number of phases in their reasoning processes. Box 5.2 outlines the different stages of reasoning when making judgements and decisions, as identified by Elstein et al (1978).

The first stage of this process is the gathering of clinical information about the patient (known as the cue acquisition stage). This information can often be collected before you see a patient; for instance you might look at a patient's notes to find out his age, medical history, what symptoms he has now (raised temperature, pain, prescribed medication) and what the doctor thinks might be wrong with him (the diagnosis).

Following this, you might generate some initial possible explanations for the clinical information you have collected (hypotheses); these are related to the data gathered, and are held in short-term memory. For instance, you might be looking after a patient who is complaining of chest pain, looks grey, and appears slightly clammy (clinical information). You think he might be having a heart attack, although he could just have bad indigestion, or he might be anxious.

The next stage in the reasoning process involves you interpreting the cues gathered during the data-gathering stage and classifying them as confirming, refuting, or not contributing to the initial explanations (hypotheses) that you have generated (cue interpretation). For instance, as part of your data-gathering exercise you might have carried out an ECG on your patient, which is normal. You would re-evaluate your hypothesis that he may be having a heart attack on the basis of this cue, together with the other signs and symptoms he is exhibiting.

Theoretical approaches

Box 5.2 Hypothetico-deductive reasoning (adapted from Elstein et al 1978)

- Cue acquisition
- Hypothesis generation
- Cue interpretation
- Hypothesis evaluation

The final stage of the reasoning process involves you weighing up the pros and cons of each possible explanation for your patient's signs and symptoms and choosing the one favoured by the majority of the evidence (hypothesis evaluation). At this stage, you might decide that none of your original hypotheses fits the data you have gathered; in this instance you would repeat the process of cue acquisition, hypothesis generation, cue evaluation, and hypothesis evaluation until you are satisfied that you can explain your patient's signs and symptoms effectively (i.e. you have reached a judgement).

A number of studies examining how nurses reason indicate that in many cases they use hypothetico-deductive approaches to reach clinical assessments and diagnoses (e.g. Lamond et al 1996, Tanner et al 1987, Twycross & Powls 2006). However, it appears that this is one of many different types of reasoning strategy that can be used by nurses in practice to make judgements and decisions. Other studies have suggested that with increasing experience and expertise nurses are more likely to use intuition (e.g. Benner 1984, Benner et al 1999, King & Appleton 1997). Alternatively, nurses can use a number of heuristics or 'cognitive short cuts' to reach judgements or decisions.

Intuition: clinical foresight or *falsae memoriae*?

No discussion of judgement and decision making in nursing can pass over the concept of intuition. It has attracted an enormous amount of interest from nurse academics, with more than 610 papers published between 1981 and 2006 (Rew & Barrow 2007).

Many authors have suggested that intuition is a legitimate basis for decision making in healthcare, especially within nursing (Benner 1984, Benner et al 1999, King & Appleton 1997). However, agreement on the definition of the concept is hard to come by (Box 5.3).

Box 5.3 Definitions of intuition used in the nursing literature

Intuition has been described as:

'Understanding without rationale' (Benner & Tanner 1987 p 23)

'A perception of possibilities, meanings, and relationships by way of insight' (Gerrity 1987 p 63)

'Knowledge of fact or truth as a whole; immediate possession of knowledge; and knowledge independent of the linear reasoning process' (Rew & Barron 1987 p 60)

'Immediate knowledge of something without the conscious use of reason' (Schrader & Fischer 1987 p 47)

'Process whereby the nurse knows something about the patient that cannot be verbalised, that is verbalised with difficulty or for which the source of knowledge cannot be determined' (Young 1987 p 52)

'Lacking underlying conscious processes and as not being able to be explained in a tangible manner' (Cioffi 1997 p 204)

Scholars often fail to distinguish between intuition as a *type of knowledge* and intuition as a way of thinking or a *mode of thought* (Sarvimaki & Stenbock-Hult 1996). If we view intuition as a type of knowledge, then we must also consider the nature of that knowledge and how it affects our decisions. A problem with intuitive knowledge in healthcare decisions is its lack of visibility. When intuitive knowledge is the basis for decisions, the beliefs and values in the decision are explicit only to the person making the decision (Pitz & Sachs 1984). This lack of explication can be seen as morally reprehensible. As Pellegrino points out:

" To resort to terms like 'art' or 'intuition' is to impede explication of a socially significant process. Whatever name we use to subsume the indefinable elements in the process, the effort to explicate them further is a moral as well as an intellectual responsibility. (Pellegrino 1979 p 187)"

Intuitive decision making is also not commensurate with the reflective learning strategies that proponents claim are the ways to unlock much of the benefit from (practice based), tacit, or intuitive knowledge of the right thing to do. If drawing on intuitive knowledge does not work out, little information is available to examine at what point(s) the decision broke down. Also lacking is insight into *how* the person reached the decision – intuition is largely invisible.

Despite the theoretical limitations of intuitive knowledge, it can be useful. Many studies highlight the accuracy of intuitive judgement in predicting risk to the patient (Benner 1984, Benner et al 1999). Cioffi (1997) illustrated this with an excerpt from a study reported by Benner and Wrubel (1982):

" Another nurse recalled having a 'bad feeling' about a patient whose observations had not changed much but who was becoming restless and vaguely complaining of not feeling good. She had called the medical officer and by the time he arrived the patient was having copious burgundy liquid stools indicative of a massive haemorrhage.' (Cioffi 1997 p 205)"

Similarly, Benner et al (1999) refer to 'clinical forethought' to describe the ability to anticipate possible clinical eventualities. These habits guide 'thinking-in-action'. Clinical forethought is embedded in particular situations and over time it becomes a habit and a patterned way of approaching clinical situations, so much so that it becomes intuitive. (Benner et al 1999 p 64).

Saint Augustine used the term *'falsae memoriae'* to refer to the phenomenon of *déjà vu*, or the sense of having been in a situation before. According to Benner et al (1999), clinical forethought shapes responses to medical diagnoses, the range of clinical interventions available, and anticipation of the unexpected. Much of the research on intuition provides similar examples of how intuitive thought benefits judgement and decision making (King & Appleton 1997, Schraeder & Fischer 1987). Many of these studies rely on the recall of 'critical incidents' by participants. However, the influence of memory and hindsight means that nurses may recall only those incidents where decision making was effective (Hastie& Dawes 2001). People are not good at recalling incidents when their intuition fails, or the times they missed patient cues altogether so that the patient suffered a worse outcome than might otherwise have been the case had a more analytic approach (e.g. using an algorithm) been available. Regardless of hindsight bias when recalling past experiences, convincing evidence shows that when faced with new evidence nurses are slow to revise their ideas – they are 'cognitively cautious'. They fail to deviate from already-held ideas or opinions (Hammond et al 1967). Relying on the sense of *falsae memoriae* of intuitive thought is insufficient for good decision making.

Heuristics and fast and frugal reasoning

Normative decision-making theories encourage an optimistic view of the world; Gerd Gigerenzer and Peter Todd sum up this optimism (1999) when they assert that decision theorists are guilty of painting a picture of a world in which humans live:

> " ... with unlimited time and knowledge, where the sun of enlightenment shines down in beams of logic and probability [the real world is] in contrast, shrouded in a mist of dim uncertainty. People in this world have only limited time, knowledge, and computational capacities with which to make inferences about what happens in the enigmatic places in their world. (Gigerenzer & Todd 1999 p 4)"

Consider seeing a patient in a clinic. The patient is grimacing, clutching her side, sweaty, and pale. When faced with this situation you are unlikely to get out a pen and paper and work though the evidence for and against a range of differential diagnoses. You are far more likely to judge (sense) that something is 'not right' and that action is required. You use shortcuts.

Heuristics are the 'cognitive shortcuts' that we use to reason and solve everyday problems. Heuristics form the basis for two influential descriptive theories of decision making: (1) the theory of heuristics and bias; and (2) fast and frugal reasoning. Both these theories represent a shortcut for formal reasoning and an alternative to probability and utility-based formulae. They are distinguished by whether heuristics are viewed as a good or bad element of decision making and judgement.

Heuristics and bias

Tversky & Kahneman (1974) suggested that individuals make use of heuristics as a way of dealing with decision complexity (given the limitations of human cognition). Mostly, these shortcuts generate decisions and judgements that are pretty close to 'optimal' solutions. However, they also generate predictable and systematic biases and errors. We will examine some of these when we look at error in Chapter 7; but as an introduction we will consider just one: overconfidence.

Individuals often overestimate the 'correctness' of their knowledge. A number of studies have shown that people are often overconfident in their decision making and judgement (Fischoff & MacGregor 1975, Lichenstein & Fischoff 1977). Overconfidence occurs at many levels, but two of the most common are: (1) in response to knowledge questions; and (2) when subjectively predicting the progress of events or individuals. Dawes (1979) examined the subjective predictions of clinicians about the outcomes for people with mental health problems and found that these were far less accurate and consistent than judgements made using objective indicators or measures of progress. Overconfidence has implications for planning intervention decisions based entirely on gut feeling or experience.

Fast and frugal reasoning

Thus far, we have encountered heuristics as a negative force in decision making and judgement. However, a school of thought exits that sees the use of heuristics as a positive side of the human condition. Gigerenzer and colleagues have suggested that we reason in ways that are both fast *and* frugal (efficient). These fast and frugal techniques bear no resemblance to normative models and yet produce good quality judgements and decisions.

Imagine a scenario in which an admitting emergency nurse practitioner must decide if a patient in the midst of a myocardial infarction merits admission to a coronary care unit (CCU) (i.e. the nurse judges the patient to be at 'high risk' of losing his life) or an acute medical ward with telemetry monitoring (i.e. the patient is at 'lower risk' of losing his life). The decision is complicated in a number of ways; the CCU might have only one spare bed and if the nurse wrongly sends this patient to the unit, that bed cannot then be used by another, more deserving, patient. The nurse probably faces making the decision under time pressure, using information cues that are only partial indicators of the true risk level. There are often many such cues: age, blood pressure, electrocardiogram patterns, presence of severe pain, etc. An 'optimal' choice would be to examine the relative predictive value of each of the cues, rank them in order of 'value' for decision making, and reach a conclusion based on the contribution of the evidence. Even if we knew the respective predictive values of the cues, this would be complicated and time consuming; there is another way.

How would you feel about making the decision based on just three pieces of information (sounds a bit counterintuitive and scary?). The information is changes in the ST segment of an ECG, a chief complaint of chest pain and the presence of any other factors (Figure 5.1). So the reasoning process consists of up to three questions at most:

1. Are there anomalies in the patient's ST segments on their ECG? If the answer is 'Yes', then stop right there and get the patient to the CCU.
2. Is the primary complaint one of chest pain? If not then the patient should go to a regular nursing bed. It 'Yes', go to 3.
3. Is there one other factor, such as the use of nitroglycerine for chest pain? If the answer is 'Yes', then the patient should go to CCU.

It might seem strange to argue that such a simple rule can be an adequate basis for decision making. However, it is important to note that it is not the myocardial infarction that is 'simple', or the patient's situation, but the judgement solution. When Green & Mehr (1997) compared the performance of this fast and frugal decision tree to both a far more complicated statistical algorithm and physicians' clinical triage judgements, they found that the fast and frugal heuristic worked best. It led to fewer myocardial infarctions and

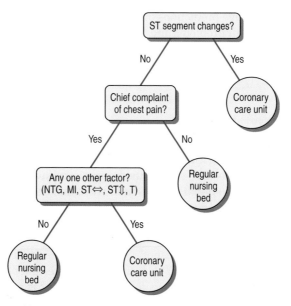

Figure 5.1 Fast and frugal algorithm for admission to coronary care unit (adapted from Green & Mehr 1997).

had higher sensitivity and lower false positive rates (see Chapter 9 for a discussion on why this matters).

There are two main groups of fast and frugal heuristics: those based on recognition and those based on reasons. Let us examine recognition-based heuristics first.

Imagine you must answer the following question for £1 million: 'Which city has more residents: San Diego or San Antonio?' If you are American, you probably got the right answer (San Diego); but if you are not from America then it was probably a bit more difficult. When this question was posed to a class full of German students though, 100% of them were correct (as opposed to 75% of American students) (Goldstein & Gigerenzer 2002). Why, when some German students had never heard of San Antonio, would more of them guess correctly?

In this case, there is a strong correlation between recognising a cue (such as a city name) and the criterion (the size of the city). When this state of affairs exists, the recognition heuristic can be summarised as (a decision rule):

    ❝ If one of two objects is recognised *and* the other is not, *then* infer that
    the recognised object has the higher value with respect to the criterion.❞

The recognition heuristic is great if one of the options is unfamiliar, but what happens if you recognise both options but still do not know the answer? The solution lies in a different heuristic: the 'take-the-best' approach. This is a reason-, rather than recognition-, based approach.

The take-the-best approach relies on a key piece of additional information: the *validity* with which each cue predicts the criterion. Suppose you were asked to look at pairs of Spanish cities and decide which had the largest population? If you did not recognise one of the cities and recognised the other then it would be best (using the recognition heuristic) to choose the one you recognise. Let us further suppose that we gave you some extra information: presence of a civic art gallery in each city, and presence of a 'la Liga' (Spanish premier soccer league) team. The take-the-best heuristic works by comparing objects (the cities) on the most valid cue available, then the second most valid cue, and so on, until a cue in which the two objects differ is found. So long as you rank the cues in order of validity, the heuristic decision rule becomes 'take the best cue and ignore the rest'. The best cue is the most valid one that discriminates: probably the la Liga football team. Many Spanish towns, as well as cities, have a civic art gallery.

An even simpler variant of the take-the-best fast and frugal heuristic describes healthcare behaviour. The 'matching' heuristic is an example of a one-reason heuristic, in that as long as cues are examined in order then the judge needs just a single reason to choose a cue. In the matching heuristic, the judge searches a small subset of the available cues and bases their prediction on the value of a single cue alone. Dhami & Harries (2001) have illustrated how a simple matching heuristic explains statin-prescribing behaviour in GPs. In this study, the fast and frugal rule associated with a single cue (is the patient's cholesterol high? If yes then prescribe statin; if not, do not) predicted more of the clinician's behaviour than a far more complex logistic regression model built around age, units of alcohol, cholesterol level, smoking status, diabetes and weight. Smith & Gilhooly (2006) found similar results in doctors prescribing antidepressants: a few key cues (presence of suicide ideation, for example) are used rather than (more complex) data such as duration of symptoms. Troublingly, these patterns are at odds to some official guidelines on managing depression (www.nice.org.uk/CG023).

Social judgement theory and the cognitive continuum

Before the 1950s, psychologists studied clinicians as a source of expertise rather than as case studies in failure of judgement. All that changed when Paul Meehl (1954) suggested that individuals' intuitive judgements were in fact less accurate than simple statistical models. Indeed, when psychologists modelled individuals' own intuitive judgements, the judgements became more accurate when removed from the clinician. This finding has been replicated a number of times, most notably by Robin Dawes (1979). After Meehl, the research community took up the explanatory challenge. What emerged was the recognition that all individuals making judgements and choices often had to deal with 'irreducible uncertainty' (Eddy 1994). The information they had to work with was often fallible, imperfect, and incomplete. Psychologists also recognised that cognition was rarely entirely rational or wholly intuitive, but occupied a kind of middle ground between these two extremes (Hammond 1986, 1996). The roots of these ideas lay in the work of Egon Brunswik, a psychologist who first considered the notion (implicit in Meehl's work) that it was necessary to understand not just the *organism* (nurse or doctor) in a judgement or decision situation but also the *environment* or *ecology* that the organism must operate in and adapt to. Brunswik proposed a model in which the relationship between decision makers and

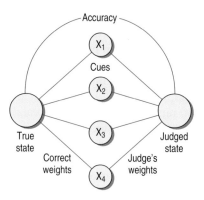

Figure 5.2 Brunswik's Lens Model (reproduced from Hammond et al 1975, with permission of K R Hammond).

the environments they operate in can be understood as a form of lens (Figure 5.2).

In the lens model, the world is uncertain and represented by fallible indicators (cues). Decision makers make sense of these indicators through their judgements. This is often done with minimal or no awareness of the process (i.e. it appears intuitive), and sometimes even with not much information involved it can be very accurate.

The easiest way to understand the model is to work our way through an example. Imagine evaluating whether an elderly patient who says, 'Everything is fine'. Is 'fine' as good as their verbal response alone implies? The lens model would represent this problem as trying to see a true (distal) state of the world through the lens of information (cues or indicators). In this case, the cues might include the fact that the patient's non-verbal facial expression does not match their verbal expression, that the patient recoils from touch, that there is a lack of eye contact, or the 'angry' tone of the patient's words. These are all signals or information cues from which we must infer the true state ('fine' or 'not fine').

Let us look at the model in a bit more detail. The left side of the model represents, and summarises, the relationship between the 'to-be-judged' state of the world (known as the criterion) and the cues that point to this state. For example, out of the cues listed above, perhaps only two – the patient recoiling from touch and lack of eye contact – are actually predictive of a patient being 'not fine'. Often the criterion causes the cues. So for example, diabetes (the criterion) causes the tangible cue of raised glycosylated haemoglobin (HbAc1) levels.

The right side of the model represents the relationship between the judgement that an individual has made (that the patient is 'not fine') and the cues that the individual has used to make this judgement (for instance, the patient recoiling from touch, a lack of eye contact, and the patient's angry tone of voice). The connecting pathways between the two sides of the model represents the judge's ability to estimate the criterion accurately (known as 'achievement'), and examine how they have used information cues to reach that judgement (for further details of how to use SJT approaches to study judgement, see Cooksey 1996).

As well as providing measures of how people perform in a judgement task, the lens model also gives us the relative weights assigned by people to the information present in decisions. This is a very powerful characteristic of the approach; suppose individuals over- or under-weight information compared with its weighting in the environment. For example, consider giving respiratory rate as a predictor of critical adverse event risk in acutely ill patients a weighting. Of routinely collected observational data, respiratory rate is the most powerful (Considine 2005) and yet respiratory rate is not weighted most heavily by many nurses when assessing risk (Thompson et al 2007). Armed with this information, it is possible to try to change the ways that individuals weight information and to try to improve their judgement performance (Thompson et al 2005).

SJT provides a powerful model for understanding the relationship between individual decision makers and their operating environments. It also reveals why individuals operate differently in differing environments. What it does not do, however, is help us predict what kinds of decision environments will lead to what kinds of judgemental performance. This idea: that a decision environment can shape decision making, judgement and reasoning, is the preserve of cognitive continuum theory (CCT).

CCT (Hammond 1996) has at its core a simple axiom, 'That human cognition is clearly capable of both intuition and analysis and that each has value' (Hammond 1996 p 89). What the theory does is elucidate in what circumstances intuition and analysis occur and where the value lies. At the heart of the cognitive continuum (Hamm 1998) is a model similar to Figure 5.3.

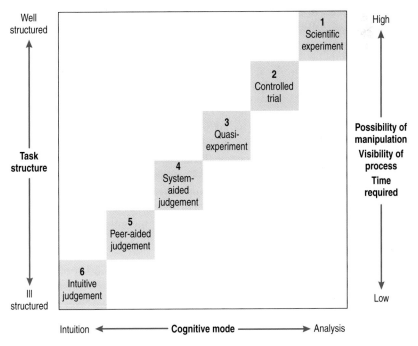

Figure 5.3 The cognitive continuum.

The main argument that leads from the model is that the way in which one approaches a judgement depends on three characteristics of the judgement task.

1. Complexity of task structure:
   a. Number of cues: when presented with lots of information a practitioner will probably utilise an intuitive approach.
   b. Redundancy of cues: the more cues help in the prediction of the presence of other cues, then the more likely that intuitive cognition will be used.
   c. The nature of an organising principle: if a simple 'averaging' approach to combining information is known to be more accurate, intuitive thought is likely to be a feature. If a complicated approach to combining evidence produces answers that are more accurate, then this will induce an analytical approach.
2. Ambiguity of the task:
   a. Whether an organising principle exists: if an organising principle exists, the practitioner is more likely to be analytical.
   b. Familiarity of the task: unfamiliarity induces an intuitive approach because the practitioner has not had time to develop more complicated ways of dealing with cue information.
   c. The potential for accuracy: if a particular approach to assessment is accurate (even if only perceived as such) then it is more likely to be used as the basis for analysis. For example, universal assessment scales for pressure sore assessment.
3. Nature of the presentation of the task:
   a. Task decomposition: if the task leads to the need to address related sub-tasks then analytic modes of thought will be used.
   b. The ways in which information is presented: if visual information is used then intuition is induced. If the information is presented as objective and quantitative then analysis is commonly a feature.
   c. Time available: the shorter the available time the more likely it is that an intuitive approach will be adopted.

The theory's predictive and explanatory abilities were tested in a classic experiment with highway engineers. Hammond and colleagues (1987) deliberately manipulated the task characteristics of a series of judgement challenges relating to road aesthetics (designed to induce analytic reasoning), safety (designed to induce quasi-analytic reasoning), and traffic capacity (designed to induce analytic reasoning). They also measured the characteristics of the reasoning employed by the highway engineers. What they found was that not only was there a significant correlation between the task characteristics and the kind of reasoning employed by the engineers but also that the engineers were more accurate in their judgements when they correctly matched reasoning to that merited by the task.

In nursing, Cader et al (2005) point to the different modes of reasoning employed by nurses (Lauri et al 1998) and the ways in which nurses evaluate internet based information as evidence of the explanatory power of the idea of a cognitive continuum. Whereas Cader and other's (Thompson 1999) analyses suggest that the model has some face validity, CCT remains largely untested in relation to nursing.

Signal detection theory

SJT and CCT present individuals as responders to the values of the information around them in order to reach judgements. In this way, they view decision makers as sensors, interpreting information in environments. One of the problems in social judgement studies is that replicating the 'noise' (irrelevant information) that is often present in the environments in which professionals operate is difficult. Individuals are also active decision makers, with varying preconceptions and thresholds beyond which they are more likely to act. Signal detection theory (SDT) is one means of incorporating such thresholds and predilections into models of how we use information. SDT is more of a statistical approach to examining communication than a decision theory per se, but it has developed into a branch of decision science.

Imagine a situation in which a nurse is required to use his or her clinical judgement to assess whether a patient is at risk of a critical event (such as a cardiac or respiratory arrest), and then to decide to take appropriate action. Table 5.1 outlines the four possible outcomes associated with this situation.

Judgement and decision making from this perspective involves the nurse cognitively 'trading-off' the various cells in the table. The nurse could maximise the correct number of 'hits' by classifying everyone as warranting intervention; a strategy that results in lots of false alarms. Conversely, the nurse might choose to apply a strict criterion for a judgement of 'at risk and needing intervention'. If this strategy is adopted, the nurse maximises his or her ability to correctly reject patients, but at the cost of risking inaction more frequently than is desirable. Such inaction amongst acute care nurses is a real and international problem (Daffurn et al 1994, McQuillan et al 1998). In both these approaches, false positives and misses are inevitable. This inability to avoid errors has been termed the 'duality' of error (Hammond 1996).

Having recognised this trade-off, we need a means to represent it. The trade-off happens within the mind of the clinician and cannot reliably be inferred simply from what people *think they do* (Thompson et al 2001). Signal detection theory (SDT) offers such a means of making such trade-offs visible.

Theoretical approaches

Table 5.1 The four possible outcomes of yes/no decisions from signal detection theory

Decision	State of the environment	
	The patient really is at risk. Should take action	The patient really is not at risk. Should not take action
Yes – take action	(1) Hit, correct outcome True positive	(2) False alarm, incorrect outcome False positive
No – Do not take action	(3) Miss, incorrect outcome False negative	(4) Correct rejection, correct outcome True negative

Consider a nurse making a decision to call a medical emergency team or to act to prevent a suicide attempt. The nurse must acquire and integrate the relevant information in a decision environment and compare this assessment with his or her personal decision criterion: the point at which to take action or not. All clinical decision situations have information present; the nurse integrates this information to yield an intuitive estimate of the 'strength of evidence', in our case the 'amount of risk'. A nurse will act if the estimate is greater than their personal decision criterion, or threshold for action. A patient at low risk of a critical event will have clinical signs and symptoms that are characteristically within a 'normal' range. A nurse's estimate of the strength of evidence for healthy patients will vary but centre on the 'normal range'. Patients at a higher risk of a critical event will have signs and symptoms that might deviate from those expected in 'low risk' or healthy patients (raised pulse, low blood pressure, reduced urine output). Estimates of strength of evidence for these patients, on average, will be higher. With the benefit of repeated contact with lots of patients with abnormal signs, observing what happens to those patients, and thus feedback on the success of our judgements nurses learn to recognise what kind of signs to look for. We often assume that the ability to acquire greater amounts of reliable information, and to integrate it more effectively, accompanies training and experience. The difference between the average estimates of the strength of evidence for normal patients and for non-normal patients will increase. This results in an increase of the chances of getting a hit or correct rejection and a reduction in the chances of making one of the two types of errors. Because nurses have varying amounts and types of clinical experience and differing approaches to 'risk', and so variable thresholds for action, they will differ in their ability to maximise correct responses and minimise errors.

Information acquisition and integration is important but different nurses will differ in the values they place on the consequences of the different types of error. Some nurses might feel that missing an opportunity to act when confronted with an 'at risk' patient is the difference between life and death. A false alarm, however, might result only in waking a doctor up in the early hours. These nurses might choose to err towards 'intervene' decisions. Other nurses might feel that waking doctors up in the night carries unpleasant consequence and that watchful waiting (a 'miss') is worthwhile; these nurses will have a tendency towards 'not intervening'. They will miss more at-risk patients but will be helping reduce unnecessary workload in a service. We can see, then, that explaining variability between nurses when intervening to prevent critical events in patients is not simply about ability to distinguish between normal and non-normal patients, but also about having differing criteria or thresholds for action.

The consequence of this interplay between the cells in Table 5.1 is that it is impossible to set a personal threshold at a level where we always spot true positives and correct rejections and avoid false alarms and misses. All nurses can do, assuming they know which information is important, is adjust the kinds of error that they make by manipulating their personal criterion; the one part of the decision equation under their control. For a more detailed overview of SDT, readers are directed to Swets et al (2000).

CONCLUSION

This is the most theoretical chapter in the book and its relevance might not be immediately obvious, especially given the focus on decision skills and practical knowledge in the other chapters. However, it is important to understand the theories that underpin our judgment and decision making for three reasons.

First, no single explanation explains fully how we *should* (normative models), *do* (descriptive approaches), or *could* (prescriptive models) make choices. To understand the phenomena of judgement and decision making it is necessary to understand a variety of perspectives.

Second, to examine and scrutinise decision making through research, the evidence-based mantra of 'right research approach for the question asked' is essential. Of course, if you are interested in whether decision makers make 'good' or 'bad' decisions then some kind of working definition of good and bad is required. Decision theories offer start points for these definitions (as discussed in Chapter 6). For example, a coherent decision can variously refer to one in which the rules of pure logic, probability and utility, means and (necessarily limited) ends, or the relationship between ecology structures and judgemental heuristics are met. It all depends on which version of rationality you employ.

Ultimately, the approaches introduced in this chapter offer us a means of making sense of the invisible activity that occurs when making judgements and decisions. Most of the activity that occurs is cognitive and the searching, synthesising, and valuing of information is largely unobservable. Without frameworks to judge, compare, and contrast then informed assessments of the worth, power, and reason associated with judgement and decision making is impossible.

RESOURCES

The temptation here is to guide readers toward 'heavy-duty' psychology texts; we have instead decided to offer two 'popular' introductions to what are essentially very heavy-going areas. Having dipped your toes into this body of work, you might decide to immerse yourself further (if, for example, you are a PhD student or academic).

One of the most accessible introductions to heuristics and intuitive reasoning is Malcolm Gladwell's 'Blink' (www.gladwell.com/blink/): Gladwell M 2007 Blink: the power of thinking without thinking. Back Bay Books, New York.

For a similarly (but a tad more technical) introduction to fast and frugal reasoning see: Gigerenzer G 2007 Gut feelings: the intelligence of the unconscious. Viking, London. His research group can be reached at: www.mpib-berlin.mpg.de/en/forschung/abc/index.htm

Those desperate to embrace the really technical should look at the *Blackwell handbook of judgement and decision making*: www.blackwellpublishing.com/Book.asp?ref=1405107464

Answers to the expected value questions: option A = 0.8 × £45 = £36; option B = 1 × £30 = £30.

Becker G 1976 The economic approach to human behaviour. University of Chicago Press, Chicago

Benner P 1984 From novice to expert: excellence and power in clinical nursing practice. Addison Wesley, Menlo Park, CA

Benner P, Tanner C 1987 How expert nurses use intuition. American Journal of Nursing 87(1):23–31

Benner P, Wrubel J 1982 Skilled knowledge: the value of perceptual awareness. Nurse Educator 7:11–17

Benner P, Hooper-Kyriakidis P, Stannard, D 1999 Clinical wisdom and interventions in critical care: a thinking-in-action approach. WB Saunders, Philadelphia.

Bernoulli D 1738 Exposition of a new theory on the measurement of risk (trans. Louise Sommer). Econometrica 22:22–36

Brennan P F, Anthony M K 2000 Measuring nursing practice models using multi-attribute utility theory. Research in Nursing and Health 23:372–382

Cader R, Campbell S, Watson D 2005 Cognitive cntinuum theory in nursing decision making. Journal of Advanced Nursing 49:397–405

Cioffi J 1997 Heuristics, servants to intuition, in clinical decision making. Journal of Advanced Nursing 26:203–208

Cooksey R 1996 Judgment analysis: theory, methods and application. Academic Press, San Diego, CA

Considine J 2005 The role of nurses in preventing adverse events related to respiratory dysfunction: literature review. Journal of Advanced Nursing 49:624–633

Daffurn K, Lee A, Hillman K et al 1994 Do nurses know when to summon emergency assistance? Intensive Critical Care Nursing 10:115–120

Dawes R M 1979 The robust beauty of improper linear models in decision making. American Psychologist 34(7):571–582

Dhami M K, Harries C 2001 Fast and frugal versus regression models in human judgement. Thinking and Reasoning 7:5–27

Eddy D 1994 Variations in physician practice: the role of uncertainty. Health Affairs 3:74–89

Elstein A S, Shulman L S, Sprafka S A 1978 Medical problem solving: an analysis of clinical reasoning. Harvard University Press, Cambridge, MA

Fischoff B, MacGregor D 1975 Subjective confidence in forecasts. Journal of Forecasting 1:155–172

Gerrity P 1987 Perception in nursing: the value of intuition. Holistic Nursing Practice 1(3):63–71

Gigerenzer G, Todd P 1999 Simple heuristics that make us smart. Oxford University Press, New York

Goldstein D G, Gigerenzer G 2002 Models of ecological rationality: the recognition heuristic. Psychological Review 109:75–90

Green L, Mehr D R 1997 What alters physicians' decisions to admit to the coronary care unit? Journal of Family Practice 45:219–226

Hamm R M 1998 Clinical intuition and clinical analysis: expertise and the cognitive continuum. In: Dowie J, Elstein A (eds) Professional judgement: a reader in clinical decision making. Cambridge University Press, Cambridge, p 78–105

Hammond K R 1986 A theoretically based review of theory and research in judgement and decision making. Report no. 260, Centre for Research on Judgement and Policy, University of Colorado, Boulder, CO

Hammond K R 1996 Human judgement and social policy: irreducible uncertainty, inevitable error and unavoidable injustice. Oxford University Press, Oxford

Hammond K R, Kelly K J, Schneider R J et al 1967 Clinical inference in nursing: revising judgments. Nursing Research 16:38–45

Hammond K R, Stewart T R, Brehmer B, Steinmann D O, 1975, Human judgement and decision processes. Article 'Social Judgement Theory,' pp 271–312, New York Academic Press.

Hammond K R, Hamm R M, Grassia J et al 1987 Direct comparison of the efficacy of intuitive and analytic cognition in expert judgement. IEEE Transactions on Systems Man and Cybernetics 17: 753–770

Hastie R, Dawes R M 2001 Rational choice in an uncertain world. Sage, London

King L, Appleton J V 1997 Intuition: a critical review of the research and rhetoric. Journal of Advanced Nursing 26:194–202

Lamond D, Crow R, Chase J 1996 Judgements and processes in care decisions in acute medical and surgical wards. Journal of Evaluation in Clinical Practice 2:211–216

Lauri S, Salantera S, Callister L C et al 1998 Decision making of nurses practicing in intensive care in Canada, Finland, Northern Ireland, Switzerland, and the United States. Heart and Lung 27:131–142

Lichenstein S, Fischoff B 1977 Do those who know more also know more about how much they know? Organizational Behaviour and Human Performance 20:159–183

March J G 1994 A primer on decision making. Free Press, New York

McQuillan P, Pilkington S, Allan A et al 1998 Confidential inquiry into quality of care before admission to intensive care. British Medical Journal 316:1853–1858

Meehl P 1954 Clinical versus statistical prediction: a theoretical analysis and a review of the evidence. University of Minnesota Press, Minneapolis, MN

Newell A, Simon H A 1972 Human problem solving. Prentice Hall, Englewood Cliffs, NJ

Offredy M 2002 Decision making by nurse practitioners in primary care. PhD theses, University of Hertfordshire, UK

Pellegrino E D 1979 The anatomy of clinical judgments. In: Engelhardt Jr H T, Spicker S F, Towers B (eds) Clinical judgment: a critical appraisal. D Reidel Publishing Company, Dordrecht, the Netherlands, p 169–194

Pitz G F, Sachs N J 1984 Judgment and decision: theory and application. Annual Reviews of Psychology 35:139–163

Plous S 1993 The psychology of judgment and decision making. McGraw Hill, New York

Rew L, Barrow E 1987 Intuition: a neglected hallmark of nursing knowledge. Advances in Nursing Science 10(1):49–62

Rew L, Barrow E 2007 State of the science: intuition in nursing, a generation of studying the phenomenon. Advances in Nursing Science 30:E15–E25

Sarvimaki A, Stenbock-Hult B 1996 Intuition – a problematic form of knowledge in nursing. Scandinavian Journal of Caring Sciences 10(4):234–41

Savage L J 1954 The foundations of statistics. Wiley, New York

Schraeder B D, Fischer D K 1987 Using intuitive knowledge in the neonatal intensive care nursery. Holistic Nursing Practice 1(3):45–51

Simon H 1971 Designing organizations for an information-rich world. In: Greenberger M (ed) Computers, communication, and the public interest. The Johns Hopkins Press, Baltimore MD

Simon H A 1983 Reason in human affairs. Stanford University Press, Stanford, CA

Smith L, Gilhooly K 2006 Regression versus fast and frugal models of decision making: the case of prescribing for depression. Applied Cognitive Psychology 20(2):265–274

Swets J A, Dawes M, Monahan J 2000 Psychological science can improve diagnostic decisions. Psychological Science 1:1–26

Tanner C A, Padrick K P, Westfall U E et al 1987 Diagnostic reasoning strategies of nurses and nursing students. Nursing Research 36:358–363

Thompson C 1999 A conceptual treadmill: the need for 'middle ground' in clinical decision-making theory in nursing. Journal of Advanced Nursing 30:1222–1229

Thompson C, McCaughan D, Cullum N et al 2001 Research information in nurses' clinical decision making: what is useful? Journal of Advanced Nursing 36:376–388

Thompson C A, Foster A, Cole I et al 2005 Using social judgement theory to model nurses' use of clinical information in critical care education. Nurse Education Today 25:68–77

Thompson C, Estabrooks C A, Bucknall T et al 2007 Nurses' critical event risk assessments: a judgement analysis. Journal of Clinical Nursing, in press

Tversky A, Kahneman D 1974 Judgment under uncertainty: heuristics and biases. Science 185:1124–1131

Twycross A Powls L 2006 How do children's nurses make clinical decisions? Two preliminary studies. Journal of Clinical Nursing 15:1324–1335

Young C 1987 Intuition and the nursing process. Holistic Nursing Practice 1(3):52–62

What is a 'good' judgement or decision?

Dawn Dowding and Carl Thompson

6

KEY ISSUES

- How we can define a good judgement or decision
- The difficulties we face in identifying good judgements and decisions
- How we define experts and expertise
- Why expertise does not necessarily equate to good decision making

In Chapter 1, we outlined why we are concerned about examining the clinical decision making and judgement of nurses. Reasons include the increasing focus on patient safety and the relationship between nurses' (and other health professionals') judgement and decision making and adverse events in healthcare. To try to improve the judgements and decisions of nurses, we need to know what 'good' judgements or decisions are. We also need to know how to measure how good they are. Equipped with this knowledge, we can identify where there are problems in nurses' judgements and decisions, and develop strategies for improving them.

WHAT IS A GOOD JUDGEMENT OR DECISION?

Defining what we mean by a good judgement or a good decision is complex. The standard we normally use for evaluating how good a judgement is, is its accuracy. To judge accuracy, we often compare individuals' judgements to some predefined standard that we consider to represent accuracy (Hastie & Rasinski 1988). For example, a nurse who identifies 90% of patients who are at risk of developing a pressure sore could be considered to make 'accurate' judgements, if we have decided that this is a reasonable measure of accuracy for this patient condition.

A nurse's ability to make accurate or 'correct' judgements is a function of a number of different elements. Cooksey (1996) suggests such factors include the predictability of the situation the individual is trying to judge, the knowledge an individual possesses about the situation, and the consistency with which an individual uses their knowledge. To illustrate this further, let us imagine that we are trying to evaluate how much pain a patient is experiencing. In this example, the nurse has to reach a judgement (how much pain the patient has). The nurse is more likely to be accurate in his or her assessment of the patient's pain if it is 'predictable' (e.g. patients who have had similar surgery in the past almost always have a certain level of pain), if he or she has more knowledge of the area (i.e. has looked after a number of similar patients with this type of pain in the past), and if he or she makes assessments about a patient's pain consistently (i.e. uses the same information in the same way each time when assessing patients' pain).

Unlike judgements, when we consider decisions we normally evaluate them as either 'good' or 'bad', rather than 'accurate' or 'inaccurate'. This evaluation often draws on the outcome of the decision. Examining decisions in healthcare is problematic because of the uncertain nature of healthcare decision environments (see Chapter 2). Baron (2000) suggests that a 'good' decision is one that achieves an individual's goals. However, as highlighted by Regher (2004):

> " Because of the probabilistic nature of patient outcomes, the most appropriate action can be associated with a poor outcome, and a suboptimal action can be associated with a good outcome."

Simply relying on the outcomes of decisions or actions to determine whether they are of good quality (Pauker & Pauker 1999, Sox 1999) is therefore problematic. An alternative to the outcomes approach is to examine the process by which a decision has been made (Pauker & Pauker 1999). This, in turn, raises the issue of what we might consider a 'good' decision process to be. One suggestion is that a good process follows the laws and logic of probability theory (Hastie & Dawes 2001) and is therefore a 'rational' approach to decision making (as discussed in Chapter 5).

Another suggestion is to identify what elements of the decision process make it 'good'. For instance Pauker & Pauker (1999) suggest that a good decision process should: define the problem, identify the goals of the decision maker, examine the consequences and relative values of each option, consider the trade-offs between the different options, include all the individuals who are involved in the decision in the process, and be explicit. Staying with our pain example, let us assume that the nurse has assessed the patient's pain (accurately) with the assistance of an appropriate pain assessment tool. The nurse then looks at the patient's prescription chart and uses the local guidelines for acute pain management to discuss different options for pain relief with the patient. They discuss whether or not the patient would prefer oral medication or an injection and the likely benefits (e.g. the likelihood of effectiveness and rapidity of pain relief) and potential costs (e.g. the likelihood of increased drowsiness) of the potential options. Having evaluated each option available, the nurse then decides what medication to use to help relieve the patient's pain. In this instance the nurse has used a good decision process (i.e. made a good decision). Despite these notable efforts, however, the patient might still end the decision process with pain (a poor outcome).

MEASURING THE QUALITY OF JUDGEMENTS AND DECISIONS

Thus far we have highlighted the need to consider criteria of quality separately for judgements and decisions. Let us move now towards considering how you might begin to measure the quality of judgements and decisions.

Patient outcomes

As we have just seen, one of the main ways of examining judgement or decision quality is to compare a judgement or choice to what actually happens to the patient (the patient outcome) after the judgement or choice has been made (Dowding & Thompson 2003). Such outcomes can be either a patient's actual outcome or condition, or a measurement of a patient's health or illness status (Dowding & Thompson 2003). Examples of this include examining how accurate nurses are at making diagnoses (Allen-Davis et al 2002, Marsden 2000, Moyer et al 2000, Rosenthal et al 1992); their ability to predict with accuracy whether a patient subsequently develops a particular outcome (Kruse et al 1988, Moore et al 1996, VandenBosch et al 1996); comparisons of nurses' assessments of patient status with either patient- or researcher-completed measurement tools (McDonald et al 1999, O'Brien et al 2001, Reid & Chappell 2000, Richardson et al 2007) and the accuracy of nurse triage decision making (Quinn et al 2000, Wennike et al 2007).

Using patient outcomes appears to be the most obvious and logical way of examining nurses' judgement or decision quality. However, it is often not a practical approach. For example, in studies examining diagnostic accuracy nurses' judgements were compared to the results of laboratory tests (Allen-Davis et al 2002, Moyer et al 2000, Rosenthal et al 1992). Such studies ask nurses to provide a likely diagnosis without the test results. In reality, it is likely that nurses would reach some form of 'provisional' diagnosis and request the test to confirm their hypothesis. In this circumstance, a better approach would be to ask at what 'threshold' of probability do nurses request the test, and how accurate (actually, sensitive and specific) is that threshold. For more detail on sensitivity and specificity, see Chapters 5 and 9.

Similarly, in studies in which nurses are asked to predict the risk of a patient developing a condition it is often difficult to assess how predictable the condition is in the first place. As highlighted by Cooksey (1996), the predictability of a situation will affect nurses' accuracy; if you can only realistically predict with any accuracy 80% of falls (Moore et al 1996), what is a realistic figure for nurses to be able to predict? In reality, in situations where nurses carry out risk predictions (such as in the area of pressure ulcer prevention) they will carry out preventive actions in situations in which they consider a patient to be at risk (it would be unethical to identify a patient as at high risk of developing a pressure ulcer and then do nothing about it). Therefore, if you are a nurse in practice trying to evaluate the accuracy of your risk judgements, you might not be able to do so using the outcomes you see because you might have altered a patient's future risk by your assessment itself. For instance, you might consider a patient to be at risk of developing a pressure ulcer and therefore instigate interventions such as providing the patient with a special foam mattress (Cullum et al 2004). The patient doesn't then develop a pressure ulcer. However, you don't know if your judgement was accurate. The provision of the special mattress might have prevented the patient from developing an ulcer. Alternatively, your judgement might have been inaccurate in that the patient would not have developed an ulcer anyway. Finally, as has already been highlighted, nurses operate in conditions of irreducible uncertainty. Therefore, relying on the outcomes of a judgement or decision where the actual process used was appropriate but the outcome occurred by chance will not provide us with adequate information on the appropriateness of nurses' decision making.

Normative approaches

Another way of examining how good nurses' judgements and decisions are is to compare them to a 'standard' or criterion derived from models of how we *should* make decisions; normative models of decision making. Normative models (which we discuss in Chapter 5) provide us with a standard for judgements and decisions when individuals conform to logical and rational ideas of quality.

In judgement research, probabilistic statistical methods, using tools such as clinical decision rules, employ large datasets to calculate the likelihood of an individual having a particular condition (Jungermann 2000). A nurse's judgement can be compared with the statistical rule to assess his or her judgement accuracy. Such statistical methods of modelling judgements are more common in medical practice than in nursing; examples include rules for managing suspected fractures of the ankle (the Ottawa ankle rules; Bachmann et al 2003) and for diagnosing conditions such as meningitis (Dubos et al 2006). A number of reviews of this actuarial approach to judgement all suggest that such methods outperform individual (clinical) judgement in terms of accuracy (Grove et al 2000, Grove & Meehl 1996).

Bayes' theorem (Hastie & Dawes 2001) is a formal normative model for handling conditional probabilities. It can be used for calculating the likelihood of an individual having a particular problem (e.g. diagnosis) given the prevalence of the condition in the population and the information (such as signs and symptoms, diagnostic test results) available to the decision maker. Bayes' theorem is discussed in detail in Chapter 9 when we consider diagnosis, so we will not provide the details of it here beyond its basic form which is, 'prior (before test) probability × value of information = posterior (after test) probability'. Bayes' theorem is capable of rationally incorporating different types of evidence or data (such as the relationship between disease frequency and diagnostic test performance) into judgement. As such, it can be used as a comparison for both the judgement process and the accuracy of its outcome. However, Bayesian and more general probabilistic models rely on the availability of datasets to provide the necessary information on the frequencies involved. Such datasets are alien to most nurses, and so the real world utility, as a comparative standard against which to compare nurses' judgements remains, for the time being, limited.

The normative model most commonly used as the basis for examining decision processes is subjective expected utility theory (SEUT). This structured approach to decision making uses decision trees to illustrate graphically the different decision options available to the decision maker. SEUT takes into account the possible outcomes that might occur as a result of each decision option, together with the probability of each outcome occurring, and the value – or utility –, the decision maker attaches to each of the outcomes (SEUT is discussed in more detail in Chapter 5 and, for a detailed overview of how it can be used to assist with decision making, see Chapter 11). It uses a logical approach to combining measures of probability and utility to arrive at the 'best' decision for the decision maker given his or her values. Like other normative models, SEUT represents a good decision process against which nurses' decisions can be compared. However, formal decision models constructed on the assumptions of SEUT are rare in nursing and, to date, we haven't been able to locate any studies that have compared nurses' decisions to those suggested by such models.

Social judgement analysis

An approach to examining both judgement accuracy *and* the appropriateness of decision making is social judgement theory (SJT; see Chapter 5 for a more detailed overview). SJT views judgement as a kind of 'lens' in which information related to the 'reality' of a given judgement or decision environment (e.g. 'what is wrong with the patient?', 'what treatment should be prescribed?') is 'focused' by the clinician to arrive at their judgement or decision (e.g. 'what is my diagnosis?' and 'what treatment would I give?'). Using the analogy of the lens, it is possible to compare how information used by the nurse mirrors the same information's relationship to the patient situation. SJT uses statistical regression to model how information is related to the actual patient situation, giving a criterion or standard against which an individual's judgements or decisions can be compared (Denig et al 2002). The strength of SJT is that it provides information about how accurate an individual's judgements are (SJT models often use data on patient outcomes to construct the regression equations) as well as a picture of how individuals use information to reach their judgements (the regression equation provides information on the weighting or importance attached to each information cue). Therefore, if an individual's judgements vary from the regression model it might be possible to tell why (e.g. they are putting too much weight or importance on a specific information cue to reach their judgement).

Such approaches have been used successfully in medicine to analyse how doctors make diagnoses and reach decisions about prescribing medications (Denig et al 2002, Harries et al 1996, Skanér et al 1998). They have also been used successfully in nursing to examine judgements of patients' risk of deterioration (Thompson et al 2007). However, not all SJT studies have an external criterion (patient outcomes) that can be used in the regression models. In such instances, studies have been carried out that aim to describe or 'capture' nurses' judgements or 'policies'. These descriptive studies can still provide some insight into why nurses vary in their judgements and decisions (e.g. Paterson et al 2007). What they cannot do is provide any insight into the quality of those nurses' judgements and decisions. To be able to use SJT as a way of measuring judgement and decision quality you need to have a large number of patient cases, some idea of how the information used in the model relates to patient outcomes, and the ability to use regression techniques to model these relationships. Although such approaches obviously have utility in nursing research, and have been able to provide interesting insights into the accuracy of nurses' judgements (Thompson et al 2007), the utility of education and training (Thompson et al 2005), and how nurses' judgements vary for the same patient cases (Paterson et al 2007), the approach probably has limited applicability in everyday nursing practice. However, once a set of patient cases has been constructed and validated it is perfectly possible that nurses can use them as a way of examining their judgement and decision proficiency for a particular decision task.

Comparison with experts

So far, we have considered comparing nurses' judgements and decisions to the patient outcomes we see at some point after a judgement or decision has been made, and to normative models of judgement and decision making. Another way to examine how good an individual's judgements and decisions are is to compare them with someone who we think already makes accurate judgements or good decisions: an expert. There are many examples in the nursing literature where nurses' judgement and decision making have been compared with a standard set by experts (e.g. Aspinall 1979, Considine et al 2000, Corcoran 1986a, 1986b, Göransson et al 2006, Gould et al 2001, Lamond & Farnell 1998, Leprohon & Patel 1995, Letourneau & Jensen 1998, Reischman & Yarandi 2002, Shamian 1991). One of the key questions to consider if we are going to use expert judgement as a standard against which to compare judgements and decisions is 'What makes someone an expert?'

Who are the experts?

Experts have been defined as individuals who 'perform extremely complex tasks almost effortlessly and without mistakes' (Rikers & Verkoeijen 2007), 'a person who is very knowledgeable about or skilful in a particular area' (*Oxford English Dictionary*), and 'one who demonstrates expertise' (Hampton 1994). Experts, therefore, are individuals who demonstrate a high level of knowledge and skill in a specific area, operating at a level of accuracy beyond the non-expert. It is the *knowledge* and *behaviour* demonstrated by an individual that defines them as an expert.

So how do you spot the expert? Despite the above definitions, the most common way of identifying experts is through their experience of and length of service in a given field (e.g. Benner et al 1992, Corcoran 1986a, 1986b, Twycross & Powls 2006). Using experience as a proxy for expertise raises problems; although experience is necessary to become an expert (Hampton 1994) it is not sufficient (Christensen & Hewitt-Taylor 2006, Ericsson 2004).

Choudry and colleagues (2005) systematically reviewed the relationship between physician experience and the quality of care the same physicians provided. Quality was measured using patient outcomes and adherence to standards of care. They concluded that those physicians who have been in practice for longer, and older physicians, possess less factual knowledge, are less likely to adhere to appropriate standards of care, and might also have poorer patient outcomes (Choudry et al 2005).

Another way of identifying experts is to ask their peers or colleagues who they consider experts in their field to be (e.g. Benner et al 1992, Bonner 2003, Corcoran 1986a, 1986b, Fisher & Fonteyn 1994). However, being considered to be an expert by your colleagues doesn't necessarily mean that you are operating at an expert level (Rikers & Verkoeijen 2007).

Combining length of experience and peer/colleague evaluation is also unlikely to identify experts in an area when the definition of expertise encompasses the performance or behaviour of that person in their chosen field of expertise (Ericsson 2004). In summary, then, to identify experts, you really need to identify individuals exhibiting superior performance in a *specific task* in a *specific context*, which can be consistently be reproduced (Ericsson 2004). Examining patient outcomes to identify expertise in health-care is difficult, as a number of individuals contribute to the overall care of a patient (Christensen & Hewitt-Taylor 2006, Ericsson 2004). We therefore need to have some idea about the actions or behaviour that experts demonstrate: their *expertise*.

What is expertise?

Expertise has been defined as 'great skill or knowledge in a particular field' (*Oxford English Dictionary*). Nursing has a long history of researching the characteristics of the skills and knowledge that 'nurse experts' seem to possess (e.g. Benner 1982, Benner & Tanner 1987, Bonner 2003, Fisher & Fonteyn 1994, Hardy et al 2006). Expert nurses can 'rapidly and accurately assess a situation, execute appropriate decisions and instigate high-quality care without consciously working through the various alternatives' (Christensen & Hewitt-Taylor 2006). The ability of experts to rapidly assess a situation and act accordingly, often without being able to explain how they reached their judgement, has been identified as a characteristic of expertise and is often referred to as intuition or 'understanding without a rationale' (Benner 1982) (see Chapter 5 for more discussion on intuition).

One of the best-known studies of expertise in nursing is the body of work carried out by Benner (1982) that used the Dreyfus and Dreyfus model of skill acquisition to explore the functioning of nurses at different levels of proficiency. Benner (1982) identified the phases that individuals go through before reaching the level of expert (Table 6.1).

What these studies highlight is the change in how more experienced nurses appear to use their knowledge, and their approach to judgement and decision making in general, which they suggest is equated with a 'better' performance in clinical practice. The Benner approach to expertise suggests that, with experience, nurses move from a reliance on abstract principles to using past (more 'concrete') experiences to inform judgements and decision.

Table 6.1	Nurses' levels of proficiency
Level	*Description*
I: Novice	Beginners who, because they have no experience with the situations in which they are expected to perform, must depend on rules to guide their actions. Following rules, however, has limits. No rule can tell novices which tasks are most relevant in real situations nor when to make exceptions
II: Advanced beginner	One who has coped with enough real situations to note (or have them pointed out by a mentor) the recurrent meaningful aspects of situations. An advanced beginner needs help setting priorities because he or she operates on general guidelines and is only beginning to perceive recurrent meaningful patterns. The advanced beginner cannot reliably sort out what is most important in complex situations
III: Competent	Typically, the competent nurse has been in practice 2–3 years. This nurse can rely on long-range goals and plans to determine which aspects of a situation are important and which can be ignored. The competent nurse lacks the speed and flexibility of the nurse who has reached the proficient level, but competence is characterised by a feeling of mastery and the ability to cope with and manage many contingencies of clinical nursing
IV: Proficient	One who perceives situations as whole rather than as component parts. With holistic understanding, decision making is less laboured because the nurse has a perspective on which of the many attributes and aspects present are the important ones. The proficient performer considers fewer options and homes in on an accurate region of the problem
V: Expert	The nurse who no longer relies on an analytical principle (rule, guideline, maxim) to connect an understanding of the situation to an appropriate action. The expert nurse, with an enormous background of experience, has an intuitive grasp of the situation and zones in on the accurate region of the problem without wasteful consideration of a large range of unfruitful possibilities

Adapted from Benner & Tanner (1987).

With experience, nurses see situations less as a compilation of equally relevant bits and more as a complete whole in which only certain parts are relevant (Benner 1982). This leads to experts having 'a different and better grasp of a situation than other clinicians' (Benner et al 1992). A project carried out in the UK has built on previous work by Benner and other researchers to identify five attributes that characterise nursing practice expertise (Hardy et al 2006). These include holistic practice knowledge (such as learning from new situations, effective use of knowledge from a range of sources), saliency (the effective use of information in a situation), knowing the patient (which refers to areas such as respecting a patient's knowledge and beliefs), moral agency (such as assisting individuals to make informed decisions), and skilled know-how (such as the ability to flexibly adapt to new situations).

What these studies identify are broad characteristics of the knowledge and skill expert nurses are thought to possess. However, they don't actually indicate whether individuals who possess these characteristics do actually function at a 'superior' level of practice to other individuals who do not possess these characteristics. Benner's work is not without its critics, who highlight that intuition can equally be explained using research carried out in the cognitive sciences (English 1993) and that it is not only experts who use intuition

(Cash 1995). Expertise is 'context specific' in that individuals might be an expert in only a very specific field of practice (Fisher & Fonteyn 1994). Cash (1995) points out that Benner acknowledges this, stating that the term 'expert' cannot be fixed on a person, but then goes on to discuss how individual experts can be characterised by a specific way of thinking.

One of the main criticisms of this body of work is how it identifies expert practice in the first place and the vested interests associated with those who do the defining:

" Determination of what constitutes expert practice is by the approval of a specific group that is empowered to do so, either by being the research team, managers or by some other legitimising groups. The concept of expertise is therefore arbitrary: it is legitimated by groups or individuals whose status is defined socially. (Cash 1995 p 532) "

In other words, the characteristics that Benner (1982) and Hardy et al (2006) have identified as expertise might not be related to superior performance (and so might not actually be expertise) at all. It is the characteristics that a group of individuals have identified as being what *they* consider to be expert practice. This could be different to what the recipients of such practice might define as expertise.

So, what other approaches can we take to identifying those who claim to possess expertise? Ericsson (2007) suggests that the focus should be on identifying individuals who show superior performance on tasks that capture the essence of expertise in a particular domain and then studying them in detail. One approach to this is to measure performance on 'simulated' tasks to identify characteristics that you would expect experts to possess. One measure taking this route is the Cochran–Weiss–Shanteau (CWS) measure of expertise (Shanteau et al 2002, Weiss et al 2006). The CWS assumes that across time experts should be *consistent* in their judgments (i.e. if they see the same patient with the same symptoms at two different points in time they should make the same judgement) and be able to *discriminate* between similar but different cases (e.g. they see two patients with similar, flu-like symptoms and are able to identify correctly the one who has meningitis). Individuals can then be given a set of simulated cases (some of them repeated) and asked to make a series of judgements and decisions. On the basis of their responses and CWS score, we can identify individuals who have an ability to both discriminate and be consistent (e.g. Weiss et al 2006). What is not yet known is how well the CWS correlates with actual clinical performance on tasks. It is possible that we are still not able to identify accurately individuals who are demonstrating expertise until we try and factor in performance.

Is comparison with experts a good measure of judgement and decision-making quality?

The discussions in the preceding sections should have highlighted the inherent problems in using 'experts' as a criterion for assessing the quality of an individual's judgements and decisions. These problems often centre on how studies identify expert individuals (often only using length of experience as a criterion) rather than the principle of expertise itself. If we can develop valid and reliable ways of identifying individuals who do indeed function as experts on *specific* tasks (so that we are happy that their performance is superior to others in the field), then using them as a comparator for other people's performance becomes more acceptable. However, to identify superior performers in the first place, we probably need to use the methods identified earlier in the chapter, such as patient outcomes or comparison against a normative decision model.

SUMMARY

In this chapter, we have highlighted some of the complexities associated with assessing the quality of judgements and decision making. We have outlined a number of ways in which we can both define and measure how 'good' judgements and decisions are, and discussed both their benefits and limitations. There is no universally correct way of carrying out such evaluations, and no method is without its problems. In practice, there are few normative frameworks nurses can use to assist them. The uncertainty associated with health, and the confounding effects of a team approach to delivering healthcare, mean it is often difficult to use patient outcomes as a benchmark for judging decisions. In these circumstances, discussion or evaluation against some form of 'expert' criterion may be all that is available to you. Hopefully, the discussions in this section will enable you to be aware of some of the problems with this approach, and adjust your evaluations and the importance of the results accordingly.

EXERCISES

As a group, find an expert (a tutor or a clinical specialist/practitioner/someone who knows what he or she is doing!). Ask the expert to develop a series of ten clinical scenarios based around his or her field of expertise. The important thing here is that the expert should be clear: (1) about the correct course of action; (2) about the information required to decide this; (3) that the solution is not a no-brainer (i.e. there should be a genuine choice with some uncertainties); and (4) that the choice is a dichotomous (binary) one (i.e. act, do not act; at risk or not at risk; condition X or condition Y). Alternatively, you could use X-rays or you could each assess a fictitious patient using the same assessment tools (such as the Waterlow pressure sore risk assessment scale).

Each individual in the group (including the expert) should make at least ten observations, judgements, and decisions (e.g. fractured or not; at risk or not).

The non-stats version

How do the group's judgements and decisions compare with the expert's? Are they different? If they are, why do you think this might be? If not, why not? (hint: ten observations is a small sample).

> ### The statistical (more advanced) approach
>
> Go to: www.cmaj.ca/cgi/reprint/171/11/1369.pdf (for a detailed overview) or www. musc.edu/dc/icrebm/kappa.html for just the basics.
>
> Construct a 2 × 2 table of agreement for each student in the group compared to the expert. Calculate the Kappa statistic. Now how does the agreement compare: beyond that expected by chance?

REFERENCES

Allen-Davis J T, Beck A, Parker R et al 2002 Assessment of vulvovaginal complaints: accuracy of telephone triage and in-office diagnosis. Obstetrics and Gynecology 99(1):18–22

Aspinall M J 1979 Use of a decision tree to improve accuracy of diagnosis. Nursing Research 28(3):182–185

Bachmann L, Kolb E, Koller M et al 2003 Accuracy of Ottawa ankle rules to exclude fractures of the ankle and mid-foot: systematic review. British Medical Journal 326:417

Baron J 2000 Thinking and deciding, 3rd edn. Cambridge University Press, Cambridge

Benner P 1982 From novice to expert. American Journal of Nursing 82:402–407

Benner P Tanner C 1987 How expert nurses use intuition. American Journal of Nursing 87(1):23–31

Benner P, Tanner C, Chesla C 1992 From beginner to expert: gaining a differentiated clinical world in critical care nursing. Advances in Nursing Science 14(3):13–28

Bonner A 2003 Recognition of expertise: an important concept in the acquisition of nephrology nursing expertise. Nursing and Health Sciences 5:123–131

Cash K 1995 Benner and expertise in nursing: a critique. International Journal of Nursing Studies 32(6):527–534

Choudry N K, Fletcher R H, Soumerai S B 2005 Systematic review: the relationship between clinical experience and quality of healthcare. Annals of Internal Medicine 142:260–273

Christensen M Hewitt-Taylor J 2006 From expert to tasks, expert nursing practice redefined? Journal of Clinical Nursing 15:1531–1539

Considine J, Ung L, Thomas S 2000 Triage nurses' decisions using the national triage scale for Australian emergency departments. Accident & Emergency Nursing 8:201–209

Cooksey R W 1996 The methodology of social judgement theory. Thinking and Reasoning 2(2/3):141–173

Corcoran S A 1986a Planning by expert and novice nurses in cases of varying complexity. Research in Nursing and Health 9:155–162

Corcoran S A 1986b Task complexity and nursing expertise as factors in decision making. Nursing Research 35(2):107–112

Cullum N, McInnes E, Bell-Syer S et al 2004 Support surfaces for pressure ulcer prevention. Cochrane Database of Systematic Reviews, vol. Issue 3, no. Art. No.: CD001735, p. DOI: 10.1002/14651858.CD001735.pub2

Denig P, Wahlström R, de Saintonge M C et al 2002 The value of clinical judgement analysis for improving the quality of doctors' prescribing decisions. Medical Education 36:770–780

Dowding D, Thompson C 2003 Measuring the quality of judgement and decision-making in nursing. Journal of Advanced Nursing 44(1):49–57

Dubos F, Lamotte B, Bibi-Triki F et al 2006 Clinical decision rules to distinguish between bacterial and aseptic meningitis. Archives of Diseases in Childhood 91:647–650

English I 1993 Intuition as a function of the expert nurse: a critique of Benner's novice to expert model. Journal of Advanced Nursing 18:387–393

Ericsson K A 2004 Deliberate practice and the acquisition and maintenance of expert performance in medicine and related domains. Academic Medicine 79(10): S70–S81

Ericsson K A 2007 An expert-performance perspective of research on medical expertise: the study of clinical performance. Medical Education 41:1124–1130

Fisher A A, Fonteyn M E 1994 The nature of nursing expertise. In: Grobe S J, Pluyter-Wenting E S P (eds) Nursing informatics: an international overview for nursing in a technological era. Elsevier Science BV, the Netherlands, p 331–335

Göransson K E, Ehrenberg A, Marklund B et al 2006 Emergency department triage: is there a link between nurses' personal characteristics and accuracy in triage decisions? Accident & Emergency Nursing 14:83–88

Gould D, Kelly D, Goldstone L et al 2001 Examining the validity of pressure ulcer risk assessment scales: developing and using illustrated patient simulations to collect the data. Journal of Clinical Nursing 10:697–706

Grove W M, Meehl P E 1996 Comparative efficiency of informal (subjective, impressionistic) and formal (mechanical, algorithmic) prediction procedures: the clinical-statistical controversy. Psychology, Public Policy and Law 2(2):293–323

Grove W M, Zald D H, Lebow B. S et al 2000 Clinical versus mechanical prediction: A meta-analysis. Psychological Assessment 12(1): 19–30

Hampton D C 1994 Expertise: the true essence of nursing art. Advances in Nursing Science 17(1)15–24

Hardy S, Titchen A, Manley K et al 2006 Re-defining nursing expertise in the United Kingdom. Nursing Science Quarterly 19(3):260–264

Harries C, Evans J S B T, Dennis I et al 1996 A clinical judgement analysis of prescribing decisions in general practice. Le Travail Humain 9(1):87–111

Hastie R, Dawes R 2001 Rational choice in an uncertain world: the psychology of judgement and decision making. Sage, Thousand Oaks, CA

Hastie R, Rasinski K A 1988 The concept of accuracy in social judgment. In: Bar-Tal D, Kruglanski A W (eds) The social psychology of knowledge. Cambridge University Press, Cambridge, p 193–208

Jungermann H 2000 The two camps on rationality. In: Connolly T, Arkes H, Hammond K R (eds) Judgment and decision making: an interdisciplinary reader. Cambridge University Press, Cambrige, UK, p 575–591

Kruse J A, Thill-Baharozian M C, Carlson R W 1988 Comparison of clinical assessment with APACHE II for predicting mortality risk in patients admitted to a medical intensive care unit. Journal of the American Medical Association 260(12):1739–1742

Lamond D, Farnell S 1998 The treatment of pressure sores: a comparison of novice and expert nurses' knowledge, information use and decision accuracy. Journal of Advanced Nursing 27:280–286

Leprohon J, Patel V L 1995 Decision-making strategies for telephone triage in emergency medical services. Medical Decision Making 15(3):240–253

Letourneau S, Jensen L 1998 Impact of a decision tree on chronic wound care. Journal of Wound, Ostomy and Continence Nursing 25(5):240–247

Marsden J 2000 An evaluation of the safety and effectiveness of telephone triage as a method of patient prioritization in an ophthalmic accident and emergency service. Journal of Advanced Nursing 31(2):401–409

McDonald M, Passik S D, Dugan W et al 1999 Nurses' recognition of depression in their patients with cancer. Oncology Nursing Forum 26(3):593–599

Moore T, Martin J, Stonehouse J 1996 Predicting falls: Risk assessment tool versus clinical judgement. Perspectives 20(1):8–11

Moyer V A, Ahn C, Sneed S 2000 Accuracy of clinical judgment in neonatal jaundice. Archives of Pediatric & Adolescent Medicine 154:391–394

O'Brien J L, Moser D K, Riegel B et al 2001 Comparison of anxiety assessments between clinicians and patients with acute myocardial infarction in cardiac critical care units. American Journal of Critical Care 10(2):97–103

Paterson B, Dowding D, Harries C et al 2007 Managing the risk of suicide in acute psychiatric inpatients: a clinical judgement analysis of staff predictions of imminent suicide risk. Journal of Mental Health (Epub ahead of print) DOI: 10.1080/09638230701530234

Pauker S P, Pauker S G 1999 What is a good decision? Effective Clinical Practice 2(4):194–196

Quinn T, Thompson D R, Boyle R M 2000 Determining chest pain patients' suitability for transfer to a general ward following admission to a cardiac care unit. Journal of Advanced Nursing 32(2):310–317

Regher G 2004 Self-reflection on the quality of decisions in healthcare. Medical Education 38:1024–1027

Reid R C, Chappell N L 2000 Accuracy of staff assessments in research: dementia and environmental characteristics. Journal of Mental Health and Aging 6(3):237–248

Reischman R R, Yarandi H N 2002 Critical care cardiovascular nurse expert and novice diagnostic cue utilization. Journal of Advanced Nursing 39(1):24–34

Richardson A, Crow W, Coghill E et al 2007 A comparison of sleep assessment tools by nurses and patients in critical care. Journal of Clinical Nursing 16:1660–1668

Rikers R M, Verkoeijen P P 2007 Clinical expertise research: a history lesson from those who wrote it. Medical Education 41:1115–1116

Rosenthal G E, Mettler G, Pare S et al 1992 Diagnostic judgments of nurse practitioners providing primary gynecologic care: a quantitative analysis. Journal of General Internal Medicine 7:304–311

Shamian J 1991 Effect of teaching decision analysis on student nurses' clinical intervention decision making. Research in Nursing & Health 14:59–66

Shanteau J, Weiss D J, Thomas R P et al 2002 Performance-based assessment of expertise: how to decide if someone is an expert or not. European Journal of Operational Research 136(2):253–263

Skanér Y, Strender L-E, Bring J 1998 How do GPs use clinical information in their judgements of heart failure? Scandinavian Journal of Primary Health Care 16: 95–100

Sox H C 1999 What is a good decision? Effective Clinical Practice 2(4):196–197

Thompson C, Foster A, Cole I et al 2005 Using social judgement theory to model nurses' use of clinical information in critical care education. Nurse Education Today 25(1):68–77

Thompson C, Bucknall T, Estabrooks C A et al 2007 Nurses' critical event risk assessments: a judgement analysis. Journal of Clinical Nursing DOI: 10.1111/ j.1365–2702.2007.02191.x.

Twycross A, Powls L 2006 How do children's nurses make clinical decisions? Two preliminary studies. Journal of Clinical Nursing 15:1324–1335

VandenBosch T, Montoye C, Satwicz M et al 1996 Predictive validity of the Braden scale and nurse perception in identifying pressure ulcer risk. Applied Nursing Research 9(2):80–86

Weiss D J, Shanteau J, Harries P 2006 People who judge people. Journal of Behavioral Decision Making 19: 441–454

Wennike N, Williams E, Frost S et al 2007 Nurse-led triage of acute medical admissions: accurate and time-efficient. British Journal of Nursing 16(13):824–827

What is a 'good' judgement or decision?

When decision making goes wrong

Carl Thompson and Dawn Dowding

KEY ISSUES

- Defining errors, slips, lapses, and mistakes
- The importance of distinguishing between individual and organisational causes of errors
- The 'duality' of error
- Skills, rules, and knowledge-based causes of errors

DEFINING ERRORS AND MISTAKES

Patient safety incidents, which have been defined as 'any unintended event caused by the healthcare that either did or could have led to patient harm' (Sari et al 2007) are thought to occur in about 20% of hospital admissions (Sari et al 2007). It is estimated that 11% of patients receiving hospital care experience some form of harm as a result of such incidents, which are known as adverse events (Sari et al 2007). To avoid patient safety incidents and adverse events, we need to know where healthcare goes wrong; we need some understanding of the causes of errors and mistakes in healthcare so that we can avoid them in the future.

Decision making – whether intuitive, evidence based, rapid, or slow – is about intention in action. When we make choices, our choices are intentional. When we assess a patient and decide that X is wrong with them and we need to consider Y or Z to rectify the situation, our choices are informed by our prior intentions and planning.

Imagine you are a nurse assisting a 68-year-old man with chronic obstructive airways disease (COPD) to wash. You notice that he appears cyanosed

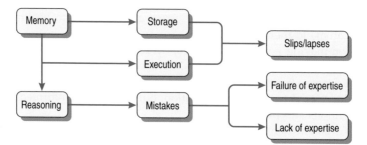

and is gasping for air and so you decide to give him some oxygen at 35%. In your experience, oxygen helps with breathlessness and so you consider this sensible. After 20 minutes, you notice that he is both breathing *more* rapidly and his oxygen saturation is *dropping* rather than improving.

What went wrong here? Perhaps the nurse didn't realise that in normal people the respiratory drive is largely initiated by Pco_2, but that in COPD hypoxia is itself a driving force for breathing. If hypoxia is corrected, the respiratory drive will be reduced. Or perhaps the nurse knew this but gambled on the fact that previous people he had cared for had responded well to O_2. In fact, what has occurred is an error or mistake in the nurse's reasoning.

How do we begin to unpack the error(s) so that we can understand and avoid them? Let us start with a definition of error. An error represents:

> " ... those occasions in which a planned sequence of mental or physical activities fails to achieve its intended outcome, and when these failures cannot be attributed to the intervention of some chance agency. (Reason 1990)"

An error, then, is a form of decision failure. There are various different kinds of error; in the example above, the nurse could have made an error of *omission* (the knowledge required for accurate planning was missing) or an error of *commission* (the knowledge was there but not used correctly).

Figure 7.1 introduces our first distinction: between slips, lapses in behaviour, and mistakes. Slips or lapses happen when we are putting our ideas into action. They occur regardless of whether there was some form of underlying plan to our behaviour (Reason 1990). A good example of a slip is walking up to a patient's family to discuss a patient's discharge and then forgetting to do so. Slips are primarily a deficiency in storing or using memory and memories.

Mistakes are deficiencies in planning and the reasoning associated with those plans. Formally, they are defined as:

> " ... deficiencies or failures in the judgemental and/or inferential processes involved in the selection of an objective or in the specification of the means to achieve it, irrespective of the actions directed by this decision scheme run according to plan. (Reason 1990)"

Mistakes happen when our reasoning goes awry and our intended actions do not proceed as planned and fail to achieve our immediate goals. Note that

Figure 7.1 Types of error.

this is not the same as initiating an intervention to achieve a longer-term goal. For example, giving analgesia and failing to relieve pain is not necessarily a mistake; as we saw in Chapter 2, healthcare is uncertain and outcomes and nursing interventions are only ever *probabilistically* related – the consequence being that not all people will respond positively to analgesia.

Mistakes are not divorced from nurses' expertise. Indeed, they can be attributed to failures of expertise itself as well as to failure resulting from a lack of the necessary expertise. We often assume that simply lacking expertise leads to a greater risk of error; however, it is not that simple. As discussed in Chapter 6, expertise is often linked to experience and training and is assumed to lead to heightened performance levels – and so fewer mistakes. However, recent systematic reviews of studies examining the *effects* of expertise, which rely on providing experts and non-experts with similar decision and practice tasks and not just self-reported behaviour or perceptions, cast doubt on these assumptions (Anders Ericsson et al 2007). Anders Ericsson et al (2007) suggest that claiming expertise on the basis of clinical experience alone does not always make for a better nurse or doctor. Choudhry and colleagues (2005) examined the clinical performance and knowledge of hundreds of doctors included in longitudinal studies and found that their quality of knowledge and decision making declined significantly over the years. Hamers et al (1994) found that experienced paediatric nurses were no more able than student nurses accurately to judge the level of pain experienced by children in video scenarios.

One of the explanations for this lack of difference is that scenarios lack the realism (internal validity) of actual practice and that experienced nurses are not able to smell, touch, and sense patients when faced with video or paper scenarios. Corcoran-Perry et al (1999), however, examined differences in the decisions of expert and novice nurses and found no differences in their reasoning on actual clinical cases *as well as* hypothetical ones. So, simply being experienced might not mean better decisions and fewer mistakes in healthcare.

Examining Figure 7.1 makes the distinction between slips, lapses, and mistakes seem clear and simple. In clinical practice, the boundaries are not so clear-cut, especially in real time while the error is happening. Hindsight is not always a force for better decisions. Let us consider the case study in Box 7.1 from the report 'to err is human' from the US Institute of Medicine (2000).

A range of possible actions that failed to proceed as intended (our working definition of error) are at play here. To get beyond this anodyne analysis we need to extend our model of what lies behind errors. 'Failure' can occur at three levels:

1. At the level of the skills of the decision maker (skills in both a practical sense and skills in terms of applying knowledge).
2. At the level of the rules that decision makers use to guide their choices.
3. At the level of the knowledge used in decisions.

Let us use these three interlinked levels to re-conceptualise our notion of error. Figure 7.2 (Reason 1990) describes this three-component system. Using this figure to examine our nurse–anaesthetist–pump case study, how might we unpack what is going on?

Box 7.1   A case study in error

A patient was undergoing a cardiac procedure. This patient had a tendency towards hypertension and the staff knew this. As part of the routine set-up for surgery, a nurse assembled three different infusion devices. The nurse was a new member of the team in the operating room; she had just started working at the hospital a few weeks before. The other members of the team had been working together for at least 6 months. The nurse was being very careful as she was setting up the devices because one of them was a slightly different model to any she had used before.

Each infusion device administered a different medication that would be used during surgery. For each medication, the infusion device had to be programmed according to how much medication would flow into the patient (in ml/h). The medications had different concentrations and each required calculation of the correct dose for that specific patient. The correct ml/h were programmed into the infusion devices.

The anaesthetist, who monitors and uses the infusion devices during surgery, usually arrived for surgery while the nurse was completing her set-up of the infusion devices and was able to check them over. This particular morning, however, the anaesthetist was running late from a previous surgery. When he arrived in the operating theatre, the rest of the team was ready to start. The anaesthetist glanced quickly at the set-up and accepted the report as given to him by the nurse.

One of the infusion devices was started at the beginning of surgery. About halfway through the surgery, the patient's blood pressure began to rise. The anaesthetist tried to counteract this by starting one of the other infusion devices that had been set up earlier. He checked the drip chamber in the intravenous (IV) tubing and did not see any drips. He checked the IV tubing and found a closed clamp, which he opened. At this point, the second device signalled an occlusion, or blockage, in the tubing by sounding an alarm and flashing an error message. The anaesthetist found a closed clamp in this tubing as well, opened it, pressed the re-start button and the device resumed pumping without further difficulty. He returned to the first device that he had started and found that there had been a free flow of fluid and medication to the patient, resulting in an overdose. The team responded appropriately and the patient recovered without further incident.

The case was reviewed 2 weeks later at the hospital's 'morbidity and mortality' meeting, where hospital staff review problems to identify what happened and how to avoid them happening again. The IV tubing had been removed from the device and discarded. The medical devices service had checked the pump and found it to be functioning accurately. It was not possible to determine whether the tubing had been inserted incorrectly into the device, whether the infusion rate had been set incorrectly or changed while the device was in use, or whether the device had malfunctioned unexpectedly. The anaesthetist was convinced that the tubing had been inserted incorrectly, so that when the clamp was open the fluid was able to flow freely rather than being controlled by the infusion device. The nurse felt the anaesthetist had failed to check the infusion system adequately before turning on the devices. Neither knew whether it was possible for an infusion device to have a safety mechanism built into it that would prevent free flows from happening.

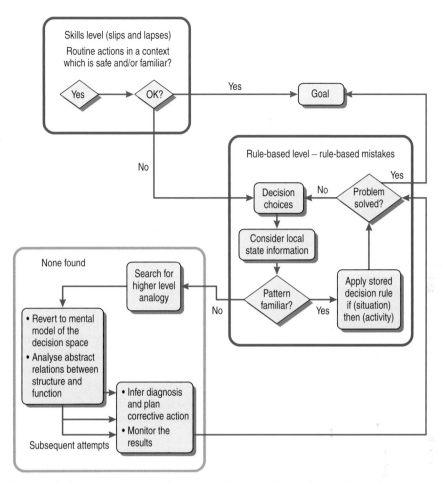

Figure 7.2 Skills, rules and knowledge failure (adapted from Reason 1990 and reproduced from Thompson et al 2002, Churchill Livingstone, with permission).

First, at the skills-based level, the nurse was both a new member of the team and had not used the exact model of infusion device before. The task involved a series of formal decision rules (e.g. if patient weighs X then calculate dose Y). As the task was unfamiliar, the use (and internalisation) of such rules will also have been new to the nurse. At the skills-based level again, the attention checks on the progress of the actions taken early on in the task (the 'set up') were likely to have been compromised by the delayed running of the operating room. At the level of knowledge deployment, the anaesthetist rapidly diagnosed the problem with the first pump and took corrective action (which provided the opportunity for the mistake with the first pump to occur). Both the main players in this error sequence were also ignorant of safe design in infusion devices that would have prevented the error regardless of the intent/actions of the nurse and anaesthetist.

What should be clear from even this briefest of decompositions of what happened is that rarely is there a single cause behind errors and mistakes. Circumstance, intent, perception, and action all interact. The chronology of events is also often confusing. Whereas there is clearly an individual focus (personal ignorance of infusion device safety characteristics, for example) to errors, these exist alongside and within a broader systemic framework (for example, organisation of workloads that allow inexperienced nurses to check medical devices). So let us introduce another distinction into our working model of errors in healthcare: a distinction between 'person' and 'system' approaches to errors (Reason 2000).

On individuals and systems

Person-based approaches see the root cause of errors as the result of flawed human beings. From this perspective, limitations such as forgetfulness, carelessness, inattention, or lack of motivation are causative factors in errors. The person-based approach is intuitively appealing because it allows us to blame an individual, or group of individuals, for mistakes and errors. However, the approach has two serious limitations.

First, when mishaps occur and are examined systematically by peers, experts, or just groups of individuals, a significant proportion are classed as 'blameless' (Reason 1990). This classification can only happen if there is a culture of reporting such mishaps. Without reporting, how can teams and individuals learn from their mistakes? However, a reporting culture will only develop if people feel that it is a just and fair system. It is far from clear that this is the case in healthcare. Sari and colleagues (2007) examined the sensitivity (the ability to detect something when it is truly present) of reporting systems in the UK NHS. They found that systems identified only 5% of actual incidents (found by scrutinising medical records).

The second major limitation of this approach is that the focus on individuals encourages us to bypass the systemic patterns and routines that are part of errors in an organisation. The uncomfortable truth (for those who see errors as the sole responsibility of individuals) is that mistakes happen to good people and that similar circumstance can provoke the same kinds of mistakes in different people (regardless of who they are). For an easy to grasp example try the following:

" Q: What do we call the tree that grows from acorns?
A: Oak
Q: What do we call a funny story?
A: Joke
Q: What sound does a frog make?
A: Croak
Q: What is another word for cape?
A: Cloak
Q: What do you call the white of an egg?
A: ?"

We bet that hardly any of you said 'albumin' – we are guessing that most of you said 'yolk'. It is that easy to respond in certain (and wrong) ways *given* the right (or wrong) set of circumstances – such as running late into an operating theatre that is waiting for you before it can begin.

So, to get to grips with errors we need to recognise that there is a strong systems dimension to them. From a systems perspective errors are not the product of a flawed human condition; rather, they result from factors that lie 'upstream' (Reason 2000) from where the error happens. These upstream factors include working conditions that constitute error traps, or organisational processes that do not allow the acquisition and deployment of the right knowledge for the tasks faced. Perhaps the most compelling reason for viewing errors as the consequence of systems rather than causes is that remedies rely on the premise that altering the human condition is very difficult (if not impossible) whereas altering the conditions under which we must work is somewhat more feasible.

'Swiss cheese', active and latent failure

Countering errors from the systems perspective relies on a series of safeguards and defences. We will examine some possible defences in Chapter 8, but for now we need to understand the role of systemic defences in the causative chain of events that lie behind many errors in healthcare organisations. Figure 7.3 represents the 'Swiss cheese' approach to explaining how mistakes occur in healthcare.

Each of the slices represents a defensive layer, each with its own holes or weaknesses. Normally, these holes in defensive layers fail to line up and so mistakes cannot pass through. Patients and professionals experience adverse events on the occasions when the holes do line up and allow the causative chain of events to continue.

> **QUESTION**
> Using our infusion device example (Box 7.1), what were the defensive layers in the scenario?

Other than chance or bad luck, what would cause the weaknesses in our model to line up? Holes in defensive layers line up because of a combination of two factors: active failures and latent conditions (Reason 2000).

Active failures are actions undertaken by those directly caring for patients. Often, these failures take the form of slips or lapses (e.g. absent-mindedly giving the medication to the wrong patient) or a deviation from

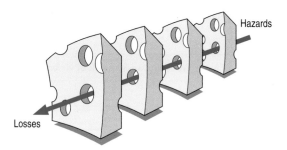

Hazards

Losses

Figure 7.3 Defensive layers, errors and Swiss cheese (from Reason 2000 © BMJ Publishing Group Ltd, reprinted with permission).

correct procedures (e.g. not bothering to calculate the drip rate in an IV infusion and just 'guestimating' the rate). Such failures are often short-lived in the system. Moreover, they often constitute the focus for those seeking a point of blame for the event. However, once unpicked, the causal history behind the active failure usually extends through time and back through the layers in an organisation (Reason 2000).

'Latent' conditions provide the backdrop for active failure. Latent conditions result from decisions made, often in the past, from managers, designers of buildings and organisational strategists. Latent conditions often lie dormant in organisations and are revealed when they combine with active failures and a trigger. Active failures (such as slips) are hard to predict, but latent conditions can be identified and managed. For example, excessive workloads, consistent time pressures, distraction, and competing calls on attention can all be altered to make errors less likely. For this reason, it is possible to be proactive in the ways that the risks of errors and mistakes are managed.

So we have established that errors are failures of intentional action due to mistakes in their planning or execution phases, that they have individual and systemic components, and that active and latent dimensions to the chain of causation lie behind them. One question that often arises is, 'can we ever avoid errors?' The simple answer is no, when human judgement plays a part. Why?

To understand the inescapable nature of some errors in healthcare it is important to reflect on the possible inputs and outcomes of a decision informed by judgement. Consider a common decision from mental health nursing practice and the judgement that informs it. The decision is whether to employ strategies for managing in-patients at a heightened risk of violence to themselves or others. The judgement that informs it is the degree of risk the patient presents. Consider the four possible states of this judgement (and there are only four – despite the seeming 'complexity' of this task) as illustrated in Table 7.1.

The two kinds of error that are possible are that we act when we should not have acted, or that we do not act when we should have. The data that 'feeds' these errors comes in the form of false positives (implying action when there is no need) and false negatives (implying no action when in truth action is required). Irreducible uncertainty as a backdrop for judgement requires that knowledge be applied (Hammond 1996). That knowledge can come from our own internal resources (memories, experiences, guesswork), which is by far the most common response to uncertainty in decision making

Table 7.1 2 × 2 tables of error types in assessing risk of violence

		Reality	
		Violent	Not violent
Judgement	At risk	True positive	False positive
	Not at risk	False negative	True negative

by nurses (Thompson 2003, Thompson et al 2004), or we can seek information from other sources. This information often comes in the form of advice from colleagues. This contains the same flaws as our own experiential knowledge. Alternatively, it can come from research information, from which many healthcare professionals are unable to extract useful messages; especially when it is presented in the 'raw' form of individual research papers (McCaughan et al 2002, McKenna et al 2004). Therefore, as all of our information-seeking options have limitations, it makes sense that in the face of irreducible uncertainty we will often have imperfect information.

This imperfection is problematic because individuals make decisions largely based on internalised rules (Hastie & Dawes 2001). These are often in the form of 'if–then' algorithms: *if* judgement = X *then* option A, *if* judgement = Y *then* option B. We call these decision *policies* and we see them in action when we think of a colleague who we might classify as a 'risk taker' or one who is 'cautious' or 'defensive'.

There are two dimensions to these rules: a judgement threshold beyond which we will act or not act (or choose option A over option B), and a criterion or 'real-world threshold' that exists but which we do not know (because uncertainty is irreducible and information imperfect). Our 'risk-taking' colleague might have a tendency towards a decision threshold higher than our more cautious colleague, who might act sooner as a result of a lower threshold for action. An example will make this clearer.

Returning to our judgement task of predicting violence, let us plot our two dimensions (the true risk of violence and the judged risk of violence) on two axes and consider the results of some hypothetical assessments. This is called a Taylor–Russell diagram. If someone was perfectly able to predict the likelihood of someone being violent (a state of perfect calibration), then the resulting graph would look like Figure 7.4, in which judged risk and actual risk are the same. However, we know that our measures of risk are imperfect, and that people's propensity for violence is individual and therefore variable. As a result, the possible plot of values of actual versus judged risk will always form an ellipse like Figure 7.5.

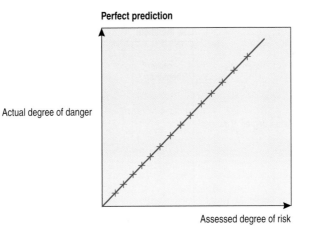

Perfect prediction

Actual degree of danger

Assessed degree of risk

Figure 7.4 Taylor–Russell diagram of perfect risk prediction (actual risk and judged risk are the same).

When decision making goes wrong

Imperfect prediction

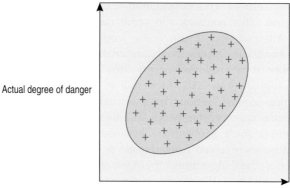

Actual degree of danger

Assessed degree of risk

Figure 7.5 Taylor–Russell diagram of imperfect risk prediction.

Suppose that the true underlying risk for a patient is just more than 50:50. We can use the Taylor–Russell diagram to illustrate how two nurses can have very different judgement policies (one risky and one cautious) and yet neither can avoid making errors. If we examine our cautious nurse's Taylor–Russell diagram (Figure 7.6) we can see that despite having a low threshold for action there is no possibility of ever avoiding some false negatives – not without having to tolerate many false-positive results.

If we then look at our risky nurse's judgement policy (Figure 7.7) applied to the same population of patients (they work on the same admissions unit) we can see that having a higher decision threshold (less likely to tolerate false positives) is at the expense of false negatives.

Regardless of where we set our decision thresholds, we will always make some mistakes. All we can hope for is that the trade-off between false positives and false negatives is acceptable to all parties involved in the decision. To determine this acceptability, we need to be explicit about the judgement thresholds that we use and the numbers of false positives and false negatives

Low threshold

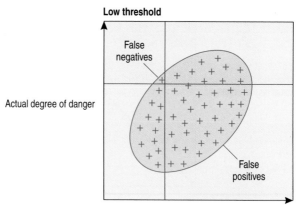

False negatives

Actual degree of danger

False positives

Assessed degree of risk

Figure 7.6 Taylor–Russell diagram for a cautious nurse (low threshold for action).

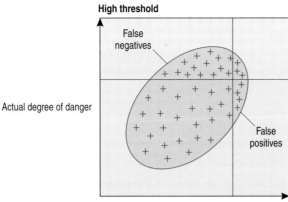

High threshold

False negatives

Actual degree of danger

False positives

Assessed degree of risk

Figure 7.7 Taylor–Russell diagram for a risky nurse (high threshold for action).

associated with our choices, as well as the possibility of altering our thresholds. This is not a comfortable prospect for many professionals as there is considerable short-term value in keeping the limitations of our judgements largely hidden from public view even if, in the longer term, we risk losing goodwill when our judgement limitations are exposed.

SKILLS- AND RULES-BASED ERRORS

This section of the chapter examines failures at the level of skills and rules in more detail and illustrates some examples of deficits in these areas.

Skills failures

Failures in the deployment of skills are associated with the amount of attention applied to task being performed. Attention, as applied to a judgement task, is a limited resource and it is easy to leave out a 'check' when making judgements. It is possible to predict when such slips are more likely (Reason 1990); they tend to occur when performing well-practised tasks in familiar surroundings, when individuals are considering departing from usual custom and practice, and when attention is compromised in some way. With these contextual factors in mind, we can further break down inattention failures into the more detailed typology in Box 7.2.

Box 7.2 Skills failures

- Inattention
- Double capture
- Omission following interruption
- Reduced intentionality
- Perceptual confusion
- Interference errors

Double-capture slips are a product of internal preoccupations or external distracters. If you think about a decision as a 'pathway' of intentions, it is possible to divert the sequence of actions contained in that pathway by replacing the schema (or pattern) associated with the desired action with a more powerful (but undesirable) schema. A classic, but not clinical, example of a double capture error is outlined by Reason (1990) in the form of a diary entry:

" I had decided to cut down on my sugar consumption and wanted to have my cornflakes without it. But the next morning, however, I sprinkled sugar on my cereal, just as I always do. (Reason 1990)"

In this example, we can see some of the predisposing factors for inattention errors at work: a change of routine (lower sugar consumption) that allowed the intrusion of an old habit (normal sugar-adding routine) into a pre-planned action sequence. Clinical examples of double capture include the novice student nurse who is so preoccupied with the cardiac monitor on coronary care that she fails to notice that the patient has removed his oxygen mask and that this is why his O_2 saturation is dropping. Another example cited by Kazaoka and colleagues (2007) is nurses' preoccupations with legal and liability issues in the administration of medications, to the extent that they make *more* – not less – errors in administration because their action sequences are interrupted by their preoccupations.

Interruptions are a common cause of lapses in clinical practice and occur when we omit checks on progress on an action or a sequence due to some external diversion. A clinical example is given by Thomas (2005):

" A 7-month-old infant with a chief complaint of vomiting is brought to the triage desk. The triage nurse does an assessment and weighs the baby. She tells the mother that the baby weighs 8 kg. The mother wants to know what that equals in pounds, so the nurse switches the scale to display pounds and tells her that the baby weighs 17.6 pounds. There is a line of patients at triage, so the nurse hurriedly documents the weight on the triage note. The chart has a space for weight in kilograms and, distracted, she writes in 17.6, failing to recognize that she did not switch the baby's weight back to kilograms."

In clinical practice, gaps exist between the planning of an action sequence and the execution of one. An example would be the nurse who, when coming on shift, knows that she must find time to talk to a patient about discharge planning and decides that she will do this after her coffee break, but at home that night realises she forgot. Unless planned action is accompanied by periodic attention checking, the planned action will be overtaken by other immediate calls on our limited attention. These kinds of slip are down to reduced intentionality (Reason 1990).

Another kind of slip that we can see in clinical practice arises from perceptual confusion. In routine actions, our attention is often reduced. The action sequences involved are almost automatic because the task is so familiar; objects that look, feel, smell, or sound familiar are pulled into the action sequence. A clinical example is the numbers of errors associated with potassium chloride in which potassium is mistakenly mixed with intravenous

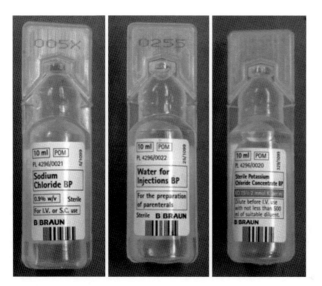

Figure 7.8 Ampoules of sodium chloride, water, and potassium.

fluids instead of sodium chloride or water. Figure 7.8 demonstrates the ease with which a perceptual slip could occur given the similarities between the three ampoules.

Rule-based failures

We have seen how decision makers when faced with information in familiar clinical environments use *if–then* rules. Over time, and with experience, nurses build up sizeable stores of such rules. How they decide to make use of a decision rule in a given situation depends on a four factors:

1. The rule needs to match a salient feature in the clinical-decision environment.
2. If a rule has been successful in the past, in similar circumstances, then it can be thought of as 'strong' and more likely to be used again.
3. If a rule is very specific to a particular decision situation then it too is likely to be used.
4. If a rule is supported by information in the clinical environment (it feels right) then it is likely to be used.

Errors due to rule failure occur in two areas: the misapplication of good decision rules and the application of bad decision rules.

Misapplying good rules

One of the characteristics of choosing to deploy a good rule is its success in the past. However, when individuals experience an exception to a generally good rule, they are prone to still employ the strong, but now wrong, rule. For example, when we start our nursing careers and having been heavily influenced by television, film, first aid at school, and a smattering of lay experience, we generally believe that giving oxygen to people who are ill is a good thing. Therefore, the decision rule is, '*If* a patient looks off colour and oxygen saturation is lower than his or her norm *then* give oxygen at 28%'. Generally, this is a good rule; however, there are some obvious exceptions. For example (as already highlighted), people with COPD, who often exhibit variable responses to high-concentration oxygen (Murphy et al 2001); very young neonatal babies whose chances of retinal damage are increased as a result of concentrated oxygen administration (Tin & Gupta 2007).

Whether we employ a particular decision rule depends on the degree of fit between the rules and the decision situation. Noise (irrelevant but influential information) in the decision environment makes it difficult to get this fit in clinical practice. A contextual factor makes deployment of the wrong rules more likely.

Decision and judgement rules with a proven record of accomplishment will, quite rightly, be given a higher weighting but individual decision makers are surprisingly resistant to discarding rules once applied. It took the systematically researched experience of thousands of neonatal babies to reveal the patterns of blindness resulting from the general decision rule that 'oxygen is good'. No doubt, individual decision makers, dealing with individual children, felt that the rule was perfectly adequate and that the blindness was simply down to bad luck or some other factor. This is one of the key roles of research evidence to reveal patterns of counterintuitive outcomes that are not easily revealed by experience alone.

Applying bad decision rules

When applying any decision rule there are two dimensions: (1) a process of making sense of a complex situation or *encoding*; and (2) planning action as a result of this encoding. Encoding throws up three common problems: (1) handling the volume of information in practice; (2) over-focusing on one dimension; and (3) the influence of perception.

There is a lot of information in clinical practice. On a decision-by-decision basis, we have a finite capacity for processing that information and for undertaking multiple judgement tasks simultaneously. Remember how it felt when you first learned to ride a bike or drive a car? Steering a straight course, keeping a steady speed, and anticipating the next required action seemed almost mutually exclusive. Human beings tend towards focusing on a single aspect of the skills set involved, placing the others on one side in a bid to keep the task manageable. This 'dislocation' of skills can be seen when novice student nurses give intramuscular injections, in the judgements and decisions that accompany the task. Asking a student to think aloud when carrying out this task invokes the following typical exchange:

“ Ermm ... I'm looking for the right upper quadrant on the buttock. Heck ... my hands are the wrong way round ... Right, so now they're the right way round ... OK, so I need to pull back the plunger ... I'm worried that if I pull it, it will fall out ... Mmm, some blood ... is it 'normal' or 'not normal'? ... OK, right ... I'm going to push in the plunger ... How quickly should I do it? ...”

Students often find themselves focusing on a single dimension of the task: safety *or* accuracy, at the expense of others, such as speed or efficiency. It is only with repeated exposure to the task and feedback on successful strategies for completion that they incorporate all of the required elements.

Nursing is a perceptual and physical activity as well as a cognitive one. When we assess patients we are often using physical sensations (skin colour, urine smell, skin 'feel', chest sounds, etc.) to sense the underlying and hidden conditions that the sounds indicate (health, pain, infection). The problem with the relationship between our senses, the stimuli we use, and our reasoning is that it is fallible. Try the following:

1. Look at Figure 7.9: imagine a ball is fired down the tube.
2. Now draw the trajectory of the ball when it leaves the tube. Was your trajectory like that in Figure 7.10 or in Figure 7.11?

If it was like Figure 7.10 – you are not alone; just over 55% of students in one experiment (in 1990) agreed with you and were also wrong. If Figure 7.11 was your choice, well done.

Another non-clinical illusion illustrates how we *construct* meaningful images from disparate stimuli. It has nothing to do with clinical practice, but is a lot of fun. Have a look at the Figure 7.12 and stare at the four tiny dots in the centre for the image for 30 seconds. Now, lean back, look at the ceiling, and blink quickly a few times. What did you see?

Of course, many nursing decisions rely on what patients tell us about *their* perceptions. For example, imagine you are a caseworker or community nurse working with teenagers to manage their diabetes. One of the key pieces of information you have to work with is the teenagers' perceptions of their condition (e.g. do they know when they are heading towards hypoglycaemia?) Obviously, it is important that they are accurate in their ability to perceive (subjectively) their objective levels of blood glucose. If we know the percentage of clinically significant errors (i.e. when the patient thinks they are 'hypo' when they are not, or when they think they are fine but are in fact hypoglycaemic) and the percentage of accurate estimates (when

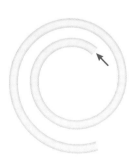

Figure 7.9   A tube.

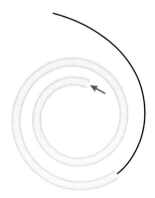

Figure 7.10   A curved trajectory.

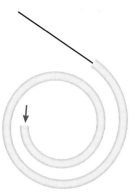

Figure 7.11 A straight trajectory.

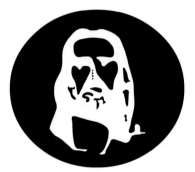

Figure 7.12 A somewhat religious experience?

subjective and objective measures coincide) it is possible to calculate an accuracy index (AI) that ranges from – 100 to 100. Positive AI scores indicate a higher frequency of clinically accurate estimates compared with clinically serious errors, whereas negative AI scores indicate more errors than accurate estimates. Figure 7.13 shows this relationship in graph format.

The average AI for adolescents with diabetes is between 7 (not so great) and 38 (better, but not fantastic). On the whole, children and adolescents' judgements are in the region of reasonably accurate (accurate 33% of the time), clinically benign errors (33%), and clinically relevant errors (33%) (Lane 2006). Alternatively, around one-third of the time, adolescents' estimates of their blood sugar are inaccurate.

Many general decision rules are wrongly 'protected' by what are called exception rules. Reason (1990) points to the social preservation of negative stereotypes as a fertile breeding ground for exceptions that serve to protect bad general rules. Often, these are manifest in statements such as 'some of my best friends are . . .', in which an individual who knows one or two people (from a population of many tens, hundreds or even millions of people) who fit their stereotypical representation of a social classification (e.g. the 'gay', or the 'immigrant'). The fact that these exceptions can be recalled 'proves' that their working stereotype has some utility and thus provides a sound basis for action.

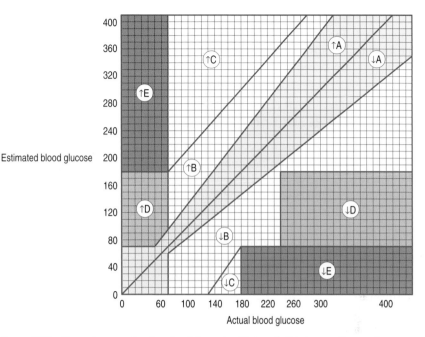

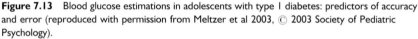

Figure 7.13 Blood glucose estimations in adolescents with type I diabetes: predictors of accuracy and error (reproduced with permission from Meltzer et al 2003, © 2003 Society of Pediatric Psychology).

A, B, C, D, E are accuracy 'zones' in an error grid.

Zone A = clinically accurate estimates leading to appropriate self-treatment.

Zone B = estimation errors resulting in benign self treatment (no harm).

Zones C, D, E clinically important errors.

    C = overcorrection of blood glucose levels.

    D = high or low blood glucose mislabled as 'normal'.

    E = dangerous errors e.g. hypoglycemia interpreted as hyperglycemia.

↑ indicates overestimates.

↓ indicates underestimates.

The key to assessing the utility of decision rules is systematic and sustained scrutiny of their effectiveness. Take as an example the issue of hand washing. Unwashed hands are a major source of hospital-acquired infections (HAI) in the UK. HAIs affect 1 in 11 patients, have a 13% mortality rate, result in patients staying in hospital for more than twice the length of time of non-infected people, and cost £3000 more per patient. Between 15 and 30% of HAIs are preventable (Grimshaw et al 2004). We confess that occasionally we also 'forgot' to wash our hands between patients. However, we did not lose much sleep over it; why? The main reason is that failure to wash outwardly clean hands is not accompanied by immediate (or even short-term) feedback on whether this was a good decision. HAIs appear later, often when we are off-shift. The causal chain between our actions and the eventual outcome is also not immediately apparent. We are not alone in our behaviour though; in the late 1990s a survey of clinical staff in six nursing homes found that the fact that complications were rarely seen was the main barrier to following hand-washing guidelines; 69% of the staff ranked it as the number 1 obstacle. If we don't get fairly rapid feedback on the quality of our decisions we very quickly 'learn' (Bandura 1969) that our actions are 'acceptable' – even when they are not.

KNOWLEDGE FAILURE: HEURISTICS AND THEIR RESULTANT BIASES

As we have seen, errors – and specifically mistakes – have a strong knowledge component to them: the knowledge informing the action to be taken; the knowledge used to make sense of the problem; knowledge about the adequacy of our own skills and internalised decision rules. This reliance on knowledge is mostly a very positive thing; assuming you have some knowledge to work with and it is fit for purpose. However, when it comes to processing and applying our knowledge, human beings have some big limitations.

Heuristics

As we saw in Chapter 5, the amount of information and the resulting complexity in our lives is far more than we are able to efficiently process and handle. We require a means of simplifying complexity, paying attention to the right information, and improving our knowledge base prior to making choices. We know from watching people make largely intuitive choices that the tools we use are cognitive. They must be, as most choices do not involve looking outside our own memory and knowledge base. We also know from listening to people describe their judgement and decision processes (thinking aloud) that these cognitive processes serve to simplify problems and reduce the amounts of information we are confronted with. We call these thought processes heuristics.

Most of the time, these heuristics are more than adequate: crossing a road, judging speed when driving, predicting aggression or conflict in social situations; we do not employ complex guidelines when carrying out these activities. However, each involves some difficult judgement calls. On an individual basis, we often see our heuristics as perfectly adequate. However, 671 people died crossing the road in 2005 and 6 people per 100,000 die in speed-related road traffic accidents (www.statistics.gov.uk/), there were also 2.4 million violent incidents recorded as crimes in the UK in 2005–06 (www.crimestatistics.org.uk/output/page63.asp). When we look at our abilities to use heuristics to manage risks in everyday life, it is clear that we are far from perfect.

Availability

The availability heuristic relies on the human tendency to assess the probability of an event by the ease with which an instance or occurrence can be brought to mind. An example is the tendency toward assessing the risk of phenomena such as heart attacks or strokes in middle age by recalling occurrences amongst our own circle of family and friends.

Availability is not always a problem because recalling large classes of phenomena is easier than less frequent classes. This is good; recall is correlated with probability, and an accurate starting point for probability assessment is a key to successful probability revision.

Factors other than frequency of occurrence, however, affect ease of recall. Moreover, what is most easily recalled is not always the correct knowledge or probability. So, for example, a study by Poses & Anthony (1991) showed that when doctors have recently cared for someone with bacteraemia they significantly overestimate the chances of the next patient they see having bacteraemia.

We tend to overuse dramatic (and often rare and/or unrepresentative) exemplars of instances as the basis for choices. Think of resuscitation attempts that you have seen. It is often easier to recall the vivid and easy to imagine than the probable but often more mundane. This susceptibility to vividness causes some problems in a profession in which knowledge transfer is primarily oral and based around stories and relayed experience (Thompson et al 2004).

Plous (1993) relays an experiment into the power of vividness in which a group of jurors (who, of course, are using their judgement) were shown 18 pieces of evidence from the prosecution and defence and asked to judge a defendant's level of drunkenness as well as his guilt or innocence. Crucially, jurors were randomised to receive either pallid or vivid versions of the evidence. A pallid version of the prosecution evidence was:

" On his way out of the door, Sanders [the defendant] staggered against a serving table, knocking a bowl to the floor. "

The vivid alternative was:

" On his way out of the door, Sanders staggered against a serving table, knocking a bowl of guacamole dip to the floor and splattering guacamole on the white shag carpet. "

What the researchers found was that although the vividness of the evidence made no difference immediately after hearing it, 48 hours after the event the group receiving the vivid information was more likely to judge the person drunk and guilty. The most likely explanation is that the vivid information was easier to recall.

Representativeness

Experts use mental representations, or prototypes, of classes of object to judge the probability that A resembles B. In diagnostic decisions, we are estimating the probability that A comes from B, where A is a pattern of symptoms and B is all of the various causes. If it is a judgement about causation then A might be the event and B a process or cause. There are two fundamental problems with this relationship, however. The first is that if our representations of a problem are wrong then our estimates of representativeness will also be wrong. The second is that the relationship between our mental constructs and underlying probabilities often break logical rules.

The classic demonstration of these tendencies is Tversky and Kahneman's 'feminist bank teller' experiment (Kahneman et al 1982). Consider the following description:

> " Linda is 31 years old, single, outspoken, and very bright. She majored in philosophy. As a student, she was deeply concerned with issues of discrimination and social justice, and participated in antinuclear demonstrations. Please select the most likely alternative:
> a. Linda is a bank teller.
> b. Linda is a bank teller and is active in the feminist movement. "

Most people judge that Linda is most likely a feminist bank teller. If you think for a moment, this cannot be the most likely alternative given the information provided. If we look at it graphically (Figure 7.14), we can see the same principle and realise why our instincts are sometimes wrong.

In a clinical setting, Brannon & Carson (2003) conducted an experiment in which 182 student and experienced nurses were provided with two sets of scenarios. In the first scenario, the patient presented with the symptoms of a heart attack: pain radiating to and down left arm, skin eruption, shortness of breath, etc. In some scenarios, these symptoms were accompanied by information that the patient had recently lost his job.

The second scenario presented a picture of a man found lying down in the emergency room (ER) waiting room and suffering a potential stroke. His assessment revealed slurred speech, uneven gait, and a right-sided weakness. Again, some of the nurses were presented with the additional information that his breath smelt of alcohol.

Of the nurses receiving the heart-attack scenario plus information on job loss, 26% attributed his symptoms to 'stress' and 76% to a physical cause. None of the nurses who received the scenario with the social context missing attributed his symptoms to 'stress'. Of the nurses who viewed the potential stroke scenario with the alcohol information present, 73% thought that the patient was drunk. Only 2% of the nurses whose scenarios did not contain the alcohol information attributed the symptoms to drunkenness.

Despite having salient information, the presence of the contextual information (job loss and alcohol) resulted in nurses dismissing serious physical diagnoses in favour of less serious situational causes. Brannon & Carson

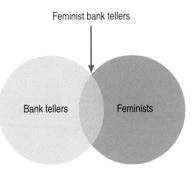

Feminist bank tellers

Bank tellers

Feminists

Figure 7.14 The conjunction fallacy.

(2003) attribute this to nurses' tendencies toward choosing less serious diagnoses because they were available via the representativeness heuristic (job loss + symptoms of heart attack = stress; alcohol + symptoms of stroke = drunk). The experiment also revealed that experienced nurses were just as prone to rely on representativeness as students.

Overconfidence

Decisions can be broken down into search behaviour and choice behaviour. A key driver for the information-seeking behaviour that accompanies decision making is an awareness of our knowledge limitations. This is a problem for human beings as we are notoriously bad at knowing what we don't know and reliably evaluating the correctness of our knowledge (Baumann et al 1991, Lichenstein & Fischoff 1977).

A quick experiment; Box 7.3 contains ten questions, which we would like you to answer. You will probably not know the answers (that is the point). For each question, we want you to give an *estimate* of the answer and a *sensible range* within which you can be *90% sure* the answer lies (i.e. saying the answer is between 0 and infinity is not allowed). For example, if asked, 'what proportion of patients in episodes of *ER* (if you are American) or *Casualty* (if you are British) are successfully resuscitated?', you might feel (with 90% certainty) that it's between 65% and 75%. In fact, it is 90%. Actually, we have no idea what the proportion is, but you get the picture. Keep your estimates sensible; in clinical practice you could hardly say to a patient, 'Your chances of being depressed are between 0% and 99% Mr Jackson'.

The answers are at the end of the chapter. How did you do? If you were correctly calibrated (i.e. you know what you do not know) and because you were supposed to be 90% sure, then you should have nine of the ten questions correct. We guess that most of you will have scored between three and six.

If we are consistently overconfident in our judgements of the knowledge used in managing patients then we will continue to deliver and prescribe

---

Box 7.3 Overconfidence questions

1. What is a healthy blood clotting time (in seconds) for an adult?
2. What is a normal chloride figure in blood plasma?
3. What is a normal pH for blood?
4. What is the specific gravity of urine?
5. How many calories do 100 g of carbohydrate provide?
6. What are the chances of an asymptomatic individual from a non-Caucasian ethnic group having organic coronary artery disease?
7. What year did Florence Nightingale return from the Crimea?
8. What is the total number of visits made by district nurses in one day in the NHS in England and Wales?
9. In which year did Iceland legalise abortion?
10. What percentage of individuals with herpes simplex virus (type 1) is asymptomatic?

suboptimal interventions. Overconfidence in our diagnostic reasoning means that we will tend towards too speedy a diagnosis and the erroneous ruling out of any further testing.

Baumann and colleagues (1991) used intensive-care nurses to illustrate the phenomenon of overconfidence. They examined nurses' abilities to recognise the uncertainty in an environment and to adjust their confidence levels (in the interventions they would carry out) accordingly. The absence of a diagnostic gold standard and the significant variations in interventions planned in the face of overt uncertainty revealed that nurses were far too confident in the choices they made.

Hindsight

When asked to predict an event in advance, people who know that such an event actually happens assign higher probabilities of it occurring than those who did not know that the event occurs (Fischoff 1975). This phenomenon, hindsight bias, leads to people changing the relative importance of influences that their judgement tells them are responsible for an event. In short, knowing the outcome of an event makes subsequent similar outcomes seem more likely. Arkes and colleagues (1981) demonstrated that physicians who knew the correct diagnoses for a series of medical conditions were more likely to assign a higher probability to those diagnoses after the event.

These findings have a number of important implications. First, when confronted with *a priori* knowledge of an event, clinicians attempt to make sense of what they know has happened rather than working with objective data. The implications of this for nurses (particularly expert nurses) can be seen in the popularity of teaching diagnosis using real clinical cases in the clinical environment. Nurses should always work prospectively from diagnostic work-up to prognostic or intervention decisions; rather than working backwards from diagnosis. If nurses already know the diagnosis, then it is likely that they will see the appropriate clinical cues. It is far better that they should work *from* clinical cues *to* the diagnosis.

Arkes and colleagues (1981) showed 15 physicians a case history accompanied by laboratory test results, and asked them to provide probabilities for four different (but possible) diagnoses. The probabilities at this stage were 44%, 29%, 16%, and 11%. Separate groups of 15 doctors were told – prior to reading the case history – that the diagnosis was one of the four possible options. Having this information changed the probabilities to 39%, 35%, 38%, and 31%, respectively. On average, then, hindsight added around 11% to the probability estimate of a correct diagnosis, regardless of whether the diagnosis is actually correct. Note that this is an average figure and includes downward shifts in estimates as well as positive revisions.

There are a number of other problems associated with hindsight, including the favourable distortion of memory (Fischoff & Beyth 1975) and (worryingly, from an author's perspective) undervaluing the original nature of thought and ideas expressed via scientific manuscripts submitted to peer-reviewed journals (Slovic & Fischoff 1977).

Base rate neglect

As nurses are increasingly asked to order (and interpret) diagnostic tests, it is essential that they understand the importance of acknowledging the base rates associated with diseases or conditions in populations. The normative rule for situations in which there are two independent probabilities of the same event (e.g. the presence of a particular disease such as depression) is to combine the two independent probabilities. The independent probabilities in this case (a diagnostic decision) are the *prior probability of having depression*, for example, and the *probability of having depression given the results of a diagnostic test*. This normative rule is known as Bayes' rule and can be expressed as: prior odds × likelihood ratio = posterior odds (see Chapter 9 for more discussion). Clinicians tend to ignore or place insufficient weight on the prior probabilities (base rates) associated with conditions or phenomena, a situation known as base rate neglect. The bias this introduces into decision making (particularly diagnostic decision making) can have important consequences (which are discussed further in Chapter 9).

Christensen-Szalanski & Bushyhead (1981) suggest that, when clinicians are encouraged to draw on experience to generate base rates, they closely approximate the normatively 'correct' way of combining probabilities. Little research into the ways nurses use diagnostic probabilities has been conducted. However, the work of Offredy (2002) shows that nurses do not appear to revise probabilities or adjust diagnostic strategies for different base rates, even when qualitatively 'rare' or 'common' conditions are presented as decision tasks.

Seeking out the positive: confirmatory biases

When gathering information to help inform our choices, we tend towards recalling and seeking information that most closely fits our preconceptions; we tend towards rejecting information that contradicts our expectations. When we are uncertain, supporting information feels good (Croskerry 2002). Information that makes us question ourselves, and perhaps start the process of thinking about a problem, diagnosis, and intervention again, feels uncomfortable. We are inveterate satisficers and, when a decision solution is found, we tend to stop search and problem-formulation activity. When the information that forms the basis of our ideas is only confirmatory, our hypotheses and start points for action will be built on weak foundations. If the foundations for actions are wrong then it is likely that the actions themselves will also fail and errors occur.

One of the areas most prone to confirmation bias is history taking on admission. Research with doctors has revealed that questions are often asked which confirm early judgements, questioning ceases when early conclusions are reached, and information gathered at the end of assessment is interpreted differently as a result of earlier judgements made (Klein 2005).

We have already seen (in the discussion of skills-based failures) how the brain has a tendency to 'fill in the gaps' and to see what it wants to see. Tuohy & Paperella (2005) show how our ability to see what we expect accounts for that proportion of drug errors in which we look at a label or packaging that confirms our ideas and so we act as if the desired drug is present even when it is not.

One of the authors (CT) took place in a debate in which he had to argue that complementary therapies had no effect on health. During the debate, a number of proponents of homeopathy argued that they had seen homeopathy work and could provide various (and moving) accounts of the effects of 'water with a memory'. The problem with homeopathic remedies is that just as patients fail to respond uniformly to treatments, they also respond positively to *no treatment*. Many illnesses are self-limiting and sometimes patients respond positively to placebos that they *think* are treatments (Crow et al 1999). Therapists tend to only remember those cases when patients seemed to improve after treatment (recall bias). Because they remember many of these instances, they seem correlated. However, when researchers systematically examined the response of thousands of patients treated with homeopathic remedies then such correlations disappeared; look at www.jr2.ox.ac. uk/bandolier/band116/b116-8.html for a fuller picture. Illusory correlation is problematic for decision making because it can act to reinforce mistaken beliefs and poor confidence calibration.

MAKING DECISIONS DESPITE OUR IMPERFECTIONS

Uncertainty, mistakes, errors, and flawed decision making will always exist in healthcare. Our knowledge, the ways in which we deploy it, and the physical actions involved in caring all contribute to patient safety, and the potential harms to which we must necessarily expose people.

This chapter may have left you with the impression that we are all doomed. The problem with clinical practice is that decisions still have to be made regardless of the uncertainty that must be managed and our flaws as decision makers, which must be contained. We have already looked at a few examples of how we can manage knowledge-based errors. The next chapter looks at some other ways in which we can manage the flaws, limitations and causes of errors in judgement and decision making.

READING AND RESOURCES

A comprehensive collection of material on errors and patient safety collated by the AHRQ in the United States: www.ahrq.gov/qual/errorsix.htm

A collection of resources and classic texts produced by the Institute for Healthcare Improvement: www.ihi.org/IHI/Topics/PatientSafety/

A series of small summaries to illustrate the problems in changing behaviour around decision making due to biases in thinking: www.changing-minds.org/explanations/theories/a_decision_error.htm

EXERCISES

The following are all fun, pretty interactive, and intended to make errors accessible.

A really nice example of illusory correlation for helping overcome prejudices and representativeness mistakes: www.jonathan.mueller.faculty.noctrl.edu/crow/ IllusoryCorrelationDemonstration.ppt

A fantastic physical demonstration of the impact of placebo (and why we should – at the very least – question the role of techniques such as therapeutic touch in nursing): http://www.pbs.org/saf/1210/teaching/teaching.htm

Have a go at: www.hondomagic.com/html/a_little_magic.htm It's a neat little trick (do you know how it's done?). This demonstrates the phenomenon by which our brain 'fills in the gaps' when representing decision problems.

SOURCES

Dingwall R, Rafferty A M, Webster C 1988 Introduction to the social history of nursing. Routledge, London

Kasner K, Tindall D 1984 Nurses' fictionary. Baillière Tindall, London

Langenberg A G, Corey L, Ashley R L et al 1999 A prospective study of new infections with herpes simplex virus type 1 and type 2. Chiron HSV Vaccine Study Group. New England Journal of Medicine 341:1432-1438

Silagy C, Haines A 1998 Evidence based primary care. BMJ Publishing, London

ANSWERS TO OVERCONFIDENCE QUESTIONS IN BOX 7.3

1. 240–600 s
2. 95–105 mmol/l
3. 7.35–7.45
4. 1002–1040 degrees
5. 400
6. 3.2%
7. 1856
8. 100,000
9. 1935
10. 60%

REFERENCES

Anders Ericsson K, Whyte J, Ward P 2007 Expert performance in nursing: reviewing research on expertise in nursing within the framework of the expert performance approach. Advances in Nursing Science 30:E58–E71

Arkes H R, Wortmann R L, Saville P D et al 1981 Hindsight bias among physicians weighing the likelihood of diagnoses. Journal of Applied Psychology 66 (2):252–254

Bandura A 1969 Social learning of moral judgments. Journal of Personality and Social Psychology 11:275–279

Baumann A, Deber R B, Thompson G G 1991 Overconfidence among physicians and nurses: the 'micro-certainty, macro-uncertainty' phenomenon. Social Science and Medicine 32:167–174

Brannon L A, Carson K L 2003 The representativeness heuristic: influence on nurses' decision making. Applied Nursing Research 16:201–204

Choudhry N K, Fletcher R H, Soumerai S B 2005 Systematic review: the relationship between clinical experience and quality of healthcare. Annals of Internal Medicine 142:260–273

Christensen-Szalanski J J J, Bushyhead J B 1981 Physicians' use of probabilistic information in a real clinical setting. Journal of Experimental Psychology 7:928–935

Corcoran-Perry S A, Narayan S M, Cochrane S 1999 Coronary care nurses' clinical decision making. Nursing and Health Sciences 1:49–61

Croskerry P 2002 Achieving quality in clinical decision making: cognitive strategies and detection of bias. Academic Emergency Medicine 9:1184–1204

Crow R, Gage H, Hampson S et al 1999 The role of expectancies in the placebo effect and their use in the delivery of healthcare: a systematic review. Health Technology Assessment 3:1–96

Fischoff B 1975 Hindsight? Foresight: the effect of outcome knowledge on judgment under certainty. Journal of Applied Social Psychology 18:93–119

Fischoff B, Beyth R 1975 'I knew it would happen' Remembered probabilities of once-future things. Organizational Behavior and Human Performance 13:1–16

Grimshaw J, Thomas R E, Maclennan G et al 2004 Effectiveness and efficiency of guideline dissemination and implementation strategies. Health Technology Assessment 8(6):1–72

Hamers J P H, Abu-Saad H H, Halfens R J G 1994 Diagnostic process and decision making in nursing: a literature review. Journal of Professional Nursing 10:154–163

Hammond K R 1996 Human judgement and social policy: irreducible uncertainty, inevitable error and unavoidable injustice. Oxford University Press, Oxford

Hastie R, Dawes R M 2001 Rational choice in an uncertain world. Sage, London

Institute of Medicine 2000 To err is human: building a safer health system. National Academy Press, Washington, DC

Kahneman D, Slovic P, Tversky A 1982 Judgment under uncertainty heuristics and biases. Cambridge University Press, Cambridge

Kazaoka T, Ohtsuka K, Ueno K et al 2007 Why nurses make medication errors: a simulation study. Nurse Education Today 27:312–317

Klein J G 2005 Five pitfalls in decisions about diagnosis and prescribing. British Medical Journal 330:781–783

Lane M M 2006 Advancing the science of perceptual accuracy in pediatric asthma and diabetes. Journal of Pediatric Psychology 31:233–245

Lichenstein S, Fischoff B 1977 Do those who know more also know more about how much they know? the calibration of probability judgments. Organizational Behaviour and Human Performance 20:159–183

McCaughan D, Thompson C, Cullum N et al 2002 Acute care nurses' perceptions of barriers to using research information in clinical decision making. Journal of Advanced Nursing 39:46–60

McKenna H, Ashton S, Keeney S 2004 Barriers to evidence–based practice in primary care. Journal of Advanced Nursing 45:178–189

Meltzer L J, Bennett-Johnson S, Pappachan S, Silverstein J 2003 Blood glucose estimations in adolescents with type 1 diabetes: predictors of accuracy and error. Journal of Pediatric Psychology 28:203–211

Murphy R, Driscoll P, O'Driscoll R 2001 Emergency oxygen therapy for the COPD patient. Emergency Medicine Journal 18:333–339

Offredy M. 2002 Decision making by nurse practitioners in primary care. University of Hertfordshire, UK

Plous S 1993 The psychology of judgment and decision making. McGraw Hill, New York

Poses R M, Anthony M K 1991 Availability, wishful thinking, and physicians' diagnostic judgments for patients with suspected bacteremia. Medical Decision Making 1:159–168

Reason J 1990 Human error. Cambridge University Press, Cambridge

Reason J 2000 Human error: models and management. British Medical Journal 320:768–770

Sari A B A, Sheldon T A, Cracknell A et al 2007 Sensitivity of routine system for reporting patient safety incidents in an NHS hospital: retrospective patient case note review. British Medical Journal 334:79

Slovic P, Fischoff B 1977 On the psychology of experimental surprises. Journal of Experimental Psychology 3:544–551

Thomas D O 2005 Lessons learned: basic evidence-based advice for preventing medication errors in children. Journal of Emergency Nursing 31:490–493

Thompson C 2003 Clinical experience as evidence in evidence-based practice. Journal of Advanced Nursing 43:230–237

Thompson C, Dowding D et al 2002 Clinical decision making and judgement in nursing. Churchill Livingstone, Edinburgh

Thompson C, Cullum N, McCaughan D et al 2004. Nurses, information use, and clinical decision making – the real world potential for evidence-based decisions in nursing. Evidence-based Nursing 7:68–72

Tin W Gupta S 2007 Optimum oxygen therapy in preterm babies. Archives of Disease in Childhood – Fetal and Neonatal Edition 92:F143–F147

Tuohy N, Paparella S 2005 Look-alike and sound-alike drugs: errors just waiting to happen. Journal of Emergency Nursing 31:569–571

Avoiding errors

Carl Thompson and Dawn Dowding

8

KEY ISSUES

- How to combat errors in reasoning and logic
- The importance of culture, leadership and communication for error reduction
- Balancing individual and system remedies for the causes of error

RATIONALE FOR THE CHAPTER

If you have got this far in the book, you will have encountered some key concepts central to the idea of mistakes and errors in decision making: uncertainty, risk, probability, errors, adverse events, decision making, and clinical judgement. Before we launch into this chapter proper, it is worth summarising the relationship between some of these central concepts:

- Due to the probabilistic world we live in, uncertainty in healthcare is 'irreducible', in that you will never be able to avoid it.
- Our responses to uncertainty lead to trade-offs between over- and undercautiousness in the judgements we use to inform our decision making – a situation known as the 'duality of error'.
- Both individuals and the systems we operate within are implicated in errors.
- As (some) errors are unavoidable, we should view them as a valuable resource from which we can learn.
- In learning from our mistakes, and the mistakes and corrective efforts of others, we might be able to prevent future errors.

So, where does this leave us? This very brief overview of progress thus far suggests that any strategy to minimise errors should be able to:

- Combat the *individual* causes of errors as much as possible.

- Combat the *systemic* causes of errors as much as possible.
- Learn from those errors that will inevitably still happen.
- Prevent those that are preventable and be theoretically *and* empirically defensible.

ERROR AND THE INDIVIDUAL

When we talk about decision making there is often the implication that it is a solo activity, or at best, shared with colleagues (sometimes) or patients (occasionally). It is perhaps not surprising then that when things go wrong we often look at the role of the individuals concerned. As human error is implicated in many adverse events, this tendency to treat individual flaws as the root cause of incidents is understandable – if not wholly defensible.

Healthcare is a complex system and, as professionals and patients, we do not act in isolation from this system and its subsystems (Department of Health 2000). Due in part to this recognition, it has become increasingly and justifiably popular to focus corrective efforts on the systems that make up the healthcare machine. Nevertheless, it would be misguided simply to ignore those causative factors that are within the control of the individual – and there are many.

Individual error in decision making amounts primarily to errors in cognition. Why so? Judgement (weighing the evidence) and decision making (choosing between those alternatives) are cognitive activities. Most judgements and decisions in practice take place primarily at the intuitive end of the cognitive continuum. Occasionally, we draw on colleagues' advice; and very occasionally, we might step outside our own internal reserves of memory, experiences, and internalised knowledge and seek support for our decision making from research evidence, guidelines or other forms of decision support. As Chapter 7 highlighted, nurses and doctors will rarely (if ever!) sit down and construct balance sheets or clinical utility analyses for the decisions they face. Instead, they rely on a series of cognitive shortcuts and strategies to make sense of the world, reach judgements, and make choices. These shortcuts, or heuristics, although often reliable, can be prone to systematic and predictable biases and errors. Chapter 7 discussed these heuristics in detail; this chapter examines the individual strategies you might be able to use to combat these negative effects.

Anchoring

One heuristic that wasn't mentioned in Chapter 7 is that of anchoring. First impressions can exert a powerful (sometimes too powerful) effect on our ability to revise our ideas in the light of new information. Forming ideas on first impressions is a risky judgemental strategy. Once an idea is formed (e.g. a diagnosis) it is often difficult to shake and often shapes a whole clinical journey and set of patient experiences. Two of the most powerful 'anchoring' effects encountered by the authors are the diagnostic label of a mother 'diagnosed' with Munchausen's-by-proxy on the basis of nothing other than hearsay and the fact that she came from a very different social class to the health visitor involved, and cases of young black male patients in a psychiatric ward whose heightened risk of violence was judged far higher than their white contemporaries with reference to nothing other than difference in skin colour (from the staff), linguistic, and cultural differences. Both of these examples lead to (erroneous) revisions of probability and changes in behaviour on the part of staff.

Simply being aware of our tendency to anchor prematurely is often sufficient to combat this bias. If possible, delay forming an impression until more complete information is available (Tversky & Kahneman 1974). Uncertainty is irreducible but being aware of the value (particularly diagnostic value) of information is a significant boost to decision making. An example of a test that is a useful anchor (because of its positive predictive value) would be the 'glass test' in relation to a child or young adult who turns up in your clinic or ER with a fever, accompanied by spots or a rash that do not fade under the pressure of a glass tumbler (see: www.meningitis-trust.org/Signs-Symptoms.html). Such patients should trigger cognitive alarm bells and constitute an emergency. Research-derived knowledge of the predictive value of the anchors that you commonly use, coupled with self-awareness that you are using them is the answer.

Availability

We judge things as more likely or frequent according to the ease with which they spring to mind. This is a good thing; phenomena that are more common are more readily recalled. As we saw in Chapter 7, however, it is not just relative frequency that leads to recall, other factors also influence how readily material is brought to bear on judgement problems: vividness and recency being the most prominent. Availability also has a (somewhat unimaginatively titled) flip-side: non-availability. Non-availability is the phenomenon by which individuals fail to pay sufficient attention to that which is not immediately apparent. Both of these variants are associated with inaccurate estimates of the base rate associated with diagnostic judgements.

Chapter 9 discusses how important base rates are for formal diagnostic judgements using test results. They are also vital for the 'informal' Bayesian reasoning we all employ when making judgements about the likelihood that a set of symptoms means that an individual belongs to a 'class' such as a disease or risk grouping. If the base rate is wrong then over- or underestimation of probability will result. The cure for availability bias is the gathering and use of objective information: accurate (research or audit based) base rates and clear clinical evidence to support or refute a particular diagnosis. An awareness of your real level of expertise in a task is also vital. Novices tend towards a reliance on available prototypes as a heuristic, whereas experts are prone to non-availability and time dedicated to atypical or rare classes or diagnoses. Asking yourself whether the estimate you first make is as robust as you perceive it to be is a good first step in combating the biases that can result from the availability heuristic (Poses & Anthony 1991, Tversky & Kahneman 1974).

An example that one of the authors (CT) often draws on is experience of cardiac arrest. Carl has 10 years' clinical experience in critical and emergency clinical settings. These have higher base rates of cardiac arrests – because people are often sicker – than many other settings. Despite this, when asked to recall cardiac arrests, Carl tends to remember those: (1) that were dramatic; and (2) in which the patient was resuscitated successfully. When he systematically tries to recall, reflect, and document them, however, it is immediately apparent that: (1) most were relatively undramatic (indeed, were often 'expected' on the part of the staff and who were ready with the arrest trolley); and (2) resuscitation attempts were mostly unsuccessful. Left to his own immediate cognition and estimates, Carl overestimated the drama and success rates of arrests in the ER.

Representativeness

Representativeness relates primarily to the strategy of pattern matching that we use as a way of making sense of the clinical world quickly. When, as students, we begin to 'learn nursing' we are often taught a series of prototypes. For example, we might be told that a patient who is having a myocardial infarction will most likely have crushing chest pain, ECG changes, pain (perhaps radiating down the left arm), will be sweating, will feel clammy, and will have a rapid or erratic pulse. These prototypes are what we compare patients against when we encounter them. The problem arises when patients don't fit these prototypes.

Normally, the heuristic works well; it does have an unfortunate property, though, that makes over-reliance on it somewhat risky. Our representative prototypes are insensitive to prior probability, prevalence, or base rates (you will have worked out by now that these are one and the same thing in decision terms). So, a representative prototype of a patient with diabetes applied to patients seen in an acute medical ward (where patients might have less-stable blood sugar levels despite a well-controlled dietary regimen) will not 'perform' as well in a community setting, where blood sugar levels might be more stable (because people are generally not as sick) but where the dietary regimen is probably more relaxed. The upshot of over-reliance on representativeness is that diagnoses and predicted response to interventions might be inaccurate or missed. An example is the 4% of patients who are sent home from the A&E unit with a myocardial infarction (Croskerry 2002). Unrepresentative groups (the young, the diabetic, females, the very old, and people with mental health problems) are over-represented in this group because they do not 'fit' the prototype of someone with an infarct.

The way to avoid the bias that arises from representativeness is awareness of its presence in our reasoning. When someone does not 'fit' a prototype we should remind ourselves of the possibilities that might exist and of the underlying prevalence. For example, the young male orthopaedic patient who returns from surgery post-fixation of a leg fracture arising from a motorcycle accident who says everything is 'fine' and 'I don't need pain killers' is: (1) atypical; and (2) should be encouraged to take the analgesia because the prevalence of pain post-orthopaedic surgery on a major limb is very high. At the very least, the nurse should take some time to discuss whether the patient is 'really fine' or just feels the need to portray this.

Overconfidence

This is an uncomfortable heuristic and one that often requires some soul searching on the part of healthcare professionals before they admit that it is something that is a feature of their reasoning. If you undertook the 10-question general health knowledge quiz in Chapter 7 (Box 7.3) how did you do? If you got less than 9 out of 10 then you have just demonstrated (for this task) how overconfident in your knowledge you are. The bottom line is that we often think we know more than we do. As a consequence, we often gather *too little* information before reaching a judgement and have *too much* faith in our opinion. Overconfidence interacts with our self-belief regarding our potential impact on health outcomes. Where we think that we will significantly impact on outcomes we tend to believe that this impact will be positive (Croskerry 2002). The major problem with overconfidence from a clinical perspective is one of too little information gathering and hasty actions. So errors of *omission* (not ordering a test that is required or not intervening appropriately) and *commission* (being too ready to dive in with unnecessary actions such as test ordering, interventions or prognostic forward projections) are common.

Asking ourselves four questions can help combat the effects of overconfidence (Croskerry 2002, Plous 1993, Yates 1990):

- Is my confidence *really* justified; why might my reasoning be wrong?
- Has the information I am using to make my choices been systematically gathered?
- If information has been gathered systematically, does it support the estimates or choices we are putting forward?
- How much reliance am I placing on anchors or information that is readily available rather than of real value?

Feedback on decisions can be a powerful means of combating overconfidence. Lichenstein & Fischoff (1980) demonstrated that students who received reports and explanations of results tended toward under-, rather than overconfidence on a one-sided probability 'rating of correctness' scale for two-choice knowledge questions. For a less academic and more accessible example, consider the good performance (on average) of weather forecasters. The reason why they are so calibrated (they constantly revise their probability estimates on the basis of what they know) is that they receive continuous feedback on the justification of their confidence levels.

The following clinical example illustrates what such calibration and feedback might look like. Imagine that you are a staff nurse working on a day-surgery unit. You have an informal analgesia protocol that you apply to most of your patients with hernia repairs. You are confident (based on a couple of years' experience) that it works and that patients are relatively pain free at home for a few hours after they have left the unit. However, you have never stopped to consider whether there are better alternatives. You realize that you receive no feedback on whether the pain relief works in the hours after discharge. You decide that if the pain relief was not effective after discharge then you would try to devise something better. You decide to 'test' whether your confidence is justified. You arrange for one of your colleagues or yourself to administer a pain measurement scale to each patient before leaving the ward and then phone them within 6 hours of discharge and simply ask them to complete it again and send it back. The findings surprise you. You realize that a large proportion of patients' pain is not well managed by the protocol after discharge. Obviously, you would not have received this information if you had not sought feedback on your initial decision choice. Clearly, you now have a solid footing for a more evidence-based approach to revision of the pain relief protocol. You can repeat the 'decision audit' later to see if this has worked.

The need for confirmation

As we saw in Chapter 7, we tend to prefer to seek out information that confirms our beliefs rather than challenges them. Confirmatory evidence simply 'feels good' when you are problem solving.

Decision problems can be conceptualised as occupying a problem *space*. Easy, well-structured problems, with very few choices occupy smaller spaces than large, ill-structured, problems with many options. Unfortunately, large problem spaces are common in healthcare; as is our tendency to settle for decisions that are 'good enough' rather than optimal (Simon 1992). In these large problem spaces there are often lots and lots of data. For an example, consider leg ulcer assessments by a community nurse. A nurse who is following best practice and guidance by systematically carrying out an 'holistic' assessment (see www.guideline.gov/summary/summary.aspx? doc_id=9830&nbr=5254&ss=6&xl=999 for an example) will have to cognitively synthesise and make sense of more than 50 separate pieces of information. During information collection, the nurse will be forming hypotheses about what might be wrong, the kind of ulcer, what sort of treatment might help, how long it could take to heal, and so on. In these complex decision environments, individuals are prone to focus on data that are most relevant to a currently held hypothesis and neglect those that don't fit.

The cure for confirmation is to search for evidence that challenges our hypotheses and hunches rather than confirms them. As Croskerry points out, 'one piece of disconfirming evidence may be worth ten pieces of confirming evidence' (Croskerry 2002). Once evidence has been gathered, then a nurse should make sure that she or he has given adequate consideration to alternative hypotheses (likely causes, potential gains from interventions, and how the patient may be in the future).

We can draw on many heuristics to make sense of information, to reach quality judgements, and to make informed choices. The list of heuristics and associated strategies for reducing the biases that are induced is too long to relay in a single chapter. Readers who wish to examine the issue in more detail should look at Plous's (1993) overview of the psychology of judgement and decision making for an accessible introduction to the range of issues that can be highlighted. Those who wish for an overview that is explicitly orientated towards healthcare should examine Croskerry's (2002) broad-ranging treatise of 'cognitive dispositions to act' (heuristics). This is based around a comprehensive typology (with healthcare examples) of all of the major heuristics that impact on healthcare delivery.

Individual contributions to errors, then, are not going to disappear, as most of our cognition is intuitive in practice and such cognition draws heavily on rules-of-thumb heuristics or 'mindlines' (Gabbay & LeMay 2004) and some guesswork. You should have grasped by now that no single individual approach to error reduction will eliminate mistakes. The best we can hope for when it comes to quality assuring our own singular contribution to error reduction is that we are open and honest about our use of such rules and shortcuts, that we link such use to research knowledge of what happens to patients as a result, and that when we have good rules that we train nurses to use them in 'disciplined and informed' ways (Gigerenzer 2007). To design interventions to combat errors we need to look not just at the individual, but toward the contexts, knowledge and systems they find themselves working with and in.

SYSTEMIC APPROACHES TO ERROR REDUCTION

Healthcare is a social activity and even the most autonomous decision maker operates in a complex network of rules, values, expected behaviours and measured performance.

The UK National Patient Safety Agency (NPSA) produces evidence-based guidance that helps organise ideas and activities for managing the complexities surrounding patient safety. Their '7 steps' approach to safer healthcare (National Patient Safety Agency 2004) provides a series of headings that anyone considering a systemic approach to prevention and reduction should consider: culture, leadership, integration of risk management, promoting reporting, communication and involvement, learning from errors, and implementing preventative solutions. We will examine each of these in turn.

Changing cultures

'Culture' is something of a buzzword in contemporary healthcare; despite the frequency of its use, there are however some fairly compelling arguments to suggest that a culture that values openness about the potential for errors, and learning from them, results in a safer environment (Reason 1990). Culture is difficult to work with and is even harder to quantify and measure. The difficulties of operationalising the notion of culture partially explain why the theoretical benefits of possessing a 'safety' culture are less easily identified in the empirical research literature (Scott et al 2003). However, the relative absence of evidence of an impact on patient safety from having a 'safety culture' should not be interpreted as evidence that having a safety culture has no effect on errors in healthcare organisations. Values, beliefs, and behaviours are so intricately linked that it would be a brave (or foolish) manager who felt no need to acknowledge their complex interplay when planning a system to improve safety and reduce errors.

What do we mean by culture?

Culture can be thought of as the, 'pattern of beliefs, values, attitudes, norms, unspoken assumptions and entrenched processes that shape how people behave and work together'(National Patient Safety Agency 2004).

Culture can be thought of as something that an organisation both *is* and as something that it *possesses* in the form of attributes or variables that can be identified and moulded (Davies et al 2000). This split is an important one; shaping values and beliefs (culture) is only a possibility if the organisation itself is not the product of that same culture. Davies and colleagues suggest ten key features of a culture that determines its ability to perform (Box 8.1).

Why does culture matter?

Culture matters because it is at the heart of good clinical governance: the framework through which healthcare is accountable for continuously improving the quality of their services and safeguarding high standards of care by creating an environment in which excellence in clinical care can flourish (Secretary of State for Health 1998). In the United States, the Agency for Healthcare Research and Quality (a federal sub-agency of the Department of Health and Human Services) is also explicitly committed to fostering evidence-based and safer healthcare. Indeed, the AHRQ has an entire collection of very high-quality resources available for free on its website (www. psnet.ahrq.gov/).

As a healthcare professional, the primary reason for placing safety high on the list of values that guides your practice is a moral one: 'first, do no harm'.

What do we mean by a safety culture?

Although Davies et al (2000) provide us with pointers to those values that might indicate a culture of performance generally, we are primarily

---

Box 8.1   Ten key features of organisational culture (adapted from Davies et al 2000)

1. *Attitudes to innovation and risk taking*: the degree to which the organisation encourages and rewards new ways of doing things or, conversely, values tradition
2. *Degree of central direction*: the extent of central setting of objectives and performance versus devolved decision making
3. *Patterns of communication*: the degree to which instruction and reporting are channelled via formal hierarchies rather than informal networks
4. *Outcome or process orientation*: whether the organisation values outcomes and results as opposed to tasks
5. *Internal or external focus*: whether the organisation looks inward and restricts itself to organisational issues as opposed to looking at the needs of customers
6. *Uniformity or diversity*: the organisational propensity towards consistency or diversity
7. *People orientation*: valuation of the human resources available to an organisation
8. *Team orientation*: does the organisation reward individualism or is it geared towards teamwork?
9. *Aggressiveness/competitiveness*: the extent to which the organisation seeks to dominate or cooperate with external competitors or players
10. *Attitudes to change*: the extent to which the organisation demonstrates a predilection for stability in preference to dynamic change

interested in what marks out a culture of safety and error prevention specifically. The Hospital Survey on Patient Safety Culture (www.ahrq.gov/qual/hospculture/) is a tool developed around 12 dimensions and indicative features (Table 8.1).

How might we measure a safety culture?

As well as the aforementioned AHRQ national hospital safety culture survey tool, various other tools exist to help measure the degree to which a culture of safety might be present in an organisation. These tools can be distinguished according to whether they are based on: (1) typologies (lists of desirable attributes pertaining to safety culture against the presence of which are

Table 8.1 Twelve dimensions and indicators associated with a safety culture (www.ahrq.gov/qual/hospculture)

Dimension	Description
1. Communication openness	Staff speak up freely if they see something that might negatively affect a patient, and feel free to question those with more authority
2. Feedback and communication about error	Staff are informed about errors that happen, given feedback about changes implemented, and discuss ways to prevent errors
3. Frequency of events reported	Mistakes of the following types are reported: (1) mistakes caught and corrected before affecting the patient; (2) mistakes with no potential to harm the patient; and (3) mistakes that could harm the patient, but do not
4. Handoffs and transitions	Important patient care information is transferred across hospital units and during shift changes
5. Management support for patient safety	Hospital management provides a work climate that promotes patient safety and shows that patient safety is a top priority
6. Non-punitive response to error	Errors are not held against staff, and mistakes are not kept in their personnel file
7. Organizational learning – continuous improvement	There is a learning culture in which mistakes lead to positive changes and changes are evaluated for effectiveness
8. Overall perceptions of patient safety	Procedures and systems are good at preventing errors and there is a lack of patient safety problems
9. Staffing	There are enough staff to handle the workload and work hours are appropriate to provide the best care for patients
10. Supervisor/manager expectations and actions promoting safety	Supervisors/managers consider staff suggestions for improving patient safety, praise staff for following patient safety procedures, and do not overlook patient safety problems
11. Teamwork across units	Hospital units cooperate and coordinate with one another to provide the best care for patients
12. Teamwork within units	Staff support one another, treat each other with respect, and work together as a team

Adapted from Davis et al (2000).

'checked'), or (2) dimensions of a safety culture against which an organisation or one of its subunits are scored.

Two examples of typology-based tools are the Checklist for Assessing Institutional Resilience (www.ihi.org/IHI/Topics/PatientSafety/Safety General/Tools/ChecklistForAssessingInstitutionalResilience.htm) and the Manchester Patient Safety Assessment Tool or MaPSat (www.pharmacy. manchester.ac.uk/cip/resources/MaPSAF/). Of those assessment tools that are based around a dimensional approach, two examples are the Safety Attitudes Questionnaire (SAQ) (www.uth.tmc.edu/schools/med/imed/ patient_safety/survey&tools.htm) and the Stanford Patient Safety Centre of Inquiry Culture Survey (Singer et al 2007). The Stanford approach looks at 16 areas linked to safer healthcare such as the degree to which reporting is rewarded, the degree of 'buy in' by senior managers, the ways in which risks are perceived by staff groups, time pressures, concordance with policies and procedures, and quality of communication (National Patient Safety Agency 2004, Singer et al 2007).

The role of leadership and support

The most open and fair reporting system in the world will fail if there is an absence of leadership. Such leadership is not always of the formal or hierarchical type. Although leadership is an expected part of the top of the organisational pyramid in healthcare (e.g. chief nurses, chief executives) the need to shape opinion within a peer group, sphere of influence, or community of practice (Wenger et al 2002) is something that all professionals engage in. Indeed, changing opinions using human-to-human interaction can be a successful change intervention in itself (Grimshaw et al 2004). Fostering motivation and good communication are also necessary elements of a culture in which safety is valued. A treatise of the elements of good leadership are beyond the scope of a text aimed primarily at those interested in decision making (although, obviously, good leaders should make more good decisions than bad). There are, however, a number of specific leadership strategies that are explicitly linked to improvements in patient safety (National Patient Safety Agency 2004 p 40):

- Appoint someone to lead on patient safety as an explicit part of his or her remit, e.g. a risk or patient safety manager. Sometimes the argument is expressed that 'safety is everyone's business' and that giving a named individual the remit for patient safety results in the marginalisation of safety. In the long term, both of these statements have some truth; but at the start of the patient safety 'journey' someone needs to communicate strategic visions; lead by example; and broker, contextualise, and translate technical and/or 'alien' language and knowledge.
- If your organisation has a management board or steering group, then nominate a board member with specific responsibility for patient safety. Responsibility in the absence of accountability is sometimes prone to dilution or lack of deployment. Having the safety remit straddle the executive and non-executive (strategic or policy making) tiers of an organisation is a crucial lever for holding executive decision makers to account for their choices and actions.

- Identify patient safety champions in every directorate, division, department, or practice.
- 'Walk-the-walk': being visible and out in the field is both valued and valuable. It is indicative of a leader who is willing to listen to staff and experience the environments in which decision making must happen (good or bad).
- By ensuring that members of your team brief (and debrief at the end of a shift or day) each other it is possible to both raise awareness and foster some sense of shared ownership of the issues that impact on decision making and patient safety. Briefings should have a clear remit and be brief, open, fair, and responsive to the ways in which the team works (small teams that work together constantly don't need to meet as often as a whole directorate of shifting interns, nurses, bank/agency staff) (National Patient Safety Agency 2004).
- Build awareness by incorporating patient safety into the staff induction programme.
- Provide general training programmes in patient safety.
- Make specialist patient safety training available for the staff with specific responsibility for the safety agenda.

Integrating risk management activity into the 'way we do things round here'

In many, hospitals the Director of Nursing is responsible for pulling together the systems and structures that deal with health and safety, clinical risk and governance, quality assurance, patient and family complaints, and clinical negligence. This pulling-together of the roles and dimensions of an organisation that are likely to influence decision making is a good thing. These dimensions of patient safety overlap and the danger in isolating them is that each operates in a kind of silo in which problems and – more importantly – solutions can only emerge from within the silo involved, be that a professional group, ward, team, or clinic. Systems-based approaches that recognise the natural overlaps are far more likely to avoid this blinkered problem and solution formulation.

Clearly, uniting previously separate roles and functions, and the organisational processes that support them, is no good if there is no way of knowing if it is having an impact. Indicators of safety within an organisation already exist (see: www.qualityhealthcare.org); commonly, outcomes such as

- surgical-site infections
- ventilator-related acquired respiratory infections
- deep vein thrombosis (DVT) and embolisms
- medication errors
- blood transfusion incidents and
- mortality rates

are used to measure internal organisational change and progress; they are also used to compare the performance of one organisation against another. Such outcomes are 'blunt' instruments with which to measure progress. However, aside from the scientific question of whether they are valid indicators of quality, they nevertheless offer a focus for the learning and interventions that team members take part in to try and reduce errors.

Promoting patient safety incident reporting

Research suggests that patient reporting systems have variable levels of sensitivity, but that even mandatory reporting of adverse events might only pick up 5% of actual incidents (Sari et al 2007). The UK National Patient Safety Agency (NPSA) suggests considering linking your local risk management system to the national reporting and learning system for reporting patient safety incidents. Moreover, by providing regular safety reports for the staff in your clinical environment, you can maintain and heighten awareness of the importance of incident reporting.

Involving and communicating adverse events and errors with patients and relatives

Over the years, we have come to realise that a major challenge to improving nurses' decision making is the need to, 'train nurses for uncertainty rather than certainty' (Luker 1998 personal communication). However, it is increasingly clear to us that there is a parallel need to train the public – users of health services – and their carers for the same uncertainties. If we foster the societal belief that the diagnostic, interventional and prognostic reasoning we employ is accompanied by too much certainty then the consequences could be severe. A loss of trust, a weakening of the social contract between professionals and patients, and increased exposure to the harmful aspects of healthcare are all possible endpoints if the public overestimate our ability to manage uncertainty.

The UK NPSA is explicit in its recommendation that patients should be involved in decision making (and the consequences of those decisions) where possible. The stance is underpinned by a key principle:

" Many patients are experts in their own condition and this expertise can be used to help identify risks and devise solutions to patient safety problems. Patients want to be involved as partners in their care. Healthcare staff need to include patients in reaching the right diagnosis, deciding appropriate treatment, discussing the risks and ensuring treatment is correctly administered, monitored and adhered to. Being open about what has happened and discussing the problem promptly, fully and compassionately can help patients cope better with the after effects when things have gone wrong. (National Patient Safety Agency 2004 p 123)"

Being open with patients and relatives following a patient safety incident is an important part of any strategy; but what of strategies that involve professional–patient partnership *before* an incident has occurred? One approach that can be useful is to recognise that the professional–patient partnership carries responsibilities on both sides: the nurse or doctor *and* the patient or his or her carers. A means of operationalising this is the SPEAK UP campaign. The acronym comes from the elements in Box 8.2, each of which is

Box 8.2 Speak up

Speak up if you have any questions or concerns and if you don't understand:

- Don't worry about being embarrassed if you don't understand something.
- Don't be afraid to ask about safety. If you are having surgery, for example, ask your doctor to mark the area to be operated on so there is no confusion.
- Don't hesitate to tell healthcare staff if you think you have been confused with another patient or if you think you have received the wrong medicine.
- Tell the staff if something doesn't seem right.

Pay attention to the care you are receiving and make sure you are receiving the right treatment and medication:

- Make sure you are clear about what treatment you have agreed to and don't be afraid to ask for a second opinion.
- Make sure you are aware of any possible risks or complications your treatment may entail.
- Expect healthcare staff to tell you who they are and look for their identification.
- Make sure staff confirm your identity when they give you medicines or administer treatment.
- Notice if staff wash their hands before and after your treatment – it's OK to remind a doctor or nurse to do this.

EDUCATE YOURSELF ABOUT YOUR DIAGNOSIS

- Ask more questions, such as: 'How does my condition affect me'? How is my condition treated? How should my condition respond to this treatment?
- Ask if there is any written information available to back up your discussion.
- Gather information about your condition from reputable sources, such as well-researched studies, journals and books, expert groups, and validated websites.
- Write down the important facts so you can easily refer to them later.
- Read all forms you are asked to sign and ask healthcare staff to explain if you don't understand anything.
- Make sure you get your test results and don't assume 'no news is good news'.
- If you have to use any equipment, make sure you understand what your role is.

ASK A TRUSTED FAMILY MEMBER OR FRIEND TO BE YOUR ADVOCATE

- Your advocate can ask questions for you if you are under stress.
- Your advocate can help remember answers to questions you asked.
- Make sure your advocate understands your preference for care.

KNOW WHAT MEDICINES YOU ARE TAKING AND WHY

- Ask what the medicine or treatment is for, if there is any written information about it, and what possible side effects, complications or risks there may be.
- If you don't recognise the medicine, verify that it is for you.
- If you are having an IV ask the nurse how long it is expected to last.
- Don't be afraid to call someone if it appears to be going too quickly or too slowly.
- Tell healthcare staff about your allergies and reactions.

Continued

Box 8.2 Speak up—cont'd

- If you are on multiple medicines, ask staff whether they can be taken together.
- Make sure you can read your prescription; if you can't read it, your pharmacist might not be able to either.

UNDERSTAND MORE ABOUT YOUR LOCAL NHS ORGANISATION

- How does your local NHS organisation perform against national targets for infection rates?
- What level of achievement does your local NHS organisation have against national targets, such as for waiting times, cancelled operations and deaths following surgery?
- What level of achievement does your local NHS organisation have for patient safety assessments, such as the clinical negligence scheme for Trusts (range 1–3)?
- Read the review of your local NHS organisation by the Commission for Healthcare Improvement (www.chi.nhs.uk).

PARTICIPATE IN ALL DECISIONS AROUND YOUR TREATMENT

- Agree with healthcare staff exactly what will be done during each step of your care.
- Know who will be taking care of you, how long the treatment will last, and how you should feel.
- Don't be afraid to ask for a second opinion at any stage – the more information you have about the options available the more confident you will be with the decisions made.
- Ask to speak to others who have undergone the procedure you are considering.

accompanied by some recommended behaviours to encourage in patients and carers (National Patient Safety Agency 2004 p 128–132).

Learn and share safety lessons and discover why an error has occurred

Adverse events and errors will always happen but one of the keys to ensuring that they are reduced wherever possible is to try to diagnose what went wrong and share the lessons learned. One approach to unpacking errors and establishing causes in a systematic way is root cause analysis (RCA). This is a retrospective review of a patient safety incident. The process of RCA helps identify areas for change, and to arrive at recommendations for future and possible solutions. RCA is a team-based approach and centres on understanding the 'what?', 'how?', and 'why?' behind an incident.

RCA is a structured process and requires some training to be deployed effectively. The UK National Patient Safety Agency has produced an excellent online (free) modular e-learning programme aimed at providing the knowledge required for you to take part in an RCA team (see: www. msnpsa.nhs.uk/rcatoolkit/course/iindex.htm).

Make changes to practice, processes, or systems to prevent harm

A number of organisations and agencies provide 'benchmarks', evidence-based advice, and guidance on how to configure, organise, and deliver services to promote patient safety. In the UK, the NPSA and the National Institute for Health and Clinical Excellence (NICE) provide alerts and guidance, which – if implemented on the ground – should reduce adverse events.

For example, a significant problem for health services is 'medicines reconciliation', the phenomenon by which patients find themselves admitted to hospital and prescribed different medications to those they were taking before admission. This matters because:

- The patient might receive the wrong dose of his or her medicine.
- The patient might not receive his or her medicine at all.
- The pharmacy could order in the wrong medication for a patient.
- There might be delays to a patient's treatment while these issues are resolved.
- The patient's stay in hospital might be extended or his or her discharge delayed.
- It fosters confusion and lack of confidence in the system, for patients, their carers and families, as well as for healthcare professionals (www.npc.co. uk/mms/FiveMinGuides/library/5m_reconciliation.htm).

National Institute for Health and Clinical Excellence, National Patient Safety Agency guidance (NICE/NPSA 2007) suggests that healthcare organisations that admit adult inpatients should have policies in place for medicines reconciliation on admission. As well as specifying standardised systems for collecting and documenting information about current medications, policies for medicines reconciliation on admission should ensure that:

- Pharmacists are involved in medicines reconciliation as soon as possible after admission.
- The responsibilities of pharmacists and other staff in the medicines reconciliation process are clearly defined; these responsibilities may differ between clinical areas.
- Strategies are incorporated to obtain information about medications for people with communication difficulties. (NICE/NPSA 2007).

For a ward or clinical manager, such guidance provides a clear focus for implementation and behaviour change.

For an international perspective, the World Health Organization (WHO) provides detailed advice for implementing patient safety initiatives via its 'Patient Safety Solutions' programme (see: www.who.int/patientsafety/solutions/en/). WHO highlights areas for improvement that impact on all health systems; for example, fostering effective and safe communication during handover. This is an important area of focus: of the 25,000 to 30,000 preventable adverse events that led to permanent disability in Australia, 11% were due to communication breakdown, by contrast only 6% of incidents were attributed to inadequate skills of healthcare professionals. Again, as with the NPSA/NICE guidance these messages are clearly presented in Box 8.3.

Box 8.3 An example of a patient safety solution from the World Health Organization

Ensure that healthcare organisations implement a standardised approach to handover communication between staff, change of shift, and between different patient-care units in the course of a patient transfer. Suggested elements of this approach include:

- Use of the SBAR (Situation, Background, Assessment, and Recommendation) technique.
- Allocation of sufficient time for communicating important information and for staff to ask and respond to questions without interruptions wherever possible (repeat-back and read-back steps should be included in the hand-over process).
- Provision of information regarding the patient's status, medications, treatment plans, advance directives, and any significant status changes.
- Limitation of the exchange of information to that which is necessary to providing safe care to the patient.
- Ensure that healthcare organisations implement systems that ensure – at the time of hospital discharge – that the patient and the next healthcare provider are given key information regarding discharge diagnoses, treatment plans, medications, and test results.
- Incorporate training on effective handover communication into the educational curricula and continuing professional development for healthcare professionals.
- Encourage communication between organisations that are providing care to the same patient in parallel (e.g. traditional and non-traditional providers) (see: www.jcipatientsafety.org/fpdf/presskit/PS-Solution3.pdf).

This wide-ranging chapter has skimmed the surface of the patient safety and error reduction agenda. Despite being primarily an overview, there are still some clear lessons to be learned (and many resources have been provided below for you to increase your depth of understanding).

First, despite working with systems, individual (person-centred) causes of errors still exist and there are strategies we can employ to reduce our propensity for being at the root cause of them. For example, we can be aware of the heuristics (and resultant biases) we use as 'short cuts'. Simply being aware of these heuristics means that we can improve our judgement.

Second, although the individual causes of errors persist, anyone who is truly serious about improving patient safety through strategic thinking and action knows that system-related causes, failures, and conditions need to be addressed. There are relatively simple ways of thinking about the complexities that we must manage and changes to the ways in which services are configured and delivered that can be made that make a difference. Moreover, resources and guidance are out there to help us make these changes. All nurses need to do is 'step up to the plate', meet the challenge, and lead by example.

SAFETY AND ERROR RESOURCES

Each link below is a gateway to other resources and organisations (governmental and professional) and as such is intended to offer a start point for exploration rather than a comprehensive list.

www.psnet.ahrq.gov/index.aspx This is the US Agency for Healthcare Research and Quality's patient safety network homepage. From here you can access classic works in patient safety sorted by target audience (such as nurses).

www.dh.gov.uk/en/Publichealth/Patientsafety/DH_081603 The UK Department of Health's key documents on patient safety page. This is something of a 'one-stop-shop' for the key policy documents pertaining to patient safety in the UK and the actions required of healthcare providers and commissioners.

www.npsa.nhs.uk/patientsafety/improvingpatientsafety The NPSA's improving patient safety home page. A key resource for accessing online training and keeping up to date with the latest integrated thinking about systems, policies, human factors, and research evidence.

www.ahrq.gov/qual/nurseshdbk/ A largely American perspective on evidence-based practice and patient safety. Well written and solidly scientific in its orientation.

REFERENCES

Croskerry P 2002 Achieving quality in clinical decision making: cognitive strategies and detection of bias. Academic Emergency Medicine 9:1184–1204

Davies H T, Nutley S M, Mannion R 2000 Organisational culture and quality of healthcare. Quality in Health Care 9:111–119

Department of Health 2000 Organisation with a memory. HMSO, London

Gabbay J, LeMay A 2004 Evidence based guidelines or collectively constructed 'mindlines?' Ethnographic study of knowledge management in primary care. British Medical Journal 329:1013

Gigerenzer G 2007 Gut feelings: the intelligence of the unconscious. Viking. London

Grimshaw J, Thomas R E, Maclennan G et al 2004 Effectiveness and efficiency of guideline dissemination and implementation strategies. Health Technology Assessment 8(6):1–72

Lichenstein S, Fischoff B 1980 Training for calibration. Organizational Behaviour and Human Performance 26:149–171

National Institute for Health and Clinical Excellence, National Patient Safety Agency NICE/NPSA 2007 Technical patient safety solutions for medicines reconciliation on admission of adults to hospital. Ref NICE/NPSA/2007/PSG001, NICE, London

National Patient Safety Agency 2004 Seven steps to patient safety. National Patient Safety Agency, London

Plous S 1993 The psychology of judgment and decision making. McGraw Hill. New York

Poses R M, Anthony M K 1991 Availability, wishful thinking, and physicians' diagnostic judgments for patients with suspected bacteremia. Medical Decision Making 1:159–168

Reason J 1990 Human error. Cambridge University Press. Cambridge

Sari A B A, Sheldon T A, Cracknell A et al 2007 Sensitivity of routine system for reporting patient safety incidents in an NHS hospital: retrospective patient case note review. British Medical Journal 334:79

Scott T, Mannion R, Marshall M et al 2003 Does organisational culture influence healthcare performance? A review of the evidence. Journal of Health Services Research and Policy 8:105–117

Secretary of State for Health 1998 A first class service: quality in the new NHS. Department of Health, London

Simon H 1992 Decision making and problem solving. In: Zey M (ed) Decision making: alternatives to rational choice models. Sage, Newbury Park, CA, p 3253

Singer S, Meterko M, Baker L et al 2007 Workforce perceptions of hospital safety culture: development and validation of the patient safety climate in healthcare organizations survey. Health Services Research 42:1999–2021

Tversky A, Kahneman D 1974 Judgment under uncertainty: heuristics and biases. Science 185:1124–1131

Wenger E, McDermott R, Snyder W M 2002 Cultivating communities of practice: a guide to managing knowledge. Harvard Business School Press, Boston, MA

Yates J F 1990 Judgment and decision making. Prentice Hall, Englewood Cliffs, NJ

Diagnosis for nurses

Carl Thompson and Dawn Dowding

9

CHAPTER CONTENTS

KEY ISSUES

- The principles of evidence-based diagnosis
- What is meant by diagnostic testing and why we use tests
- What to look for in a test:
  - What is meant by sensitivity, specificity, likelihood ratio, predictive value and how to use this information
  - How to interpret an ROC curve
- How to put diagnostic thinking into practice

EVIDENCE-BASED DIAGNOSIS

Diagnosis means using a patient's clinical history, physical examination, laboratory test results, imaging studies, and other tests to identify the disease or condition responsible for the patient's complaint or current state. If we know the causes of a condition and can give it an accurate label, we can make informed decisions about treatment or intervention and give patients more accurate information on their prognosis. More generally, it involves answering the question, 'what is going on here?'

Clinicians (indeed, all human beings) use a variety of mechanisms for making diagnostic judgements (Sackett et al 1991):

We would like to acknowledge the explanatory power of Tom Sensky, Professor of Psychological Medicine at Imperial College. London.

- *Algorithmic*: using flowcharts and algorithms to guide decision making. An example of an explicit algorithm would be the use of the Ottawa Ankle Rules to decide if a patient requires a diagnostic X-ray for a suspected fractured ankle. Often, though, such rules are internalised in the form of 'if–then' rules. These take the form of, '*if* pattern X *then* classify as Y'. An example of this kind of reasoning is, '*If* cloudy urine *and* positive urinalysis *and* painful micturition *then* consider urinary tract infection'.
- *Pattern recognition*: 'instant recognition' of a disease. A 55-year-old male patient comes into A&E complaining of chest pain on exertion relieved by sitting down and resting. Most nurses would place heart disease high on a list of possible causes.
- *Exhaustive*: gathering every possible piece of data before trying to make sense of it. An example here would be the comprehensive, but somewhat mechanistic, clinical examination, medical, and social histories gathered by junior doctors and inexperienced nurses. There is often little attempt to make sense of information during the data collection and the analysis of patterns, signs, and symptoms comes after the examination and history.
- *Hypothetico-deductive*: generating and rejecting hypotheses on the basis of data collected and the balance of probabilities.

Each approach has something to offer *in particular clinical contexts*. For example, algorithmic approaches are useful for conditions in which the information we collect from patients is discrete and accurate, such as the role of blood counts in diagnosing anaemia.

Pattern recognition is commonly used by clinicians for the diagnosis of common conditions such as urinary tract infection (UTI) or diabetes, and is a very efficient style of diagnosis.

The exhaustive approach is appropriate for unusual presentations of illness when the other modes of decision making have failed. It is commonly used by nurse consultants, specialists, and doctors in tertiary care, where patients have already received a basic assessment. The exhaustive approach is generally inappropriate and inefficient in primary care settings where initial evaluations have to be undertaken in limited timeframes.

Finally, the hypothetico-deductive style involves: (1) proposing a differential diagnosis (from a list of what might be wrong with the patient); (2) asking questions of the data available or applying a diagnostic test; (3) using the results to refine the differential diagnosis; (4) applying other tests; and (5) further refining the differential, and so on until a final working diagnosis is obtained. It is generally held up as the 'gold standard' in terms of approaches to clinical diagnosis. It is comparatively rare.

For each of these styles of diagnosis, it is important to use the information that we gather from patients accurately. This means understanding how much each symptom, sign, or test result increases or decreases the likelihood of a given disease; a process known as, 'revising the probability of disease'. Unfortunately, this is something that human beings aren't very good at (Hammond et al 1967).

Before we look at diagnostic information in more detail, try to answer the clinical problem in Box 9.1. If you cannot work it out don't worry, just go with your intuition.

Box 9.1 Test results and probabilities

You are a primary-care nurse practitioner. You have a 45-year-old woman in for a smoking-cessation clinic appointment and she tells you that she has had a mammogram last week. She also tells you that the radiologist said something about 'suspicious for malignancy'. The patient asks you: 'Does this mean I have cancer?', and you (correctly) answer 'No, the doctors have to do more tests.' Your – very sensible – patient then asks, 'OK, I understand the mammogram isn't the final answer, but given *what we know now*, what are the chances that I have breast cancer?' Assume that the overall risk of breast cancer in any 45-year-old woman, regardless of mammogram result, is 1%. Assume also that mammography is 90% sensitive and 95% specific.

What is the answer? (see the end of the chapter for the correct answer)
1% 15% 60% 85% 95%

Were you surprised by the answer? Don't beat yourself up if you got it wrong, most people do. It is important, however, that you learn to get it right, because diagnosis is associated with instigating treatment, and treatments carry risks of harm as well as benefits. If you incorrectly believe that a patient's chances of a given disease are higher than they really are, then your chances of exposing that person to potentially harmful treatments are also higher than they need be. This chapter is about learning how to handle information like this in clinical practice.

So, how can we make our use of diagnostic test results (even basic ones like signs and symptoms) more rational and accurate? The answer lies in understanding that tests and information are not perfect predictors of underlying diseases or conditions. Concepts such as sensitivity, specificity, predictive value, and likelihood ratios highlight the limitations and strengths of information. Being able to apply them to making choices is a key part of being a good clinician.

DIAGNOSIS AS PROBABILITY REVISION

We can classify what we know or believe about a patient before we have applied any diagnostic tests as a 'prior' probability; prior in this sense means before (prior to) any testing. This could – and in fact should – be made up of knowledge of the prevalence of a disease in particular groups of patients and your (quantified) subjective opinion of the likelihood of the various diseases you are considering. What we know after we have tested for various possibilities, or just gathered more clinical data, is known as our 'posterior' probability.

There is a normative rule for revising your opinions; it is called Bayes' rule [after the reverend Thomas Bayes (1702–1761) the amateur mathematician and polymath who formulated it]. Simply stated, Bayes' rule is:

Posterior odds = Prior odds × Likelihood ratio

In even simpler form, we can express it as:

Your belief after gathering evidence
= Your belief before you gathered evidence
× The strength of the evidence you are faced with.

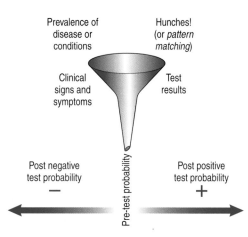

Figure 9.1 Diagnosis as probability revision.

This chapter focuses on the idea of diagnosis as probability revision, as this is an 'evidence-based' means of making a diagnosis (remember, the theorem states that the decision is a function of your beliefs *and* the strength of the evidence).

Before looking at ways of incorporating Bayesian reasoning into our diagnostic decisions using simple mathematical and other tools, let us stick with the idea that for diagnostic thinking to operate you need some basic information. What kinds of information are you likely to need? First, we need to know something about the patients themselves (clinical data to work with). Second, we need to know how common (or not) the diseases or conditions we are considering are in *similar kinds of patients*. Finally, we need to know something about the accuracy of the 'tests' that we are using to check our hunches and to provide more data with which to work (Figure 9.1).

COLLECTING DATA: THE CLINICAL EXAM AND HISTORY TAKING

The first data often collected by the nurse seeking to diagnose a patient's condition are generated from history taking and clinical examination. These two elements of the diagnostic process are very important and far more powerful than many people assume. As an example, consider that you are a sister on a coronary care unit. You have one bed available and the medical wards would like to admit two patients to the unit because the staff nurses involved are concerned about them. It is 3 a.m. and there are no doctors around. Patient 1 is a 60-year-old man who has come through A&E with a history of chest pain on exertion that passes after around 5–15 minutes. Patient 2 is a 30-year-old woman with non-anginal chest pain. You can obviously gather more information, but for now where does your hunch lead you? If you said the 30-year-old woman you might be surprised to learn that the man has a 94% chance of coronary stenosis and the woman only a 1% chance (Sackett et al 1991). The fact that you are in a coronary care unit matters; the higher prevalence of coronary stenosis on a

Box 9.2   The clinical examination (and a clinical example)

1. CHIEF COMPLAINT

Why is the patient seeking our help (e.g. frequency of urination and smelly urine)?

2. HISTORY OF PRESENT ILLNESS

Description of symptoms: what are they? When did they start? Where are they located (e.g. urine smells 'fishy', slightly painful on voiding, not feeling 'fully empty')?

3. PAST MEDICAL HISTORY

Previous illness, operations, mediations, and allergies. This includes over-the-counter medications and herbal or complementary medicines. (e.g. takes St John's wort for 'depression', type 2 diabetes, no allergies or operations, frequently uncontrolled blood glucose levels).

4. FAMILY AND SOCIAL HISTORY

Hereditary illness, habits and activities, diet, etc. This includes factors such as IV or recreational drug use, homelessness, poor diet or absence of any medical knowledge of family (e.g. lives with parents, relatively poor diet – mainly 'chips' and soft drinks – no significant family history).

5. REVIEW OF SYMPTOMS

Review of all the possible symptoms relating to all bodily systems. (e.g. night sweating for a week, has lost a kilo over the past week).

6. PHYSICAL EXAMINATION

This is an attempt to gauge whether there are any objective signs of disease. Physical examination usually helps to confirm or deny the physician's suspicions based on the history (e.g. examination normal and no loin pain or suprapubic discomfort).

coronary care unit affects your evaluation of the information with which you are faced.

There are six elements to the history and clinical examination (Box 9.2).

GENERATING IDEAS (HYPOTHESES) ABOUT WHAT'S WRONG AND DIFFERENTIAL DIAGNOSES

The history and clinical examination generates hypotheses about what's wrong with the patient. Some causes will be more likely than others. The aim at this stage is to order this list accurately. An accurate list will be one that, at this stage, reflects the probability of a given disease in similar patients to yours. As you have not yet done any 'testing' of your ideas about what's wrong with the patient, you are still at the prior probability stage.

Let us take the example of a 27-year-old man presenting to a primary-care nurse practitioner with a severe, rapid-onset headache (he describes it as 'I wanted to pull my hair out') and mild neck stiffness while performing press-ups at the gym. His neurological examination is fine but the symptoms are still present 2 hours after they began. This could be a migraine (common, with around 17% of the population suffering them at any one time) or a tension headache (even more common, with around 38% prevalence), or it could be indicative of some underlying serious, but far less common, cause such as a subarachnoid haemorrhage. How worried should you be that this is something more serious than a migraine? Would you refer to a doctor? Or put him straight into the practice's neuroimaging protocol? What would be your pretest probability for subarachnoid haemorrhage?

The fact that the man has a very severe headache with a rapid onset (known as a thunderclap headache) means that in this case he has a pre-test probability of 43% of having a subarachnoid haemorrhage (Detsky et al 2006); enough for most nurses to decide that he needs to see a doctor urgently.

What about another example? A 38-year-old woman presents complaining of 'pulsating', one-sided headaches lasting around 8 hours each time, they are 'crippling' and she needs to sleep to relieve them. She experiences no visual auras and her neurological exam is normal. Is this a migraine or something more serious? In this case a simple mnemonic (POUNDing) can help and provides us with some very useful information. POUNDing stands for headaches that are:

Pulsating
Duration of 4–72 hours
Unilateral
Nausea
Disabling.

A person with four or more of these features is 24 times more likely to be having a migraine than someone with less than four (Detsky et al 2006). In the absence of any other clinical features to suggest any underlying pathology, you could safely assume that this woman's characteristics were indicative of migraine and treat accordingly.

When working up a list of differential diagnoses, it is useful to think systematically. You will remember from Chapter 7 why selective recall of information is such a problem when you think unsystematically. We have already come across one mnemonic (POUNDing) but another that helps organise our ideas is VINDICATE (Box 9.3).

Box 9.3 VINDICATE: a useful mnemonic for organising ideas about disease for a list of differential diagnoses

V	vascular
I	inflammatory and/or infectious
N	neoplastic and/or neurological or psychiatric
D	degenerative and/or dietary
I	intoxication and/or idiopathic and/or iatrogenic
C	congenital
A	allergic and/or autoimmune
T	trauma
E	endocrine and metabolic

Table 9.1 'Rough and ready' pre-test probabilities and their interpretation			
Pre-test probability		Action	Interpretation
Low	< 1%	Off the list (for now)	Rare disease but rare presentation
	1%	Cannot exclude, but very unlikely (effectively ruled out)	Rare disease but common presentation
	10%	Should be ruled out	Common disease but rare presentation
	25%	Possible	
Moderate	50%	50–50: it's a toss-up	
	75%	Probable	
High	90%	Very likely	Common disease and common presentation
	99%	Almost certain: ruled in	
	99.9%	Pathognomic: no other disease presents in this way, It is a unique presentation of the disease and so the patient can only have this disease	

When you have created a list of differential diagnoses, assign each of the diseases or conditions on the list a pre-test probability. Table 9.1 provides a list of rough pretest probabilities to use, their qualitative expressions of likelihood, and some recommended courses of action.

WHAT DO WE MEAN BY A DIAGNOSTIC 'TEST'?

Tests come in all shapes and sizes in healthcare, and not all tests are expensive or involve exotic laboratory equipment. For example, when taken together, the following three questions constitute a 'test' known as the Ottawa Ankle Rules. The test is for ruling in the need for an ankle X-ray in the A&E department:

- Is the patient unable to bear weight immediately and in the Emergency Room?
- Is the ankle tender on the lateral malleolar tip or posterior aspect of lateral malleolus?
- Is the ankle tender on the medial malleolar tip or posterior aspect of medial malleolus?

A positive answer to any of the three questions means that an X ray is warranted. Expressed alternatively, the probability that the foot is broken is high enough to warrant further (harmful) investigation. For more details on the application of the Ottawa Ankle Rules see: www.gp-training.net/rheum/ottawa.htm

Similarly, the questions in Box 9.4, when taken together, constitute a 'test' for alcoholism (Bush et al 1987).

There are other tests for alcoholism (some more elaborate, detailed, and/or invasive) but the question we need to know the answer to is: do they make a worthwhile difference to our estimated probabilities of alcoholism (see www.emedicine.com/med/topic98.htm for more tests)?

Box 9.4 The CAGE alcohol screening test

Have you ever felt the need to	**C** ut down on drinking?
Have you ever felt	**A** nnoyed by criticism of your drinking?
Have you ever had	**G** uilty feelings about your drinking?
Have you ever taken a morning	**E** ye opener?

Reasons for testing

There are four reasons why we might want to carry out a diagnostic test on a patient. First, to establish what's wrong in a patient with clinical signs and symptoms. For example, a culture and sensitivity test in a urine sample from an otherwise fit young woman with urine that is cloudy, smelly, and discolored, and who is suffering mild abdominal pain. Second, screening for disease in people who are asymptomatic; for example, looking for prostate-specific antigen in healthy men to screen for prostate cancer, or screening for depression in the adult population. Third, diagnostic tests can be used to provide prognostic information on people with established disease. For example, the viral load diagnostic test in people with HIV infection provides an indicator of the risks of opportunistic infection. Finally, diagnostic tests also help in some cases when monitoring existing interventions, therapy or treatments. For example, examining the prothrombin times of patients undergoing treatment with warfarin helps to monitor anticoagulation and helps to prevent too high or too low a level.

Is a test useful or not: a rough guide

It is vital that we know something about the usefulness of a test. For a diagnostic test to be clinically useful it should be able to correctly identify (rule in) and exclude (rule out) cases, the results should be interpretable and you must actually be able to apply the test with patients. Pearl (1999) suggests six criteria (Table 9.2) for a useful test. The more criteria are met, the more useful the test. This is not an exhaustive or particularly technical critical appraisal list; for a fuller treatise, visit the excellent website: www.cebm.utoronto.ca/practise/ca/diagnosis/

USING TEST PROPERTIES AND RESULTS IN DECISION MAKING

Two decision rules for using tests

Use a test only when that test:

1. *Is valid in the setting to which it is to be applied*: by valid we mean positive or negative results will *truly* be positive or negative, and it will help correctly identify those people with and without the condition.
2. *Will change the probability of the condition, leading to a change of clinical strategy*: if the results will not affect what you do, do not apply the test.

Table 9.2 Six key questions to ask of diagnostic tests	
Criterion	*Questions*
Technical aspects of the test – is it easy to perform? Are the results reliable?	*Reliable and precise?* Does the paper or the test suggest whether the results would be the same if repeated on the same individual under the same conditions? Even 'objective' tests, such as X-rays or analysis of tissue samples, involve some subjective interpretation and risk reductions in reliability and precision *Accurate?* Does the test produce the same results as the gold standard and a standardised specimen? *Operator dependency?* Does the test need specialist skills or expertise to deploy it accurately? *Feasibility and acceptability?* Is the test easy to employ or does it require specialist or expensive machinery? Expensive tests that no one can afford are not good *Cross-reactivity?* Will commonly occurring substances in the body or environment cause false results? A classic example is the eating of poppy-seed bread before a drugs urine test *Inter- and intra-observer reliability?* Do the results of clinicians over time and between each other correlate on the same patients? How do they demonstrate this?
Diagnostic accuracy	*Validity?* Does the test discriminate between those with and those without the condition? Does it have good criterion validity (i.e. does it correlate well with other tests for the same condition?) *Gold/reference standard?* Was the test compared to a gold standard? If so, how good a standard is it?
Diagnostic thinking	Will the results of the test make any difference to your probability of the patient having the condition? If not then don't do it?
Therapeutic thinking	Will the results make any difference to your management of the person with the condition? If not, then why bother?
Patient outcomes?	Will the test results make the patient feel, or actually be, better?
Societal outcomes?	Is the test good for society? Sometimes cheap tests applied excessively can be expensive at a societal level. A good example would be routine prostate screening via prostate-specific antigen, when the (very risky and expensive) treatments might not be worth the positive results

So far, we have established that the prevalence of a disease or condition, coupled with a patient's examination and history, lead to a rough idea of the likelihood of the diseases that you are considering: the *prior probability*. After doing a test, we revise our ideas of the likelihood of a given condition or disease in order to arrive at a *post-test* or *posterior probability*.

THE RESULTS OF TESTS

There are two kinds of test result: dichotomous (yes/no; positive/negative), such as X-rays, and continuous, where there are more than two possible values [such as glycosylated haemoglobin (HbAc1) measurements]. However, when test results are continuous they are often transformed into dichotomous results by virtue of the fact that clinicians set thresholds or *cut-off points* where results above or below these are classed as normal or abnormal, positive or negative (more on thresholds in a bit). How can we use the properties and results of a test in our decision making? We are going to look at five ways of making sense of what we know about a given test and the data it generates in the form of results.

Technique 1: natural frequencies

Most of us find graphical representations of decision problems easier to handle than raw numbers and percentages. Here is one way of representing diagnostic information visually:

You are a school nurse. The prevalence of urinary tract infection (UTI) among children at your school is 4%; the test you are using is 75% (0.75) sensitive and 93% (0.93) specific. If someone tests positive, what are the chances of that person having a UTI? The natural frequencies method can help you visualise what this might mean.

Start by imagining 100 typical children. Some of these children will have a UTI and some will not. The child you are worried about is one of these 100 children (Figure 9.2).

The next stage is to visualise the sensitivity associated with the test (Figure 9.3).

Like sensitivity, we need to visualise what the specificity of the test might mean for our 100 children (Figure 9.4).

Sensitivity tells us the chances of the test being positive given that the patient has a particular condition. This is *not* the same as the chances that a patient has a condition or disease given that he or she has tested positive. It is this latter probability that is of most use to us.

Although sensitivity tells us something about the test when we know that a patient has a condition, the whole point of diagnosis is that we do not know whether a patient actually has a condition. The limitations of sensitivity for clinical decision making are down to a central tenet of Bayes' theorem: that the probability of A given B does not equal the probability of B given A (written as $PA \mid B \neq PB \mid A$).

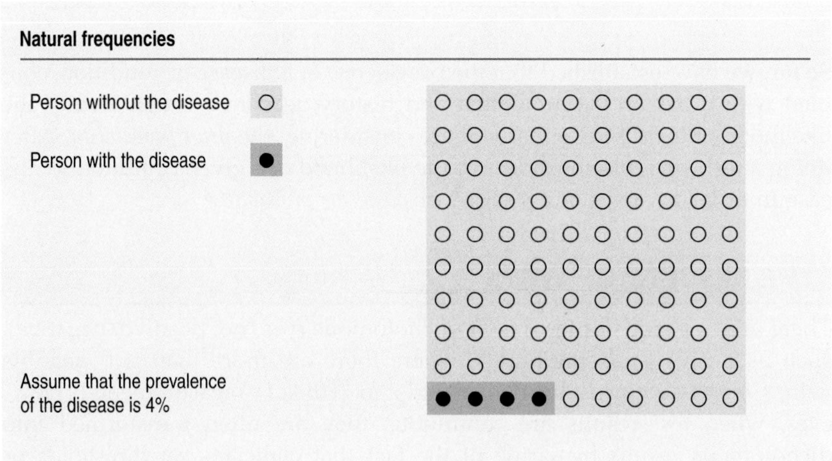

Natural frequencies

Person without the disease ○

Person with the disease ●

Assume that the prevalence of the disease is 4%

Figure 9.2 Natural frequencies stage 1.

Sensitivity

Person without the disease	○
Person with the disease	●
Person who tests positive	▨
Person who tests negative	▨
True positive on the test	●
False positive on the test	○
True negative on the test	○
False negative on the test	●

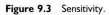

- SENSITIVITY is the proportion of people with the disease correctly identified by the test
- It measures the proportion of false NEGATIVES
- In this case 3 people out of the 4 who test positive actually have the condition so sensitivity = $^3/_4$ or 75%

Figure 9.3 Sensitivity.

Specificity

Person without the disease	○
Person with the disease	●
Person who tests positive	▨
Person who tests negative	▨
True positive on the test	●
False positive on the test	○
True negative on the test	○
False negative on the test	●

- SPECIFICITY is the proportion of people without the disease correctly identified by the test
- It measures the proportion of false POSITIVES
- In this case 7 of the 96 people who don't have the disease also test positive. Specificity = (96–7)/96 = 93%

Figure 9.4 Specificity.

You can test this for yourself. Imagine the possibility that all bank robbers (call them set A) are men (call them set B). Is this the same as saying that all men are bank robbers? These kinds of cognitive misunderstanding have serious health implications. For example, during the reduction in measles, mumps, and rubella (MMR) vaccinations that followed the supposed link between autism and the triple vaccine, it was clear that many parents (and quite a few health professionals) failed to recognise that the probability of developing autism given that your child was vaccinated (virtually nil) was not the same as the probability of being vaccinated given that you had autism (quite high as nearly all children – whether autistic or not – had been vaccinated). The more clinically useful measure of the strength of a test is the positive predictive value (PPV).

The PPV tells us the *chances of having a disease given a positive test result*; which – after all – is what we want to know. Looking at our frequency grid again (Figure 9.5), we can see that a total of ten people tested positive, of which three actually had the disease. The PPV then is 3/10 or 30%.

Conversely, we can ask what the chances are of the patient not having the disease given that he or she has tested negative. This is the negative predictive value or NPV. In the frequency grid (Figure 9.6) you can see that of a total of 90 people who tested negative, one had the disease (was a false negative) and that 89 didn't have the disease. The NPV then is 89/90 or 99%.

Technique 2: Gigerenzer and the frequency tree

People are generally pretty bad at handling ratios and percentages when making decisions. Gigerenzer (2002) argues that one way of combating these flaws is to present problems with real numbers (integers like 1, 2, 3, etc.) rather than percentages. Let us try this with our UTI example again.

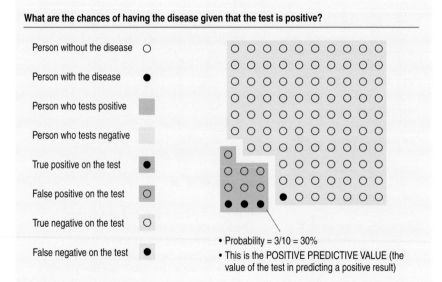

What are the chances of having the disease given that the test is positive?

Person without the disease ○

Person with the disease ●

Person who tests positive ▨

Person who tests negative ▨

True positive on the test ●

False positive on the test ○

True negative on the test ○

False negative on the test ●

- Probability = 3/10 = 30%
- This is the POSITIVE PREDICTIVE VALUE (the value of the test in predicting a positive result)

Figure 9.5 Positive predictive value.

What are the chances of not having the disease given that the test is negative?

Person without the disease	○
Person with the disease	●
Person who tests positive	▨
Person who tests negative	▨
True positive on the test	●
False positive on the test	○
True negative on the test	○
False negative on the test	●

- Probability = 89/90 = 99%
- This is the NEGATIVE PREDICTIVE VALUE (the value of the test in predicting a negative result)

Figure 9.6 Negative predictive value.

Once again, assume a prevalence of 4% of UTIs in our population. Because whole numbers are easiest to work with, let's again express this as 4 patients out of 100 people at risk of a UTI.

First, use the sensitivity and specificity information (sensitivity = 75%, or 0.75; specificity = 93%, or 0.93). Of the 4 people likely to have the disease (our pretest probability of 4%) the test will most likely identify 3 correctly (4 × 0.75). Our test's specificity was 93%, meaning that of the 96 people without the UTI, the test will correctly identify 89 (96 × 0.93) people as not having a UTI (Figure 9.7).

So, of 100 people, 10 are likely to test positive but only 3 are truly positive (Figure 9.8).

So, as before, the positive predictive value is 30% (3/(3 + 7)), meaning a 30% chance that someone testing positive on our urine test has the disease. Remember that our prior probability (before the test) was only 4%, so it has gone up quite a lot.

Among the 96 people without the disease, 7 will test positive

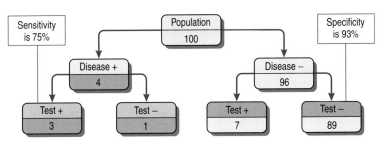

Figure 9.7 Sensitivity and specificity with real numbers.

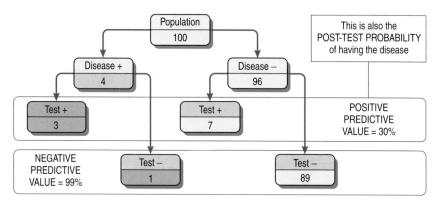

Figure 9.8 Positive and negative predictive values using real numbers.

What if the patient was negative on the urine test? Let us stick with a prior probability of 4%. Of the 90 (1 + 89) patients who were tested as negative, only 1 has a false result (i.e. has the UTI when we thought he or she did not) and so the negative predictive value is 89/(1 + 89) = 99%.

What happens to this 'real-world' probability (i.e. the probability of a disease *given* a positive test) when the prevalence increases or decreases? Let us reduce the prevalence from 'reasonably common' (4 in every 100 patients) to a 'bit rarer' (4 in every 1000 patients). We can see from Figure 9.8 that the sensitivity and specificity remain the same (75% – or the test still spots 3 of the 4 disease-positive patients and 93% of those who are disease negative). But the positive and negative predictive values are now radically different. Of the 73 patients who test positive, only 3 are truly positive. So the PPV of the test when the prevalence (our pretest probability) is lower is now only 4% (rather than the 30% it was when the prevalence was 4 in every 100 patients). The negative predictive value is still pretty high (926/1 + 926) at 0.99 or 99% (Figure 9.9).

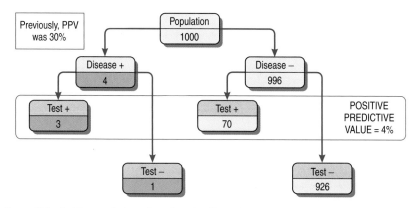

Figure 9.9 Positive predictive value when the disease is rarer.

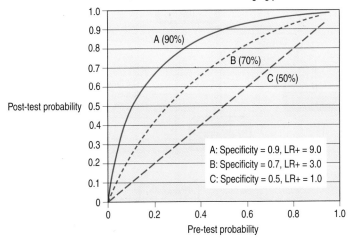

Figure 9.10 Changing test performance as pre-test probability changes.

It is important to realise that even the best (most specific) test, when applied to diagnostic situations in which the condition being considered is very rare, yields high numbers of false-positive results. The PPV of specific tests for rare events is low. The impact of low prevalence on the negative predictive value is far lower, however. Figure 9.10 highlights the changing performance of useful (high-specificity) and less useful (low-specificity) tests at various levels of pretest probability.

Thus far, we have dealt with concepts of sensitivity and specificity. An alternative approach is to use the notion of likelihood alongside our frequency tree (Figure 9.11).

The relationships between the likelihood of positive results given that you have the disease and the likelihood of a positive test given that you don't have the disease can be expressed as a ratio: called the likelihood ratio (LR+) (again, see Figure 9.10). A likelihood ratio of 1.0 indicates a test that gives us no information for clinical decision making. This occurs when sensitivity and specificity are both 50%; or just as likely to generate false positives and negatives as true positives and negatives. The higher the likelihood ratio, the better the test (all other factors being equal).

Bayes revisited and the likelihood ratio

Remember Bayes' theorem? (post-test odds = prior odds × likelihood ratio)? We can now use the likelihood ratio to complete this equation. However, to work with Bayes' formula we need to work with probability expressed as odds. Odds are just another way of expressing probability (with slightly different mathematical properties). Odds are the ratio of chances of an event (or disease) to chances against an event (or disease). Probability, however, is the chance of an event or disease divided by the total number of chances of a given disease.

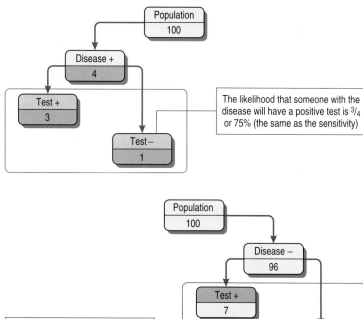

Likelihood ratio

Likelihood of positive
test given the disease
─────────────────────
Likelihood of positive test
in the absence of the disease

$$= \frac{\text{Sensitivity}}{1 - \text{specificity}} = \frac{0.75}{0.07} = 10.7$$

Figure 9.11   Likelihood and the likelihood ratio.

This time, let us assume a prevalence of 10% of UTIs (this is artificially high but makes the maths easier) and a likelihood ratio for our test of 10.7. Box 9.5 outlines how we would calculate the PPV using likelihood ratios and odds.

The principle and process for the likelihood ratio for a negative test (or LR−) is the same. This time let us assume that the LR− for our urine test is 0.61 and prevalence 10% again. Post-test odds = 0.11 × 0.61 = 0.067. So our post-test $P = 0.067/1.067 = 0.063$ or 6%. Our probability of having a UTI has gone from 10% to 6%. This is the false reassurance rate (FRR). It is the number that tells us how many children (6 out of 100) we would falsely tell to 'not worry'. 1 − FRR is the negative predicted value, which in this case is 0.94 or 94%, or 94% of children testing negative are in fact free of UTI. So, likelihood ratios give an indication of how much to revise your probability by for positive and negative test results. But what is a good likelihood ratio?

> **Box 9.5 Converting probabilities to odds and odds to probabilities**
>
> 1. Convert probability (P) to odds: pretest $P = 0.1$. So pretest odds $= 0.1/(1 - 0.1)$ $= 011$.
> 2. Apply Bayes: multiply the pretest odds by the likelihood ratio for a positive test. In our case, the likelihood ratio is 10.7 (which is good) and so the test is a powerful one if positive. So: $0.11 \times 10.7 = 1.17$.
> 3. Convert odds back to probability: post-test $P = $ odds/(1 + odds) $= 1.17/2.17 =$ 0.53 or 53%.
> 4. Interpret the result: the post-test probability is 53%. So, a positive urine test means our probability has leapt from 4% to 53% – quite a jump (*Note*: most tests are not this good!)

Table 9.3 Likelihood ratio (LR) values and the strength of tests

Strength of test	LR+	LR−
Excellent	10	0.1
Very good	6	0.2
Fair	2	0.5
Don't bother	1	1

Table 9.3 gives qualitative expressions of how 'strong' various likelihood ratios are.

Technique 3: the 2 × 2 table

First, let us introduce one of the most useful concepts in decision making: the 2 × 2 table (Figure 9.12). Think of a diagnostic test and the possible relationships between the states of the patient and the test results. There are four possible conditions:

1. The patient can test positive and truly have the disease (a true positive or cell A in the table).
2. The patient can test positive and not have the disease (a false positive or cell B in the table).
3. You could test negative but in truth actually have the disease (a false negative or cell C in the table).
4. You could test negative and in truth not have the disease (a true negative or cell D in the table).

We can represent these possibilities as a 2 × 2 table (Figure 9.12 and Figure 9.13). The 2 × 2 table in Figure 9.12 allows us systematically to represent these possible outcomes. Again, work with an easy-to-think-of sample of 100 people. To calculate the sensitivity, look at cells A and C (the column of those who actually have the disease). For specificity, look at the disease absent column (cells B and D).

Just as with the frequency-tree approach, we can work out the pre- and post-test odds for positive and negative tests.

	Have the disease	Do not have the disease
Test positive	**A**	**B**
Test negative	**C**	**D**

(A)

Sensitivity

	Disease		
	Yes	No	Total
Test Yes	a b	7	10 $a + b$
No	c d 1	89	90 $c + d$
Total	96 $a + c$	100 $b + d$	$a + b + c + d$

False negatives

(B)

Specificity

	Disease		
	Yes	No	Total
Test Yes	3 a b	7	10 $a + b$
No	c d 1		90 $c + d$
Total	4 $a + c$	$b + d$	100 $a + b + c + d$

False positives

(C)

Figure 9.12 The 2 × 2 table – sensitivity and specificity. (A) Key. (B) Sensitivity. The proportion of people with the diagnosis ($n = 4$) who are correctly identified ($n = 3$), sensitivity = a/(a + c) = 3/4 = 75%. (C) Specificity. The proportion of people without the diagnosis ($n = 96$) who are correctly identified ($n = 89$), specificity = d/(b + d) = 89/96 = 93%.

Technique 4: the receiver operating curve

The receiver operating curve (ROC) is a graphical way of representing the performance of a test. By examining the area under the curve we can learn something about the test's performance. The area under the curve (AUC) is a function of plotting sensitivity (the true positive rate) against the false positive rate (1 − specificity). The greater the AUC value, the stronger the performance (high sensitivity and low false-positive rate). As with our frequencies grid in technique 1, sometimes it is easier to visualise the area under the curve in order to understand the concept.

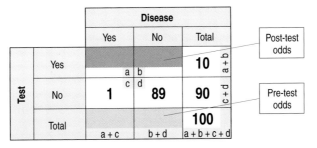

Figure 9.13 Pre- and post-test odds with 2 × 2 table. In the sample as a whole, the odds of having the disease are 4 to 96 or 4% (the pre-test odds). In those who score positive on the test, the odds of having the disease are 3/7 or 43% (the post-test odds). In those who score negative on the test, the odds of having the disease are 1/89 or approximately 1%.

Figure 9.14 illustrates what the area under a curve will look like for a perfect test (there isn't one) and a useless test (there are a surprising number). Note the area under the curve of 0.8. How best can we interpret this figure? Consider (hypothetically) two patients drawn randomly from the DISEASE+ and DISEASE− groups, respectively. If the test is used to guess which patient is from the DISEASE+ group, and the area under the ROC curve is 0.8, then it will be right 80% of the time.

Receiver operating curves (like positive predictive values) change their shape and area as a function of the pre-test probabilities in the setting to which the test is to be applied. If you don't believe me, look at the curves for a dementia screening tool (Flicker et al 1997) in Figure 9.15. One of the curves was generated applying the tool in the community (ACAT, lower prevalence) and one from being put to work in a memory clinic (MC, higher prevalence). Again, the message here is think about where the tests you are using come from and where they are going to be applied.

ROC curves might look complicated but the best way to get to grips with using them is to try plotting one. Table 9.4 gives some data associated with the CAGE questionnaire again. Follow the activity in Box 9.6 to plot on ROC curve.

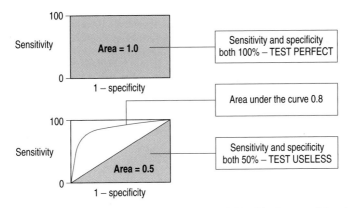

Figure 9.14 The area under a receiver operating curve (ROC) will be between 0.5 and 1.0.

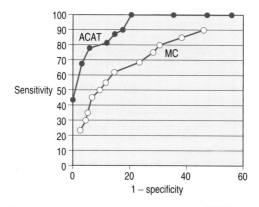

Figure 9.15 Changing areas under a receiver operating curve (ROC) because of differing pre-test probabilities (prevalence). This study compared the performance of a dementia-screening test in a community sample (ACAT) and a memory clinic sample (MC).

Table 9.4	CAGE sensitivity and specificity table			
Number of 'Yes' answers	Alcoholic (events/cell total)	Non-alcoholic (events/cell total)	Sensitivity: true-positive ratio	1-specificity: false-positive ratio
> 3	56/294	56/527		
> 2	130/294	516/527		
> 1	216/294	482/527		
> 0	261/294	428/527		

Box 9.6   Activity: plot a receiver operating curve

- Photocopy Figure 9.16.
- Work out the sensitivity (true-positive ratio) for each row in Table 9.4.
- Work out 1 − specificity (false-positive ratio) for each row in Table 9.4.
- Plot the curve on the graph (you might want to print it out; the 'chance' diagonal has been drawn on for you, as have the 'good' and 'excellent' curves). *Note:* ROC curves always start at 0,0 and end at 1,1.
- What do you think? The CAGE has an AUC of around 0.89 (divide-up the graph into squares and count the number under the curves if you need confirmation).
- How often does this mean that a randomly selected alcoholic will have a higher CAGE score than a randomly selected non-alcoholic?

(The answers to these questions appear at the end of this chapter.)

Technique 5: the quick and user-friendly approach – the nomogram

We have saved probably the easiest way to make use of Bayes' theorem in diagnostic decision making until the end. The Bayes nomogram (Figure 9.17) can be used to work out the post-test probability of our child with a possible UTI given a positive test. The process is very simple and involves next to no mathematics (Page & Attia 2003).

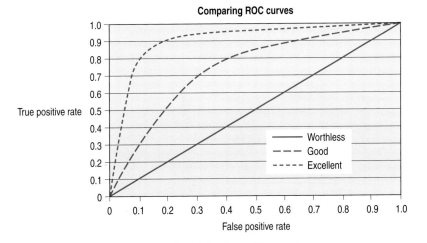

Figure 9.16 Receiver operating curve (ROC) for the CAGE example.

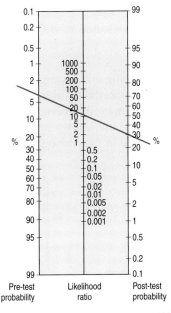

Figure 9.17 Bayes nomogram (reproduced from Page & Attia 2003, © BMJ Publishing Group Ltd, with permission).

1. Find the pretest probability (lets stick with our 4% prevalence).
2. Find the likelihood ratio of 10.7 (say 10 or 11).
3. Connect the points and continue the line until it crosses the post-test probability line.
4. Read the post-test probability of that line (in this case it is around 30%).

In clinical practice, there is usually a degree of 'uncertainty about our uncertainty'. For example, you might not know the exact prevalence of a condition (a very common scenario). Let us say, for example, that we are 95% sure that

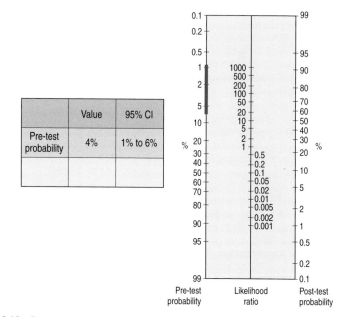

	Value	95% CI
Pre-test probability	4%	1% to 6%

Figure 9.18 Bayes nomogram sensitivity analysis (for range of prevalence).

the prevalence of UTIs in our population is somewhere between 1% and 6%. With the nomogram, incorporating this information into our reasoning is easy.

Figure 9.18 represents our uncertainty about the prior probability with a range rather than a single estimate. However, it is quite likely that we are uncertain about the strength of the test we are using. Again, we can represent our uncertainty as a range in the nomogram. Figure 9.19 demonstrates

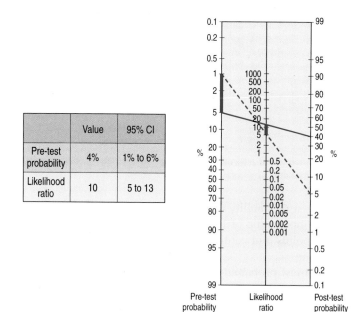

	Value	95% CI
Pre-test probability	4%	1% to 6%
Likelihood ratio	10	5 to 13

Figure 9.19 Bayes nomogram and uncertainty about the strength of a test.

that we are 95% sure that the likelihood ratio for the urine test we are using is between 5 and 13. We can represent this as a vertical line in the likelihood ratio column. By drawing lines that pass through the upper and lower ranges of the likelihood ratio estimate it is clear that our post-test probability is somewhere between 5% and 40%; considerable uncertainty and probably not enough to instigate treatment in this case. We might want to undertake further testing with a new pre-test probability of between 5% and 40% as our starting point.

PUTTING DIAGNOSTIC THINKING INTO PRACTICE

Diagnostic thinking is at the cutting edge of nursing roles and service developments. Nurses are rarely formally taught diagnostic reasoning or receive practice or mentorship in clinical environments. This chapter has tried to introduce some of the key techniques and ideas for thinking about the uncertainties that you will encounter as a nurse – that is, as someone faced with diagnostic uncertainty and the need to appropriately revise their ideas about, 'what is wrong here?'

If you have the time and the inclination, you could try and do the calculations and techniques here for yourself with real patients and tests and in real time. In truth, though, such thinking is unlikely. However, diagnostic thinking and probability revision is one area in which information technology can make life much easier. Visit www.cebm.utoronto.ca/practise/ca/statscal/ and download it onto your PDA/PALM. These kinds of calculator require little or no statistical or mathematical expertise; all you need to do is be able to understand the meaning of the numbers.

What if you don't have a PDA to hand and time is limited? As well as needing to think about numbers and probability, there are some decision rules you should apply. Moreover, these rely on no mathematical prowess whatsoever:

1. If the pre-test probability (your strength of belief) of a condition is high and the test is positive then you should intervene or treat.
2. If the pre-test probability is low (you are really sceptical) and the test is negative then you should not treat.
3. If you are faced with a high pre-test probability and a negative test then test again (use a different test). If the second test is positive then you need to investigate further as a kind of tie-break. The process is the same in the face of a low pre-test probability and a positive first test.

ANSWERS

The answer to the mammogram question in Box 9.1 is 15%. Using the frequency-tree method, the positive predictive value is $9/(9 + 49) = 0.15$ or 15%.

The answer to the ROC question in Box 9.6 is you would expect a randomly selected alcoholic to have a higher CAGE score than a randomly selected non-alcoholic 89% of the time.

RESOURCES AND FURTHER READING

The people at Bandolier have produced an excellent (detailed) essay on diagnostics, evidence and bias at: www.jr2.ox.ac.uk/bandolier/Extraforbando/Diagnostic.pdf

The diagnosis collections at the evidence-based journals (BMJ publishing) provide accessible and concise summaries of the value of various tests for diagnosing conditions. For example: www.ebm.bmjjournals.com/cgi/collection/diagnosis

The Centre for Evidence-based Medicine at Toronto has produced an excellent mental health scenario, completed worksheet, and CATs (critically appraised topics) for evidence-based nursing: www.cebm.utoronto.ca/syllabi/nur/diagnosis/

EXERCISE

You are a practice nurse/nurse practitioner working in primary care. It is winter and the surgery is full of people sniffling and coughing and looking miserable! Consider the following data on the likelihood ratios (positive and negative) for common symptoms. Some of your patients are young (less than 30 years) and some are older (greater than 65 years). You know that the prevalence of influenza is lower in younger people (7%) and that it much higher in older people (40%). What is the post-test probability (*hint*: don't forget to convert post-test odds to post-test probabilities) for:

1. a young patient with a cough
2. an older patient with a cough
3. a young patient with a cough and fever
4. an old patient with a cough and fever

Test	Positive likelihood ratio	Negative likelihood ratio
Fever (37.8–38.5°C)	1.8	0.40
Cough	1.1	0.42
Myalgia	0.93	1.2
Headache	1.0	0.75
Sore throat	1.0	0.96
Sneezing	1.2	0.87
Nasal congestion	1.1	0.49
(Adapted from Call et al 2005)		

Bush B, Shaw S, Cleary P et al 1987 Screening for alcohol abuse using the CAGE questionnaire. American Journal of Medical Science 82:231–235

Call S A, Vollenweider M A, Hornung C A et al 2005 Does this patient have influenza? Journal of the American Medical Association 293:987–997

Detsky M E, McDonald D R, Baerlocher M O et al 2006 Does this patient with headache have a migraine or need neuroimaging? Journal of the American Medical Association 296:1274–1283

Flicker L, Loguidice D, Carlin J B et al 1997 The predictive value of dementia screening instruments in clinical populations. International Journal of Geriatric Psychiatry 12:203–209

Gigerenzer G 2002 Reckoning with risk: learning to live with uncertainty. Penguin, London

Hammond K R, Kelly K J, Schneider R J 1967 Clinical inference in nursing: revising judgments. Nursing Research 16:38–45

Page J, Attia J 2003 Using Bayes' nomogram to help interpret odds ratios. Evidence-Based Medicine 8:132–134

Pearl W S 1999 Hierarchy of outcomes approach to test assessment. Annals of Emergency Medicine 33:77–84

Sackett D, Haynes B, Guyatt G et al 1991 Clinical epidemiology: a basic science for clinical medicine, 2nd edn. Little, Brown and Company, London

Diagnosis for nurses

Prognosis in nursing

Dawn Dowding and Carl Thompson

KEY ISSUES

- What is prognosis?
- The difference between prognostic and risk factors
- Ways in which prognosis is described
- The nature of prognostic decisions
- The role of clinical prediction rules in helping reduce prognostic uncertainty

WHAT IS PROGNOSIS?

As nurses, we have to think about the (uncertain) future all the time in practice. Yet, prognosis – predicting what will happen to a patient, either with or without treatment – is an often-overlooked area of decision making in nursing. As nurse educators, we were not introduced to prognostic thinking until well into our careers and the need to use evidence to inform our prognostic decisions came even later. Prognosis has been defined as:

" The effects of a disease or condition over time and the estimated chance of recovery or ongoing associated morbidity, given a set of variables, which are called prognostic factors or prognostic indicators. (Fineout-Overholt & Melnyk 2008)"

Estimates of a patient's prognosis often inform our decision making. For instance, in a recent study of decision making by British heart-failure specialist nurses (HSFNs), one of the choices reported by HFSNs was deciding whether a patient with heart failure had reached a point where referral to palliative care services was warranted. This decision was based (in part) on a nurse's assessment of the patient's prognosis: the nurse had to judge how much longer the patient was likely to live (Thompson et al 2008). The interventions and treatments that we recommend to patients often draw on our estimate of their prognosis with or without that treatment. In addition, patients will often want to know what is likely to happen to them with or without treatment, so that they can decide what to do. Prognosis is an important and inescapable element of nursing practice.

PROGNOSTIC AND RISK FACTORS

A patient's prognosis is affected by variables known as 'prognostic factors'. Prognostic factors predict which patients are likely to do better or worse over time. These are different to risk factors, which are patient characteristics associated with the likelihood of a patient developing a disease in the first place. For example, a family history of heart disease is a *risk* factor for having a myocardial infarction (MI). Having had an MI, the likelihood that an individual dies in the 7 years following the MI will depend on medical, psychosocial and behavioural factors, such as whether a person is depressed, has a stable partnership, and smokes (Pfiffner & Hoffmann 2004); these are known as *prognostic* factors.

It is important to distinguish between risk factors and prognostic factors. Nurses often provide patients with advice on how to adjust their behaviour and lifestyle to reduce their chances of developing ill health on the basis of risk factors. As a practice nurse, you might be advising patients to reduce weight or stop smoking because this reduces their risk of developing diseases such as diabetes or heart disease. You therefore need to understand both the risk factors for certain diseases and an individual person's risk. This is different to counselling a patient who has developed type 2 diabetes about the management of the condition. In this instance, a factor such as obesity was previously a risk factor for the development of the disease. Once a person has developed type 2 diabetes, however, obesity becomes a prognostic factor that can greatly influence long-term survival. Your role will include trying to ensure that the patient keeps his or her blood sugar levels within a certain range using diet (and possibly medication) and helping him or her to make lifestyle modifications to reduce weight in order to reduce the risk of developing long-term complications from their diabetes (i.e. improving their prognosis). This set of judgement and decision challenges requires knowledge of their likely course of the patient's disease with well-controlled blood sugars and a healthier weight, compared with uncontrolled blood sugar and a less healthy weight. Crucially, you also need some way of communicating these differences to the patient.

DESCRIBING PROGNOSIS

Prognosis is closely related to the concept of risk, and so most of the terms used to describe risk are also used in the description of prognosis. For the purposes of this chapter, we will define risk as, 'the likelihood or chance of a specified event occurring'. We can describe risk and/or prognosis in a number of different ways. These include measures such as absolute and relative risk and odds ratios. Prognosis is also often demonstrated using graphical representation in the form of 'survival curves' (see: www.graphpad.com/www/Book/survive.htm).

In its simplest form, the risk of an outcome occurring after a period of time can be described in terms of a percentage. For example, in a systematic review of the effectiveness of exercise-based cardiac rehabilitation in patients with coronary heart disease, the risk of a patient who had received rehabilitation dying within the follow-up period (15 months) was 7.6%, compared with 9.2% for patients who had not received exercise-based cardiac rehabilitation (Taylor et al 2004).

Another way of expressing these figures would be as an *absolute risk*, which is the arithmetic difference in the rates of the outcome between the experimental (people who received exercise-based rehabilitation) and control (those who did not get any rehabilitation) groups (Sackett et al 2000). In this instance, the absolute risk associated with receiving exercise-based cardiac rehabilitation is:

$$9.2 - 7.6 = 1.6\%$$

That is, a 1.6 lower risk with rehabilitation than without it. The results of a study are also often reported in terms of *relative risk*, which is a proportional measure of the reduction or increase in the rate of outcomes between the experimental and control groups in a trial (Sackett et al 2000). For the Taylor et al (2004) study, we would work out the relative risk associated with the potential benefits of exercise-based cardiac rehabilitation as:

$$9.2 - 7.6/9.6 = 17.4\%$$

As you can see from the above two figures, the way in which you calculate the effectiveness of an intervention will impact on the figure that you get; 17.4% makes the intervention (exercise-based cardiac rehabilitation) look much more effective than 1.6%. The way in which we describe the risks and benefits of different interventions to patients is described further in Chapter 14.

You can also see the chances of an individual developing a disease or condition (when exposed to a certain risk or preventative factor), or their prognosis (when exposed to a prognostic factor) expressed in 'odds' – sometimes in the form of an odds ratio. As we saw in Chapter 3, odds are the ratio of the chance of an outcome occurring in one group compared with the chance of it not happening in another group. If you are considering the effectiveness of cardiac rehabilitation in heart-failure patients, for instance, it would be the odds of heart-failure patients receiving cardiac rehabilitation dying relative to the odds of a heart-failure patient not receiving cardiac rehabilitation dying. Taylor et al (2004) report the odds ratio in this instance to be 0.80 [95% confidence interval (CI) 0.68–0.93]. This can be interpreted as the odds of dying as a heart-failure patient if you receive cardiac rehabilitation being 0.8 compared with those not receiving rehabilitation. An odds ratio of 1 indicates no difference between two groups. In this example, odds below 1 indicate a positive effect of the intervention (less chance of you dying) and above 1 a negative effect (more chance of you dying).

You will find information about prognosis and prognostic factors reported as measures of risk or odds over a specified time period. What these figures cannot provide you with, however, is any idea of the disease trajectory. For instance, you might have a patient who has had an MI who wants to discuss with you the benefits of following an exercise-based cardiac rehabilitation programme. On the basis of the data from the systematic review by Taylor et al (2004), you could tell him that, after 15 months, approximately 8% of patients who receive rehabilitation will have died compared with the 10% who did not receive rehabilitation. He may then ask you if his chances of surviving over time change at all. So, although he might consider his risk of dying to be relatively high immediately after his MI, will that change after 15 months? The use of absolute or relative risk measures will not enable you to answer this type of question. For this reason, information about prognosis is often represented graphically as a 'survival curve'. A survival curve is a graph of the number of events you are interested in over time (or alternatively, the chance of being free of these events over time) (Sackett et al 2000). To construct a survival curve, you need discrete events (such as death, recurrent MI, stroke) and you need to know precisely when those events occurred (Sackett et al 2000).

An example of a survival curve is given in Figure 10.1. Along the bottom of the curve (the *x*-axis) is the time after the start of patients being monitored in years (so, for instance, the number of years after their first MI). The vertical part of the graph (the *y*-axis) gives the proportion or percentage of patients who are alive (survival) at each point in time. In this example, after 1 year, 75% of patients are still alive. When interpreting a survival curve, you should look at the *x*-axis (time) as this could be given in years, months, or days. Also, the vertical (*y*-axis) might be reporting a number of different types of event, such as death, recurrence of a disease, number of patients who are disease free, which will alter your interpretation of the results (Dunn 2004).

The *shape* of a survival curve also provides information. Look at the four different survival curves in Figure 10.2. Each of the curves provides a different picture of a patient's potential prognosis. Curve A shows that over a period of 6 years there is a decrease in the number of patients who are alive. However, after 6 years the curve flattens, which suggests that if a patient is still alive after 6 years he or she is likely to remain disease free for the condition represented in the curve. Curve B also flattens after 6 years, but in this instance the drop in the curve is steeper than that in curve A. Therefore, your chances of being alive after 6 years in curve B are around 10%, compared with the 75% expressed in curve A. Both curves A and B show that if you are alive after 6 years you are likely to remain that way (until, of course, you die at a grand – but natural – old age).

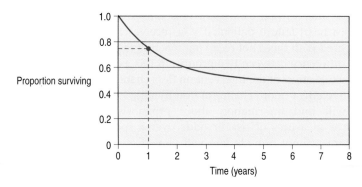

Figure 10.1 A simple survival curve.

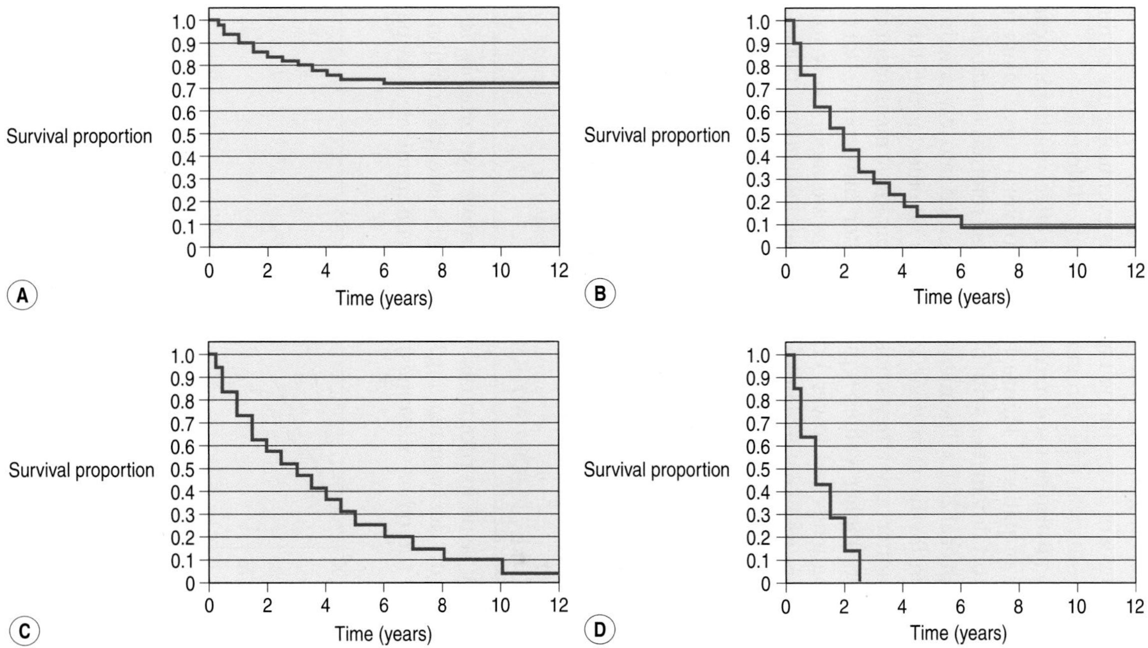

Figure 10.2 Different types of survival curve. (A) The likelihood of survival after 6 years is 75% before curve flattens. (B) The likelihood of survival after 6 years is 10% before curve flattens. (C) The consistent drop in survival over 12 years. (D) An acute drop in survival: after 3 years, all the individuals with the condition are dead.

Curves C and D represent patient conditions in which, after a period of time, there are no survivors (the graph drops to 0). Again, the picture of survival portrayed in the two graphs is very different. In curve C there is a consistent drop in the number of patients surviving, so that after 3 years about 50% of patients are alive; after 12 years all the patients have died. By contrast, the condition represented by graph D shows a worse prognosis for patients compared with graph C, with over 50% dying after 1 year, and all dead in less than 3 years. Even though all patients eventually die of the condition, the relative survival time (prognosis) is very different.

Survival curves can also be used to compare the effect of prognostic factors in different groups of patients. Figure 10.3 is a survival curve taken from a study examining mortality in men with heart disease referred for cardiac rehabilitation (Kavanagh et al 2002). The men were classified into low-, medium- or high-risk groups on the basis of their Vo_2(peak), whether or not they were on digoxin, and whether or not they smoked. Vo_2(peak) is a measure of cardiorespiratory function; higher values represent better cardiorespiratory function. Higher-risk patients had lower Vo_2 scores, were more likely to be on digoxin, and were more likely to smoke (Kavanagh et al 2002). The survival curve indicates the proportion of men surviving in each group over a period of 15 years. What is interesting to note on this graph is the influence of time on survival; after 5 years there are few prognostic differences between the three groups (although the low-risk group does have a higher chance of survival). However, after 15 years it is clear that the men in the high-risk group have a significantly higher chance of dying than men in the low-risk group.

PROGNOSTIC DECISION MAKING

For nurses, the key issue in prognosis is how can we use prognostic information to assist with decision making? Although some information about potential survival (or other outcomes) can be communicated to patients

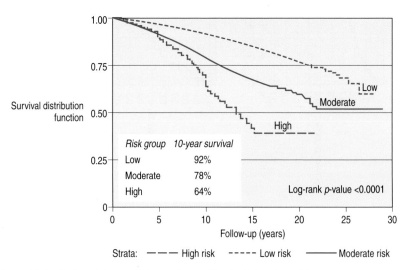

Figure 10.3 Kaplan–Meier survival curve for cardiac death based on risk score group (reproduced from Kavanagh et al 2002, with permission WoltersKluwer Health).

by discussing absolute or relative risks (see Chapter 14 for further discussion of this issue), this type of information often fails to provide the whole picture to patients. Using survival curves as a way of exploring a patient's prognosis might be more beneficial; you can discuss with a patient what the likely disease trajectory might be (is it a disease which has a high initial mortality rate that then plateaus, or are the chances of dying relative stable over a period of time?). Patients might also find it useful to see that not everyone will die (or suffer another alternative outcome). For instance, the survival curve might illustrate that after 10 years 75% of patients are still alive.

Often, prognostic information is used as the basis for clinical prediction rules or decision rules, defined as:

" A clinical tool that quantifies the individual contributions that various components of the history, physical examination and basic laboratory results make toward the diagnosis, prognosis or likely response to treatment in an individual patient. (McGinn et al 2002) "

Clinical prediction rules are used to help clinicians decide on future clinical events (McGinn et al 2002). These provide information in the form of a probability or likelihood ratio of an event occurring. An example of a prognostic decision rule is given in a paper by Haukoos et al (2004), who examined the factors most likely to predict both 'survival to hospital discharge' and normal neurological function or moderate impairment following an out-of-hospital cardiac arrest. The study suggests that patients who have a cardiac arrest that is witnessed, and who are under 78 years of age, are more likely to be discharged from hospital and have a Glasgow Coma Score of more than 13 than patients who do not fulfil these criteria. The chances are 5% (95% CI 3–8) compared with 0% (95% CI 0–0.9). This decision rule needs to be validated in a different population to ensure that it is robust (McGinn et al 2002). However, with this information, if you were faced with a family whose relative had just had an out-of-hospital cardiac arrest that had been witnessed and who was under the age of 78, you would be able to use the rule to provide a more accurate evaluation of their relative's prognosis, or at the very least would be more aware of it yourself.

SUMMARY

Prognostic decisions tend to be overlooked when we examine how nurses make decisions; although patients often want answers to questions that are prognostic in nature. Providing patients with such information is often difficult because of a lack of data and omnipresent uncertainty and unpredictability. To help make decisions about the potential benefits of interventions, you need to have an understanding of how we can use and interpret information about patients' survival or disease trajectory, at the same time being aware of the often wide-ranging uncertainty surrounding that information. Using graphical illustrations of prognosis, such as survival curves or clinical prediction rules (if they exist), can be helpful to both nurses and patients as a way of assisting with decision making in this area.

EXERCISES

As a group of individuals, go to the website www.qrisk.org/ and work out your risk of heart disease or stroke given your own risk factors. Discuss your scores with the group (assuming you feel happy to do so).

Have a look at the prospective cohort study that underpins the QRisk tool: www.bmj.com/cgi/content/full/bmj.39261.471806.55v1.

Read Ellen Fineout-Overholt & Bernadette Melnyk's (2004) article. How does the QRisk study stack up in terms of its validity, results and applicability?

REFERENCES

Dunn S 2004 Survival curves: the basics. Cancer Guide Statistics

Fineout-Overholt E, Melnyk B 2004 Evaluation of studies of prognosis. Evidence-Based Nursing 7:4–8

Fineout-Overholt E, Melnyk B 2008 Evaluation of studies of prognosis. In: Cullum N, Ciliska D, Haynes R B et al (eds) Evidence-based nursing: an introduction. Blackwell Publishing, Oxford, p 168–178

Haukoos J, Lewis R, Niemann J 2004 Prediction rules for estimating neurologic outcome following out-of-hospital cardiac arrest. Resuscitation 63:145–155

Kavanagh T, Mertens D, Hamm L et al 2002 Prediction of long-term prognosis in 12,169 men referred for cardiac rehabilitation. Circulation 106:666–671

McGinn T, Guyatt G, Wyer P et al 2002 Clinical prediction rules. In: Guyatt G, Rennie D (eds) Users' guide to the medical literature: a manual for evidence-based clinical practice. AMA Press, Chicago, p 471–483

Pfiffner D, Hoffmann A 2004 Psychosocial predictors of death for low-risk patients after a first myocardial infarction. Journal of Cardiopulmonary Rehabilitation 24:87–93

Sackett D, Straus S, Richardson W et al 2000 Evidence-based medicine. How to teach and practice EBM, 2nd edn. Churchill Livingstone, Edinburgh

Taylor R, Brown A, Ebrahim S et al 2004 Exercise-based rehabilitation for patients with coronary heart disease: systematic review and meta-analysis of randomised controlled trials. Americal Journal of Medicine 116:682–692

Thompson C, Spilsbury K, Dowding D et al 2008 Do heart failure specialist nurses think differently when faced with hard or easy decisions: a judgement analysis. Journal of Clinical Nursing 17:2174–2184

Evidence-based decisions: the role of decision analysis

Dawn Dowding and Carl Thompson

CHAPTER CONTENTS

KEY ISSUES

- What is a decision analysis?
- How to undertake a decision analysis:
  - structuring a question
  - designing a decision tree
  - extracting probabilities
  - gathering utilities
  - combining information on probability and utility in the process of 'rolling back' a decision tree
- The strengths and weaknesses of decision analysis

INTRODUCTION

The components of an evidence-based decision include the results of research, a patient's values or preferences for particular choices, an awareness of available resources, and the experience and expertise of the decision maker (DiCenso et al 1998). Having made it this far in the text, you will have grasped that making evidence-based decisions in practice can sometimes be difficult; requiring the use of complex, often incomplete information, and with uncertain decision outcomes (Hunink et al 2001, Tavakoli et al 2000). Paying attention to and integrating the volume of information in practice can often seem overwhelming. Nurses, like all human beings, have limited capacity to manage all of the different components of a complex decision at the same time (Hunink et al 2001, Sarasin 2001). Decision analysis is one approach that can help systematically combine the elements required for an evidence-based decision.

WHAT IS DECISION ANALYSIS?

Decision analysis is based on the normative expected utility theory (EUT; see Chapters 2 and 5; Elwyn et al 2001, Tavakoli et al 2000, Thornton 1996). Decision analysis is used prescriptively as a way of assisting decision makers with their choices. Underpinning the process is the assumption that humans are rational, logical decision makers. A rational decision, in the context of decision analysis, is one that results in the outcome with the greatest usefulness to the individual (Elwyn et al 2001).

Carrying out a decision analysis involves breaking a decision problem down into its component parts. For decision analysis, these component parts are the probability of different outcomes occurring and the value or preference an individual attaches to those outcomes. Synthesising the value of these component parts guides you toward the 'best' decision option (Dowie 1993, Tavakoli et al 2000) given your goal to maximise the decision maker's utility (more on utility in a moment). Breaking the decision problem down in this way provides an explicit and transparent map of how a decision has been taken:

" Decision analysis is a systematic, explicit, quantitative way of making decisions in healthcare that can ... lead to both enhanced communication about clinical controversies and better decisions. (Hunink et al 2001 p 3) "

Decision analysis is not a suitable tool to be used for all decision situations. It is, however, a technique particularly suited to *complex* decision situations: those choices in which the 'best' option is not readily available. Complexity can be due to different options carrying different risks or benefits, or because how a patient views different outcomes is particularly important.

THE STAGES IN A DECISION ANALYSIS

The stages involved in carrying out a full decision analysis are outlined in Box 11.1.

Structuring the decision

The first thing that you need to do when planning or managing patient care, is to outline the decision problem you are faced with; a process known as *structuring* the decision problem. Structuring a decision involves translating an ill-defined problem into a set of well-defined elements (von Winterfeldt 1980). As a starting point, take the clinical scenario described in Box 11.2.

Box 11.1   Stages in carrying out a decision analysis

- Define the decision problem
- Structure the decision: construct a decision tree
- Assess the probability of different outcomes: add probability to the decision tree
- Measure patient utility: add utility to the decision tree
- Calculate the 'expected value' of a decision tree: identify the 'best' option
- Assess the sensitivity of the decision model

Box 11.2 Clinical scenario

You are a practice nurse who runs a women's health clinic. You provide advice to women on a variety of different health issues, including women who are experiencing menopausal symptoms. In your clinic this morning, you see a 51-year-old woman who is experiencing considerable distress from a number of menopausal symptoms. You discuss at some length with the woman the potential choices available to her to aid the symptoms, including taking hormone replacement therapy (HRT), non-HRT therapies, and doing nothing. There are associated risks and benefits with all of the different choices that she has open to her, and no particular option seems to be the most appropriate.

In this instance, you are faced with an uncertain and complex decision situation. The woman has a number of choices available to her. You are aware that there are risks and benefits associated with those decision choices and need to help the woman make a decision about what to do.

Balance sheets

One strategy to help define the decision problem is to list all the different options or actions you can think of that the woman could choose, and consider the possible benefits and risks of each choice; an approach known as constructing a 'balance sheet' (Hunink et al 2001).

Identifying the options for a particular decision can be made easier by examining the research literature. Using the '5S' approach to looking for evidence, the first place we might look are decision support systems (Haynes 2006). Systems such as NHS Clinical knowledge summaries (CKS) (http://CKS.library.nhs.uk/home) and Clinical Evidence (www.clinicalevidence.com), which provide evidence-based guidance on interventions, also illustrate common management options for conditions. In this instance, both Clinical Evidence and CKS provide guidance on the management of menopausal symptoms. The options available to the woman are: (1) do nothing or receive/provide lifestyle advice; (2) taking hormone replacement therapy (HRT); (3) non-hormonal alternatives to HRT. Clinical evidence also gives details on the benefits and risks of the different interventions. You could use this information to construct a balance sheet like the one in Table 11.1.

Decision trees

Another way of structuring the decision is to represent the choices in the form of a 'decision tree', which provides the structure for a decision analysis. A decision tree represents both the decision options you have available to you (represented in a tree as a square node between branches) and the uncertainty associated with each decision option (represented in a tree as a circular node) (Dowie 1993). When structuring a decision problem in the form of a tree, the model needs to be complex enough to represent all the important events that might happen to an individual, whilst simple enough

Table 11.1 Balance sheet for menopausal decision

Intervention	Benefit	Harm
Provide lifestyle advice	Might be sufficient to help manage hot flushes and anxiety symptoms	None from intervention itself. Long-term consequences of the menopause: increased risk of osteoporosis, urogenital atrophy, cardiovascular disease, stroke
Hormone replacement therapy (provision of oestrogen with a progestogen in women with a uterus)	Relief of menopausal symptoms; hot flushes, night sweats, urogenital atrophy Decreased risk of osteoporosis Decreased risk of colorectal cancer	Increased risk of breast cancer Increased risk of stroke Increased risk of venous thromboembolism
Non-hormonal alternatives that contain phytoestrogens (e.g. soy foods)	May reduce symptoms such as hot flushes	None known

to be understandable (Detsky et al 1997). The decision tree will always be a simplified model of the actual decision situation, but should still incorporate the risks and benefits associated with the decision you are faced with (Detsky et al 1997). Figure 11.1 shows the information in the balance sheet of Table 11.1 as a decision tree.

The structure of the tree reflects the key elements of the decision problem: the choices available to the woman and the risks and benefits of each option. To simplify the model, only the most important potential benefits and risks of different interventions have been included: relief of menopausal symptoms, decreased risk of osteoporosis, and increased risk of breast cancer. If we modelled all of the potential risks/benefits for each option, then the model might better reflect the decision situation but might not be so understandable.

The importance (to the person making the choice) of the different elements in a decision will determine the shape of the tree. For some decisions, just identifying the different options available, and their associated benefits and risks, might provide enough of a structure to make a decision on the best option for this particular individual.

Assessing the probability of different outcomes

An important dimension of any decision is the likelihood that events you would like to see happen actually happen. Rejecting a decision option on the basis that there is a one in a million chance of an outcome occurring might not be that rational, but we can only judge the adequacy of a choice if we make such information explicit.

Having structured the decision problem and identified the *potential* benefits and risks associated with each option, we need to consider in detail how

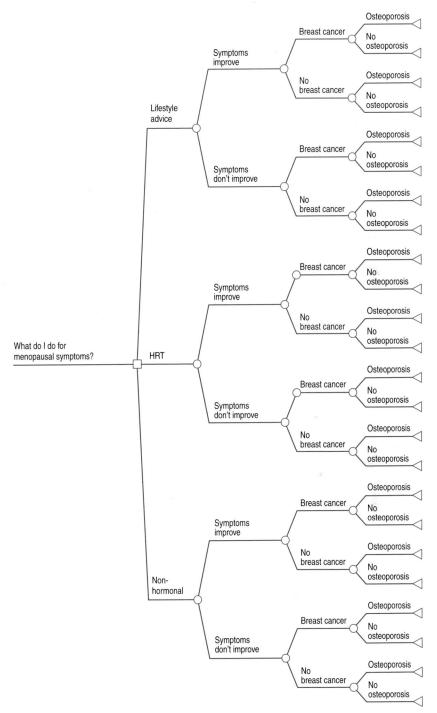

Evidence-based decisions: the role of decision analysis

Figure 11.1 Structure of a decision tree.

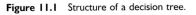

likely those outcomes are to occur. As decision analysis is commonly associated with decisions to intervene or treat, then the data needed to estimate such probabilities should come from good quality research evidence. The best kinds of research design to provide unbiased treatment or intervention probabilities are well conducted randomised controlled trials (RCTs) or – preferably – meta-analyses of good-quality RCTs (Richardson & Detsky 1995a, 1995b). Whereas research-based estimates are preferable to experience for ascertaining probabilities, even experience expressed explicitly in the form of a numeric estimate is preferable to keeping such estimates implicit and hidden from patients and colleagues when making choices.

Using research evidence

For each potential outcome within your decision problem, we need the probability of that outcome occurring for your patient or patient group, together with an estimate of the uncertainty surrounding this probability. The less confidence you have in your estimate of probability (i.e. the greater the uncertainty), the wider the range of your estimate of uncertainty should be (Naglie et al 1997).

To find these probabilities, we conduct a search for research evidence (see Chapter 4). As with any evidence-based decision, any evidence we find needs to be appraised critically. If, following our search, we find one study that is better in terms of its methodological quality than the other retrieved studies (it might be a good-quality systematic review/meta-analysis as opposed to a single, small trial), then this can be used to provide our probability estimates. If we find several relevant studies, then we need to assess them for methodological quality, eliminate those of poor quality, and use the average of the results of the remaining studies to estimate our values (Naglie et al 1997).

Study results can be reported as dichotomous or continuous measures. For the purpose of basic decision analysis, you need an estimate of how likely an outcome is to occur *or* not occur. This dichotomous outcome can be expressed as a probability, percentage or fraction (see Chapter 3). Sometimes, papers give raw figures for the number of participants who experienced an outcome. In this case, you can calculate the probability yourself.

However, studies sometimes report outcomes as continuous measures (i.e. the mean decrease in pain as measured on a pain score). Results presented in this way provide the overall effect of an intervention (e.g. giving pain relief decreased mean pain scores compared to control), but do not tell you the number/percentage of individuals experiencing the outcome (i.e. it doesn't whether 40% or 60% of the subjects in the intervention group had improved pain). This is the information we need to estimate the likelihood of an event occurring within a decision model.

One way to convert continuous probability data into a format you can use in a decision model is to use 'mean effect sizes' (Tickle-Degnen 2001). The effect size (*d*) is the difference between mean outcomes for two conditions in *standard deviation units*. An effect size that is reported in standard deviation units can be used to calculate the proportion of individuals for whom an intervention succeeded or failed (Tickle-Degnen 2001). We will

Table 11.2 Effect sizes and success rates

Magnitude of effect	d	Success rates			r	Success rates		
		Control (%)	Intervention (%)	Change (%)		Control (%)	Intervention (%)	Change (%)
Zero	0	50	50	0	0	50	50	0
Small	0.20	46	54	8	0.10	45	55	10
Medium	0.50	40	60	20	0.24	38	62	24
Large	0.80	34	66	32	0.37	32	69	37
Very large	2.00	16	84	68	0.71	15	86	71

From Tickle-Degnen 2001, copyright ©. Reprinted by Permission of SAGE Publications, Inc. All calculations and estimations are based on the assumption of a binomial distribution of the outcome measure, with approximately equal number of cases and approximately equal variances within each condition. All rates here are success rates. To calculate failure rates, subtract any success rate from 100%.

not discuss how to calculate mean effect sizes (for an outline and Excel spreadsheet, see: www.cemcentre.org/renderpage.asp?linkID=30325015) and Table 11.2.

What if there is no evidence?

You will not always be able to find research studies that provide you with probabilities for the outcomes you are interested in. Despite this, a decision still needs to be made (Hunink et al 2001). The most common solution is to ask an expert or experts in the clinical area to provide estimates of the likelihood of different outcomes. As highlighted in Chapter 8, expert estimates based on experience can be subject to bias and a lack of consensus (Naglie et al 1997). Because of this, it is important to ensure that your estimates of the range of uncertainty around the expert-derived probabilities reflect this uncertainty. Reflecting this uncertainty might involve using the range of estimates provided, or creating your own personal 'confidence intervals' around the estimates.

Adding probabilities into the decision model

Having identified the likelihood of different outcomes occurring, together with an estimate of the uncertainty around this figure, you need to add it to your decision model. Sometimes it helps to list all of the possible outcomes that may occur within the decision situation together with your probability estimates and their source in a table. An example of this for the menopause decision is given in Table 11.3. The probability estimates in this table were identified from CKS or from references in Clinical Evidence. We have assumed that the woman will be considering using HRT that contains both oestrogen and progestogen (combined HRT therapy) as she still has a uterus. All the data are given for a 5-year period. The likelihood of developing osteoporosis is measured by the likelihood of having a fractured

Table 11.3 Probability table for menopausal decision

Outcome	Probability estimate	Range
Symptoms improve with lifestyle advice*	0.55	0.2–0.705
Symptoms improve with HRT	0.86	0.706–0.96
Symptoms improve with non-hormonal treatment	0.43	Not known
Risk of developing breast cancer over 5 years with no treatment	0.014	0.013–0.014
Risk of developing breast cancer over 5 years with HRT	0.028	0.028–0.031
Risk of developing breast cancer over 5 years with non-hormonal treatment	0.014	0.013–0.014
Risk of hip fracture (osteoporosis) over 5 years with no treatment	0.0015	0.0005–0.0025
Risk of hip fracture (osteoporosis) over years with HRT	0.0012	0.0002–0.0022
Risk of hip fracture (osteoporosis) over 5 years with non-hormonal treatment	0.0015	0.0005–0.0025

There is no evidence to suggest that using non-hormonal therapies for menopausal symptoms affects either the overall risk of developing breast cancer or osteoporosis, so the incidence rates for women who don't take hormone-replacement therapy (HRT) have been used.
*The values for this outcome were the ones for the placebo group.

neck of femur (which is the most common outcome associated with osteoporotic disease).

Having listed the likelihood or probability of different outcomes occurring in this way, the values can then be added in to the decision tree (Figure 11.2). For each branch in the tree, the probability values should add up to 1. This is because the outcomes are mutually exclusive; meaning that you cannot have more than one outcome for each branch simultaneously. For example, if there is a 25% chance that the menopause will lead to a fractured neck of femur there is a complementary 75% chance that it will not. You cannot have a fractured neck of femur on one leg, and at the same time *not* have one.

Assessing patient values or preference: measuring utility

A key challenge for evidence-based decision makers is incorporating a patient's preferences for different decision options (DiCenso et al 1998) into the decision-making process. In decision analysis, patient values or preferences are explicitly considered in the form of measures of utility. Utility is a numeric or quantitative measure of the value an individual or group place on the different outcomes or consequences of a decision (Richardson & Detsky 1995b). The aim of many decisions in healthcare is to improve an individual's state of health. For this reason, utility might also be referred to as 'health state preference' and reflects how an individual values a given state of health. This is not the same as measures of quality of life, which focus on the characteristics of that health state (Hunink et al 2001).

Utility is measured on an interval scale, from 0 to 1 (or 100). Zero equates to the worst possible health state *for that individual* and 1 or 100 represents the best possible health state *for that individual*. You might find in some publications that 0 is equal to death and 1 or 100 perfect health. The problem

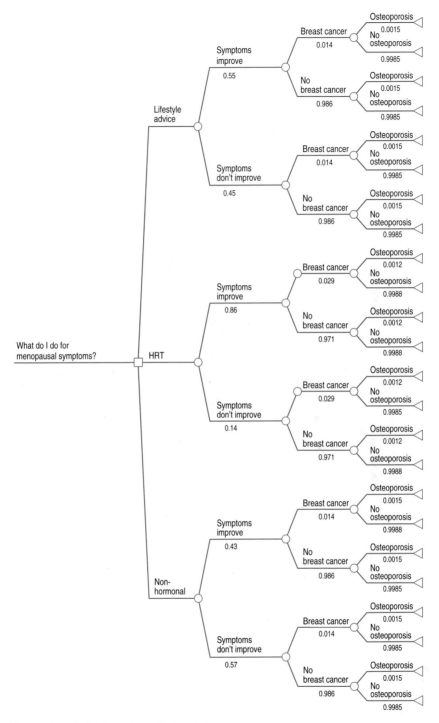

Figure 11.2 Probability values added to decision tree.

with this convention is that it fails to recognise that, *for some individuals*, there are health states that are worse than death *for them*; far *better* to refer to them as 'worst' and 'best' health states (Drummond 1993). Utility can be measured at the individual patient level for individual clinical decisions, or at a population level for societal decisions. This chapter focuses on individual-level decisions between patients and professionals.

Utilities can be estimated in a number of ways:

- Arbitrarily assign a value according your own judgement: this is by far the most common approach in healthcare. For example, statements such as, 'there is no point in discussing compression (therapy) for his leg ulcer as he won't tolerate it' represent an arbitrarily assigned value statement.
- Ask a group of experts to reach a consensus on their estimates of utility.
- Use relevant utility values published in the literature.
- Measure utility values directly using reliable and valid measures (Naglie et al 1997, Sarasin 2001). Methods for measuring utility directly include rating scales, the use of a technique known as the 'standard gamble' and 'time-trade off'.

Rating scales

With a rating scale, an individual is asked to evaluate the utility of different outcomes on a line between 0 and 10 or 100. The scale is anchored with the most preferred health state at one end and the least preferred at the other. The remaining health states are placed on a line between them, reflecting differences in the preferences of the individual (Drummond 1993).

Standard gamble

The standard gamble involves examining an individual's valuation of health states compared with death. The individual is offered two alternatives: a gamble with two possible outcomes (death or return to normal health), or the certain outcome of remaining in the health state being valued for the rest of his or her life. The probability of the outcomes occurring in the gamble is altered until the individual is 'indifferent' (has no clear preference). This state of indifference represents the preference value (Thornton et al 1992).

Time trade-off

In the time trade-off approach the individual is asked to consider the relative amounts of time he or she would be willing to spend in a given health state. For each health state for which you need a utility, the individual is offered a choice: to stay in this health state for the rest of his or her life, or return to perfect health but for a shorter period of time. The amount of time the patient is willing to 'trade' is used to calculate the value for the health state (Drummond 1993).

An example of how the same health state would be elicited from an individual using the different methods is shown in Box 11.3.

Different methods of eliciting utility use different approaches, and produce different values for the *same health state* in the *same individual*

Box 11.3   Examples of utility elicitation using different methods

RATING SCALE

On a scale where 0 represents death and 100 represents excellent health, what number would you say best describes how you would feel about developing breast cancer over the next 5 years (Figure 11.3)?

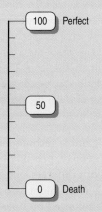

Figure 11.3   Rating scale.

STANDARD GAMBLE

Imagine that you will develop breast cancer over the next 5 years. You are told that there is a new treatment available to you, which has a 50% probability of completely curing you of cancer. However, the treatment also has a 50% probability of causing immediate death. Would you have the treatment (Figure 11.4)?

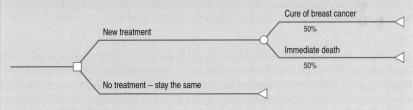

Figure 11.4   Standard gamble.

DEPENDING ON YOUR ANSWER

If your answer was 'No', would you be prepared to have the new treatment if there was a 60% chance of the cure and a 40% chance of death?

If your answer was 'Yes', would you be prepared to have the new treatment if there was a 40% chance of the cure and a 60% chance of death?

Alter the values up or down until the person is at a point where she cannot decide (i.e. both options are equal). The person's utility for having breast cancer is the probability of having a cure for breast cancer. So say, for instance, that the patient would accept the treatment when it had a 90% chance of cure and a 10% chance of death, her utility for breast cancer is 0.9.

Continued

Evidence-based decisions: the role of decision analysis

> ### Box 11.3 Examples of utility elicitation using different methods – cont'd
>
> **TIME TRADE OFF**
>
> Imagine that you have 40 years of life expectancy, living with breast cancer. Now imagine that someone can give you a cure for your cancer but you will only live 20 more years, instead of 40. Would you take the cure?
>
> Depending on the answer, alter the amount of time traded. So if the answer is 'No', would they accept the treatment if it cured them and they lived 39 years? If the answer was 'Yes', would the patient accept the treatment if she lived 10 more years?
>
> Continue until the two options are the same (living with breast cancer or being cured). At this point, the utility for breast cancer would be the ratio of the length of life in perfect health to the length of life in the health state being evaluated.

(Drummond 1993). Standard gamble techniques produce higher values than other methods of utility measurement, possibly because they ask individuals to consider the risks associated with different outcomes when making choices in the gamble (Drummond 1993). They might also be subject to 'framing effects', in which the preferences are influenced by how the information and trade-off is presented. Rating scales, although easy to use, might result in values being distorted as individuals tend to avoid the extremes of the scale (Thornton et al 1992).

You also need to take into account *whose* preferences or values you are considering. Often, studies in healthcare will ask a clinician how they think their patients feel about different health states. Clinician's evaluations and a patient's own views might actually be very different (Brand & Kliger 1999). Wherever possible, the utilities for each of the health states should be elicited from the person who is going to be affected most by the decision. This is not without its problems; often, patients will be asked to evaluate a health state of which they have no personal experience. Alternatively, it could be a 'hypothetical' state that could happen to them in the future; the implications of which for the here-and-now are sometimes difficult to grasp (Hunink et al 2001). Preferences or values attached to health states are not always stable. They vary across time and can alter when an individual actually experiences the health state being valued (Hunink et al 2001).

Using utility measures in a decision tree

For many decision models, the outcomes of a decision will be a combination of different health states. For instance, we could evaluate how a woman feels about taking HRT (i.e. taking a tablet for a period of time), her symptoms improving, developing breast cancer, and having osteoporosis. In these circumstances, utility can be measured as a whole, or in parts, which are then combined to provide an overall evaluation (Naglie et al 1997). If you are estimating utility for different outcomes as a whole, then you would use a utility measure to do this. If you are using a 'decomposed' approach, you would firstly assess the utility of each separate outcome (e.g. utility for symptoms improving, utility for taking a tablet, and utility for developing breast cancer) and then combine them. Naglie et al (1997) suggest that, to combine

Table 11.4 Calculation of utility scores for menopausal decision

Short-term outcomes	Utility value	Disutility
HRT*	0.98	0.02
Non-hormonal therapy*	0.99	0.01
Symptoms improve	I	0
Menopausal symptoms (Brazier et al 2005)	0.81	0.19
Long-term outcomes	Utility value	
Breast cancer	0.8 (CEAR)**	
Fractured hip	0.63 (CEAR)[†]	
Lifestyle branch – outcomes	Utility	
Symptoms improve, breast cancer, fractured hip	$(0.8 \times 0.63) - 0 = 0.504$	
Symptoms improve, breast cancer	$0.8 - 0 = 0.8$	
Symptoms improve, fractured hip	$0.63 - 0 = 0.63$	
Symptoms improve	I	
Symptoms the same, breast cancer, fractured hip	$(0.8 \times 0.63) - 0.19 = 0.314$	
Symptoms the same, breast cancer	$0.8 - 0.19 = 0.61$	
Symptoms the same, fractured hip	$0.63 - 0.19 = 0.44$	
Symptoms the same	0.81	
HRT branch – outcomes	Utility	
Take HRT, symptoms improve, breast cancer, fractured hip	$(0.8 \times 0.63) - (0.02 + 0) = 0.484$	
Take HRT, symptoms improve, breast cancer	$0.8 - (0.02 + 0) = 0.78$	
Take HRT, symptoms improve, fractured hip	$0.63 - (0.02 + 0) = 0.61$	
Take HRT, symptoms improve	0.98	
Take HRT, symptoms the same, breast cancer, fractured hip	$(0.8 \times 0.63) - (0.02 + 0.19) = 0.294$	
Take HRT, symptoms the same, breast cancer	$0.8 - (0.02 + 0.19) = 0.59$	
Take HRT, symptoms the same, fractured hip	$0.63 - (0.02 + 0.19) = 0.42$	
Take HRT, symptoms the same	$I - (0.02 + 0.19) = 0.79$	
Non-hormonal therapy branch – outcomes	Utility	
Take non-hormonal therapy, symptoms improve, breast cancer, fractured hip	$(0.8 \times 0.63) - (0.01 + 0) = 0.494$	
Take non-hormonal therapy, symptoms improve, breast cancer	$0.8 - 0.01 = 0.79$	
Take non-hormonal therapy, symptoms improve, fractured hip	$0.63 - 0.01 = 0.62$	
Take non-hormonal therapy, symptoms improve	0.99	
Take non-hormonal therapy, symptoms the same, breast cancer, fractured hip	$(0.8 \times 0.63) - (0.01 + 0.19) = 0.304$	
Take non-hormonal therapy, symptoms the same, breast cancer	$0.8 - (0.01 + 0.19) = 0.6$	
Take non-hormonal therapy, symptoms the same, fractured hip	$0.63 - (0.01 + 0.19) = 0.43$	
Take non-hormonal therapy, symptoms the same	$I - (0.01 + 0.19) = 0.8$	

*This is 'author judgement' on the assumption that having both will be worse than either by themselves.
**Five studies had examined the utility of breast cancer. Three used time trade-off (TTO) and two used clinician/author judgement to estimate utility. The value given is the mean of the five values.
[†]Nine studies estimated the utility of fractured hip, some after 1 year, others after 2 years. Two studies used standard gamble, one time trade-off, and one a mixture of TTO and rating scales. The other studies were all author judgement. The value given is the mean of the nine values.

utilities, you first need to divide them into short-term and long-term outcomes. You would then convert the utilities of all your short-term outcomes into 'disutility' values, by subtracting them from 1. For each branch of the tree, you would then multiply the utility values of all the long-term states together, before subtracting the disutility values for the short-term states to provide you with your overall utility rating. Finally, you should rank the utility values for each tree branch, to ensure that they make sense.

An example of how to do this is given in Table 11.4, for the possible outcome states for the decision model given in Figure 11.1.

Where possible, the utility values for each individual health state have been taken from the Cost Effectiveness Analysis Registry (CEAR) at the New England Medical Centre (www.research.tufts-nemc.org/cear/default. aspx) and a study estimating the utility of menopausal symptoms (Brazier et al 2005). The CEAR gives the preference scores derived from empirical studies for a number of health states, listed by disease. This is a useful resource to estimate utility measures for health states when eliciting utility measures from individual patients is not possible. We failed to find published utility values associated with taking HRT and non-hormonal therapies, therefore these values are the authors' own estimations.

For each branch of the decision tree in Figure 11.2, we calculated the utility value, using the approach suggested by Naglie et al (1997). For instance, the outcome for the top branch of the tree is not having an intervention, symptoms improving, but over the long term developing breast cancer and osteoporosis. The short-term states in this case are symptom improvement (with a disutility score of 0) and long-term states of breast cancer and fractured hip (with utilities of 0.8 and 0.63 respectively). The overall utility for the outcome of this branch is therefore:

$$(0.8 \times 0.63) - 0 = 0.504$$

Once you have calculated the utility for each outcome in your decision model, you can add the values to your decision tree at the appropriate point. An example of how to do this for the menopausal decision is given in Figure 11.5.

Identifying the 'best' option

When both probabilities and utilities have been added to the decision tree, the 'expected utility', or value of each decision option, needs to be calculated. The eventual value represents both the probability of an outcome occurring and the value/utility the decision maker attaches to that outcome. If you are a logical, rational decision maker, you would select the decision option that has the highest numerical value. The expected utility represents the option that maximises the decision maker's values and the likelihood of a particular outcome occurring (Hunink et al 2001).

Calculating the decision tree

Calculating the expected utilities is called 'folding back' a tree. Starting from the left hand side of the tree, for each branch you multiply the probability by the utility, and then add each result together, at each stage, until you reach the decision branch. Figure 11.6 shows the full calculation for the menopausal decision tree.

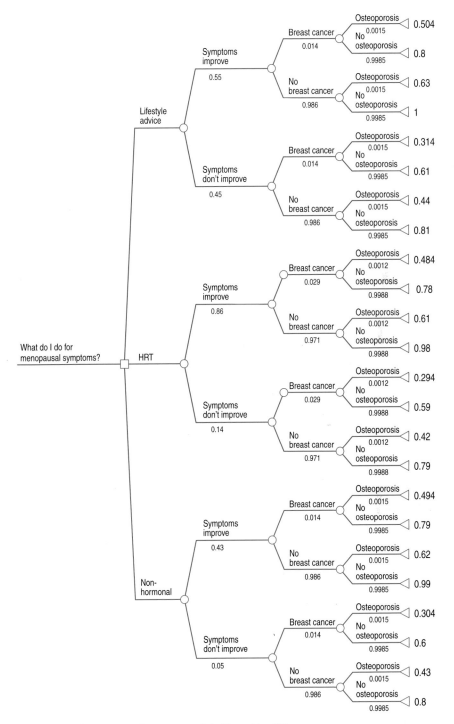

Figure 11.5 Decision tree for menopausal decision with utilities.

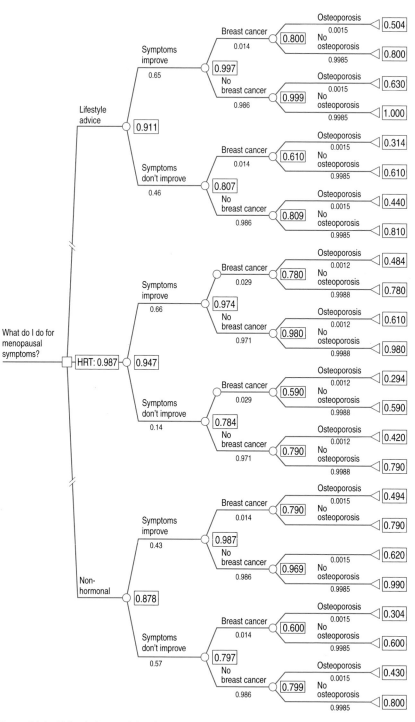

ESSENTIAL DECISION MAKING AND CLINICAL JUDGEMENT

Figure 11.6 Full calculation of the decision tree.

An example of how to calculate the expected utility (EU) for each branch is given for the lifestyle part of the tree as follows:

1. Multiply the utility of the outcome for the top branch (0.504) with the probability of osteoporosis (0.002), which equals 0.001.
2. Multiply the utility of the outcome for the second branch (0.8) with the probability of no osteoporosis (0.999), which equals 0.799.
3. Add these figures together (0.001 + 0.799 = 0.8) and multiply this by the probability of having breast cancer (0.8 × 0.014 = 0.011).
4. Follow the same procedure for the next two end points of the tree branch: ((0.63 × 0.002) + (1 × 0.999)) × 0.986 = (0.001 + 0.999) × 0.986 = 0.986.
5. Add the results of c) and d) together: 0.011 + 0.986 = 0.997.
6. Multiply this by the probability of symptoms improving (0.997 × 0.55 = 0.548).
7. Follow the same procedure for the 'symptoms don't improve' branch, starting from the furthest branches and working backwards:
   a. (0.314 × 0.002) + (0.61 × 0.999) = 0.61
   b. (0.44 × 0.002) + (0.81 × 0.999) = 0.809
   c. (0.61 × 0.014) + (0.809 × 0.986) = 0.807
   d. 0.45 × 0.807 = 0.363.
8. Add together the two values from the symptoms improve (0.548) and symptoms don't improve (0.363) branches to give the overall expected value for the lifestyle advice option (0.548 + 0.359 = 0.911).

Carry out the same calculations for each branch of the decision tree, folding back from right to left, until you have an overall value for each decision option in the model. In this instance, the option with the highest value, of 0.947 (or 0.95) is HRT, so (if she were a logical, rational decision maker) the woman should choose to take HRT for her menopausal symptoms.

Sensitivity analysis

Sensitivity analysis is a way of assessing the 'robustness' of your decision analysis (Dowie 1993). Like all models, the results are dependent on the numbers that go in. There are some situations where either the research evidence is very uncertain (perhaps the estimates of likelihood of certain outcomes have a wide range) or individual values/preferences for certain outcomes vary considerably. In these instances, if you alter the probability or utility estimates in the model, the results might be different. This is important, as you might want to use the decision model with another individual. Different patients might have different probabilities (due to differing prognostic factors) or have varying values/preferences for outcomes.

When you carry out a sensitivity analysis, you alter the probabilities and/or utilities in your decision model to explore the impact these alterations have on the expected value of different branches and whether the optimum decision changes as a result. The point at which the optimum decision switches given the probability or utility values is known as its 'threshold'. If you subsequently have a patient with probabilities above or below that threshold then *their* optimum decision might be different from the initial model.

Let us alter the probability and utility values for the variables in our menopausal treatment decision analysis. The probability values were altered using the estimates of uncertainty in Table 11.3. Utilities were altered at points between 0 and 1. The results of the analysis can be seen in Figure 11.7. These two graphs illustrate that our decision model is sensitive to changes in the probability of symptoms improving with non-hormonal therapy, and the utility of taking HRT and symptoms improving. The threshold for the probability of symptoms improving with non-hormonal therapy is 0.8. This means that if the probability of this therapy improving symptoms is above 0.8 (i.e. if 80% or more of individuals who take the therapy experience an improvement in symptoms), then this becomes the preferred decision option. The threshold for the utility of taking HRT and symptoms improving is 0.9. This means that if a woman has a utility value of above 0.9 for taking HRT *and* having improved symptoms, then HRT is her preferred option. However, if her utility value is below 0.9, then lifestyle advice is her preferred option.

If the decision model is relatively insensitive to changes in either probability or utility, then you can be confident with the preferred options it suggests

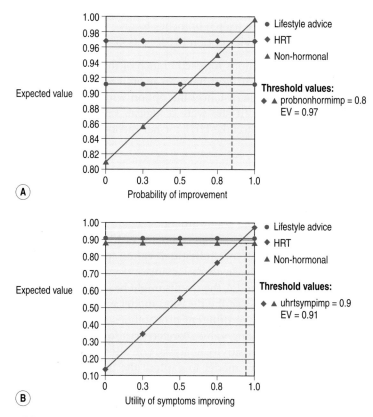

Figure 11.7 Results of one-way sensitivity analysis on menopausal decision tree: a) sensitivity analysis on probability of improvement with non-hormonal therapy, b) sensitivity analysis on symptoms improving with HRT.

(Naglie et al 1997, Richardson & Detsky 1995b). If the model is extremely sensitive to changes in these values then there is a high degree of uncertainty surrounding the decision and the recommendations of the model should be treated cautiously (Naglie et al 1997). In those situations in which the decision model is sensitive to utilities alone it is important to ensure that the utilities used accurately reflect the views of the individual making the decision.

BENEFITS AND LIMITATIONS OF DECISION ANALYSIS

Decision analysis is clearly not an approach for handling uncertainty in all clinical decisions. However, it is a useful technique for assisting complex and uncertain decisions, where the best option is not immediately obvious. By specifically including the results of research studies in the decision model, it can help a practitioner make evidence-based decisions. Often, the decision models used in a decision analysis are based on a wider range of information than would be used in a more unstructured approach to decision making (Elwyn et al 2001).

Decision analysis provides an explicit and systematic approach to decision making, which enables clinicians to explain both to patients and colleagues how a particular decision has been reached (Elwyn et al 2001, Richardson & Detsky 1995b, Tavakoli et al 2000). By incorporating patient values into the decision model, it also enables patients to be more involved in the decision process and to directly influence the final decision (Elwyn et al 2001).

Decision analysis has some potent limitations. Sometimes the probability estimates necessary to populate a tree do not exist in the research literature; a situation that necessitates using subjective estimates of probability (Naglie et al 1997). Such estimates are subject to a number of forms of bias (see Chapter 7).

Utility measurement itself may also be questioned as an approach. Is it possible, or indeed appropriate, to try and quantify something which is so subjective and emotional (Tavakoli et al 2000)? As we saw earlier, utility values depend on the method by which they are measured and are subject to framing. Asking individuals to evaluate a health state of which they have no experience, and might not be able to understand (Dowding & Thompson 2002), is not only counterintuitive but also fundamentally flawed. Hastie & Dawes (2001) highlight the anomaly whereby individuals asked to rate a health state before diagnosis (e.g. being HIV positive) were more negative about the state than when asked to rate the same state a year after being diagnosed. People adapt.

Decision analysis is often criticised for being too time consuming and artificially simplifying complex decision problems (Tavakoli et al 2000). However, all forms of decision making are open to criticism and limited by the amount of data available to the clinician. What makes decision analysis a different approach is that these weaknesses are explicit and open to debate (Dowding & Thompson 2002).

CONCLUSION

When faced with a decision situation in which complexity, uncertainty and the lack of an optimum choice are all present, decision analysis may help. Decision analysis helps structure your evaluation of the evidence base and relate it directly to the decision options you face. Perhaps the biggest contribution decision analysis makes is the explicit and systematic incorporation of the preferences of the patients whose lives will be most affected by the decisions taken.

Combining preferences for outcomes *and* the likelihood of those outcomes occurring goes a long way to answering the frequently asked question, 'How exactly do I practice evidence-based decision making? Although there is no escaping the fact that for many clinicians decision analysis represents a 'black-belt' decision technique, it should be part of the armoury for those nurses who strive to be truly advanced decision makers.

EXERCISES

Exercise 1. Structuring decisions

Try to identify a recent decision that you have made in practice that you found difficult. Perhaps this was because it was very complex or uncertain, or because you and your patient had different views about what might be the best thing to do. (Remember a *decision* is made when you have to choose between different options):

1. Write a description of the decision situation, trying to identify the key features that made it difficult.
2. Now list all the different options you had open to you, and the risks and benefits associated with each option. You might need to think about whether there are options available to you for that decision which you didn't consider at the time.
3. Put this into a balance sheet (see Table 11.1)
4. Now try to represent your decision situation as a decision tree (see Figure 11.1).
5. Remember that decision nodes in a tree are represented by a square box, and chances by a circle node. You might need to simplify the decision situation by focusing on the key outcomes that might happen as a result of different actions you could take.

For help structuring the tree, refer to the article by Detsky et al (1997).

Exercise 2. Assessing the probability of different outcomes

Take the decision tree that you constructed in Exercise 11.1:

1. List all of the possible outcomes in a table like the probability table in Table 11.3.
2. Carry out a search to try and find research evidence to tell you what the probability or likelihood of each of those outcomes happening might be. Places you could look include:
   a. published evidence-based guidelines
   b. systematic reviews of available evidence

c. pre-appraised studies (such as those available via evidence-based nursing: www.ebn.bmjjournals.com/)

d. searching for randomised trials/research studies in available databases (such as CINAHL and Medline).

3. Summarise the evidence you have found. Discard poor-quality studies where appropriate. Use the average result of studies to give you your overall estimate. Remember that you might need to convert the figures for continuous outcomes into a probability estimation using mean effect sizes.

4. Put in estimates of the range of uncertainty (probability) for your figures into the table – this could be confidence intervals from published studies, or the full range of estimation from a number of published studies.

5. If you can't find any evidence for your probability estimations then you will need to estimate them. You could do this by asking an expert (if you have access to one) or carry out an estimation based on your own experience. Remember that this type of estimation may be open to bias, so perhaps put in a broader probability range.

6. Put your probability estimates into the decision tree you constructed in Exercise 1. Make sure that the probabilities for each branch add up to 1.

Exercise 3 Measuring utility

Take the decision tree you have constructed from learning Exercises 1 and 2:

1. List all the possible outcomes that could occur to the person who is making the decision.

2. Separate the outcomes into short-term outcomes (which could happen to the person straight away, such as side effects from a drug therapy) and long-term outcomes (which might happen over a longer period of time, such as developing an illness such as heart disease).

3. Try to estimate the value or preference individuals attach to these health states. Ask a friend or colleague to evaluate your different health states, using a rating scale approach, or a standard gamble (see Box 11.3). See if you get different responses using different methods.

4. If you estimate values from different people, then take the average utility, and give each outcome a utility value.

5. List all of the possible combinations of outcomes that could occur in your decision model in a table (like the list in Table 11.4)

6. Calculate the 'disutility' of all of your short-term health states, by subtracting your utility value from 1.

7. Calculate the utility for each possible combination of outcomes. Multiply the utility values of all the relevant long-term states together, and then subtract the disutility values for the short-term states.

8. You should have a utility value for each possible health state for each branch of your tree – add these values to your decision tree.

Continued

Evidence-based decisions: the role of decision analysis

EXERCISES – CONT'D

Exercise 4 Calculating a decision tree

Take the decision tree with both your probability and utility values that have been constructed following learning Exercise 3:

1. Calculate the 'expected utility' for each choice option in your tree. You do this by working systematically back from left to right, multiplying utility by probability and then adding branches together. Use the example calculation in the chapter to help you.

2. When you have calculated the values for each branch, look to see which branch has the highest value. This is the option that you should choose, if you are a logical rational decision maker.

3. How does this option compare with the decision you actually took? Is it the result you expected? Why?

4. Identify the branch of the tree where your probability estimates are the most uncertain. Alter these values, perhaps first to represent the lowest possible value you think is reasonable, and then the highest value. Recalculate your values for each branch.

5. How does this affect what you should do? Has the decision option you should choose altered? How? What do you think this tells you about your decision model?

Did one particular outcome cause disagreement between individuals (or where the value someone else gave you and your value were different) when you were measuring utility? Alter the values in your tree for this utility value and see if it affects what decision you should take. What does this tell you about your decision model?

RESOURCES

www.treeage.com/ A decision analysis software package that can be used to construct and calculate decision trees. Has a 30-day trial download that students can use to help them with the process. Students do need to be reasonably computer literate to make full use of the program.

SOURCES

Clinical knowledge summaries (http://cks. library.nhs.uk/menopause) 2008.

Detsky A S, Naglie G, Krahn M D et al 1997 Primer on medical decision analysis: Part 1 – getting started. Medical Decision Making 17:123–125

MacLennan A, Broadbent J, Lester S et al 2004 Oral oestrogen and combined oestrogen/progestogen therapy versus placebo for hot flushes. In: Cochrane Database of Systematic Reviews, Issue 4

Morris E, Rymer J 2006 Menopausal symptoms. Clinical Evidence 15. Mean value of the trial results reported in the guidance

REFERENCES

Brand D A, Kliger A S 1999 Planning for a kidney transplant: is my doctor listening? The Journal of the American Medical Association 282:691–694

Brazier J E, Roberts J, Platts M et al 2005 Estimating a preference-based index for a menopause specific health quality of life questionnaire. Health and Quality of Life Outcomes 3:13

Detsky A S, Naglie G, Krahn M D et al 1997 Primer on medical decision analysis: Part 1 – getting started. Medical Decision Making 17:123–125

DiCenso A, Cullum N, Ciliska D 1998 Implementing evidence based nursing: some misconceptions. Evidence Based Nursing 1:38–39

Dowding D, Thompson C 2002 Decision analysis. In: Thompson C, Dowding D (eds) Clinical decision making and judgement in nursing. Churchill Livingstone, Edinburgh

Dowie J 1993 Clinical decision analysis: background and introduction. In: Llewelyn L, Hopkins A (eds) Analysing how we reach clinical decisions. Royal College of Physicians of London, London, p 7–26

Drummond M. 1993 Estimating utilities for making decisions in healthcare. In: Llewelyn L, Hopkins A (eds) Analysing how we reach clinical decisions. Royal College of Physicians of London, London, p 125–143

Elwyn G, Edwards A, Eccles M et al 2001 Decision analysis in patient care. Lancet 358:571–574

Hastie R, Dawes R M 2001 Rational choice in an uncertain world. Sage, London

Haynes B R 2006 Of studies, syntheses, synopses, summaries, and systems: the '5S' evolution of information services for evidence-based healthcare decisions. Evidence-Based Medicine 11:162

Hunink M, Glasziou P, Siegel J et al 2001 Decision making in health and medicine. Integrating evidence and values. Cambridge University Press, Cambridge

Naglie G, Krahn M D, Naimark D et al 1997 Primer on medical decision analysis: Part 3 – estimating probabilities and utilities. Medical Decision Making 17:136–141

Richardson W S, Detsky A S 1995a Users' guides to the medical literature VII: how to use a clinical decision analysis A. Journal of the American Medical Association 273:1292–1295

Richardson W S, Detsky A S 1995b Users' guides to the medical literature VII: how to use a clinical decision analysis B. Journal of the American Medical Association 273:1610–1613

Sarasin F P 2001 Decision analysis and its application in clinical medicine. European Journal of Obstetrics and Gynecology and Reproductive Biology 94(2):172–179

Tavakoli M, Davies H T O, Thomson R 2000 Decision analysis in evidence-based decision making. Journal of Evaluation in Clinical Practice 6:111–120

Thornton J G 1996 Decision analysis. Clinical Obstetrics and Gynaecology 10:677–695

Thornton J G, Lilford R J, Johnson N 1992 Decision analysis in medicine. British Medical Journal 304:1099–1103

Tickle-Degnen L 2001 From the general to the specific. Using meta-analytic reports in clinical decision making. Evaluation and the Health Professions 24:308–326

von Winterfeldt D 1980 Structuring decision problems for decision analysis. Acta Psychologica 45:73–93

The economics of clinical decision making

Jo Dumville and Marta Soares

KEY ISSUES

- What the results of economic evaluations mean
- Key concepts in the economics of decision making
- The critical appraisal of economic evidence

INTRODUCTION

Decision making as a healthcare professional differs from our everyday judgement calls and choices. In healthcare systems, budgets are finite and money spent on one choice constitutes resource that, by-and-large, cannot be spent on something else. In healthcare often, many interventions are effective (or ineffective) *to some extent*. This chapter deals with selecting a choice from a plethora of potentially effective treatment options in which our choices have economic as well as clinical impacts.

Clinicians and policy makers are often required to make difficult decisions regarding the health technologies they use. Increasingly, governmental bodies, such as the National Institute of Health and Clinical Excellence (NICE) in the United Kingdom, produce national clinical guidelines and technology assessments to direct practice (NICE 2004). These assessments often consider not only the benefits conferred by alternative treatment choices but also the costs.

It is vital that nurses have a clear understanding of why economic evaluations are needed, what the result of such evaluations mean, and how these findings can inform allocation decisions. We will start by introducing key ideas before illustrating these with examples. We then go on to outline the critical appraisal of specific types of economic evaluation.

ECONOMIC EVALUATION IN HEALTHCARE

Central government or federally funded services must deliver healthcare within fixed and limited budgets (Box 12.1). Decisions made to spend money in one way will incur an *opportunity cost* in terms of investment in other health services that are foregone. For example, investment in a new cancer centre might mean that a new spinal rehabilitation centre is not set up. Alternatively, the delivery of an expensive treatment to one patient might mean that ten other patients cannot be treated with a cheaper health technology.

In general, economic evaluation is the, 'comparative analysis of alternative courses of action in terms of both their costs and consequences' (Drummond et al 1997). In other words, an economic evaluation compares two or more health technologies in terms of the costs incurred (or resources used) against the resulting benefits (or consequences). The aim of such evaluations is to inform understanding about the return on money spent. Such understanding assists health policy makers' choices about which healthcare technologies to fund (Briggs 2006). Economic evaluation can be conducted in several ways (Table 12.1). Of these, the most widely used are cost-effectiveness and cost-utility analyses.

Box 12.1

Economics is the study of allocating scarce or limited resources (i.e. labour, land, raw material, or capital). Whatever the type and volume of resource available, society will always have more wants than can be met. Economic decisions aim to maximise benefits for the costs incurred. However, for every decision made regarding resource use, there is an opportunity cost – the cost of failing to use a resource for the next best alternative.

Table 12.1   Different types of economic evaluation

Cost-minimisation analysis	Benefits obtained are assumed to be equal for all treatments. Decision based solely on difference in costs between treatments. Rarely used
Cost-benefit analysis	Costs and benefits are valued in the same unit (normally monetary) to establish to what extent benefits may outweigh costs for different treatments
Cost-effectiveness analysis and cost-utility analysis	In cost-effectiveness analysis, outcomes are measured in natural units i.e. disease-free days or survival time. The incremental cost versus incremental benefit of one treatment over others is the main outcome estimated. In cost-utility analysis, benefit is based on a weighted measure of mortality and morbidity for example the Quality Adjusted Life Year (QALY)

Adapted from Shiell et al (2002).

Resource use

The results from an economic evaluation will be relevant to different decision makers depending on the perspective from which it is conducted. If the cost perspective is that of the healthcare provider, all costs incurred by this provider must be measured and included. These resources may include staff time, equipment used, drugs prescribed, hospital length of stay, transport costs, and overheads incurred. If relevant, the perspective might also include resources utilised from wider state-care services, such as social care services. In the UK, the NICE guidelines advocate a National Health Service (NHS) and personal social services perspective on costs, as NICE's interest is predominantly in cost to the public purse (NICE 2004). In other countries, a wider societal perspective is taken; this might include indirect costs that impact on wider society, i.e. time away from paid employment, as well as the direct costs to patients, such as private treatment.

Health benefit

Table 12.1 shows that health benefits can be measured in a number of ways depending on the evaluative approach being undertaken. The more common methods are the use of *effectiveness* measures (cost-effectiveness analysis) and the use of *utilities* (cost-utility analysis).

Effectiveness measures include 'natural' units such as life years, disease-free days, or even surrogate outcomes (i.e. cancer biomarkers in wound area). Although such measures are useful when assessing the cost-effectiveness of two or more treatments for a particular disease, they do not allow comparison between health technologies or diseases when the natural units are different.

Economic evaluations should aim to help decision makers allocate resources to maximise patient benefit across the whole of society. Thus, the outcome measures most useful for decision makers are those inviting comparisons between conditions and health technologies. Mortality is the most generic and common measure; however, for many diseases improvement in morbidity is the main treatment aim. Because we are all interested in how long we will live and whether we will spend that time in good (enough) health, having measures that capture both quantity *and* quality of life in a single index is desirable.

A common index used in economic evaluation is the Quality Adjusted Life Year (QALY) (Box 12.2, Figure 12.1). This measure adjusts the 'amount of time lived' by a measure of utility (utility weight) that expresses the impact of morbidity. Data required for the calculation of QALYs can be collected from patients using questionnaires, such as the EuroQol-5D (EQ-5D). The EQ-5D (www.euroqol.org/) is a widely recognised and validated means of describing and measuring health-related quality of life (Kind 1996). It has five questions, each relating to a different health dimension: mobility, self-care, ability to undertake usual activity, pain, and anxiety/depression. Each question has three possible response levels: no problems, moderate, and severe. Based on their answers to the EQ-5D questionnaire, participants can be classified into one of 243 possible health states. Each of these health

> ### Box 12.2 What is a QALY?
>
> A QALY is a measure of time lived (mortality) weighted by health-related quality of life during this period (morbidity). Being in perfect health for 1 year has the maximum weight of 1 QALY. However, if the individual has not lived the year in full health, the associated QALY will be reduced, via a lower utility weight. QALYs can be used to assess improvements in mortality and morbidity that a health technology brings about (see Figure 12.1).

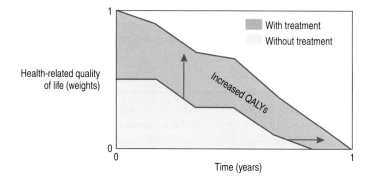

Figure 12.1 Increased QALYs with treatment are due to increase in life lived ($\rightarrow$) and improved quality of life during the period lived ($\uparrow$).

states has an associated utility weight, denoting the impact this state will have on health-related quality of life. Thus, perfect health has a weight of 1; a weighting that decreases as health becomes impaired.

There are two methods of evaluating the impact of quality of lived life in different health states to generate utility weights; both rely on the elicitation of individual's preferences (Neumann et al 2000). The first is a form of 'trade-off' between quality and quantity of life where individuals record the amount of life lived they would be willing to sacrifice to live in perfect health. The second is a gamble in which individuals record the risk of death they would accept in return for restoring perfect health (called a *standard gamble*). The tariff of weights for the EQ-5D questionnaire was based on a time trade-off exercise in a sample of the UK population (Dolan et al 1995). Examples of other questionnaires used to generate utility indices are the Health Utilities Index (McCabe et al 2005) and SF-36 (through the SF-6D) (Brazier & Roberts 2004).

Conducting cost-effectiveness and cost-utility analyses

Broadly speaking, there are two approaches for undertaking cost-effectiveness or cost-utility analysis. The first is a single source of data collected via primary research, i.e. a randomised controlled trial (RCT); the second is the synthesis of data from multiple sources in the form of a decision analytic model (DAM). The aim of both is to calculate and relate average costs and the consequences of different health technologies.

The growing demand for cost-effectiveness information about health technologies means cost-effectiveness and cost-utility analyses (known as cost-effectiveness analyses, or CEA, for ease) are increasingly being conducted within RCTs. Trial-based CEA uses statistical models to evaluate costs and consequences using data collected during the trial. A well-conducted trial-based CEA provides useful data with high internal validity (i.e. it measures what it is supposed to measure); however, there are also limitations. Where multiple strategies to treat a disease or illness exist, individual RCTs provide only partial information. Time, expense, and feasibility limit the number of health technologies that can be assessed in a single study. These same factors can also limit trial duration. Additionally, basing decisions on a trial-based CEA alone means that other relevant evidence might be excluded (Sculpher et al 2006).

As we have seen, an optimal (and rational) decision about how we use health technologies requires us to use all the available evidence on all relevant competing strategies. If the evidence comes from multiple data sources, it can be synthesised using a DAM (Siebert 2003). DAMs represent a simplified version of 'real-world' decision making, which identifies and relates important states associated with a condition. The most common designs for DAM are decision trees, state-transition models (e.g. Markov models; Sonnenberg & Beck 1993) and simulation models (Brennan et al 2006). Decision-tree models do not explicitly account for time, thus are not usually adequate for modelling chronic disease patient pathways. Markov models can model time; but sometimes more complex scenarios require the use of simulation models.

Figure 12.2 shows a decision tree used to conduct a cost-effectiveness and cost-utility analysis for zanamivir in the treatment of influenza (Burls et al 2002). The white square represents the decision being evaluated: in this case the use of zanamivir or not, to treat influenza. The decision tree then describes possible patient pathways and assigns benefits and costs to each. This process allows the calculation of average estimates for the different health technologies of interest.

Figure 12.3 shows a Markov model used to investigate the life-time cost effectiveness of combined therapy with interferon-α and ribavirin compared with no treatment for patients with mild chronic hepatitis C (Wright et al 2006). For Markov models, costs and consequences are assigned to each state and the transition of patients between states is modelled. In this case the model starts with a cohort of 1000 hypothetical patients, who have mild disease. These patients can then move to different health states (i.e. from having mild disease to having moderate disease) over time, progressing through the disease. The authors considered general mortality in the Markov model, although this is not clear from Figure 12.3.

Outcome of economic evaluation

The results of cost-effectiveness or cost-utility studies can lead to one of four scenarios. The graph shown in Figure 12.4 is described using compass points. Of the four scenarios, the northwest (NW) quadrant of the

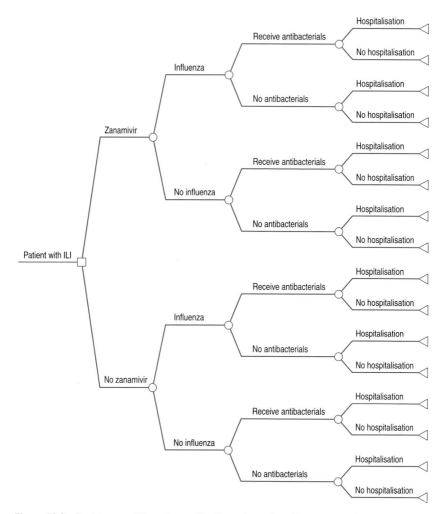

Figure 12.2 Decision tree; ILI = influenza-like illness; (reproduced from Burls A, Clark W, Stewart T et al, 2002, with permission).

cost-effectiveness plane implies that a new health technology is *dominated* (i.e. not as good) because its cost is higher and its benefits lower than the comparison technology. In this case, the decision regarding the new treatment is straightforward: one should not adopt it. The decision is also straightforward when the cost-effectiveness measure is positioned in the southeast (SE) quadrant. The new health technology is *dominant* (i.e. better) as it is less costly and more beneficial than the comparator and should therefore be implemented.

However, for the scenarios positioned in the northeast (NE) or southwest (SW) quadrants, a decision is more difficult to make. Here we must evaluate whether the increased cost of the new health technology is worth the increased benefit (NE scenario); or if the reduced benefit conferred by the new health technology is justified by the reduced costs (SW). To do this, a measure combining the two components (costs and benefits) is required so that a decision rule can be applied.

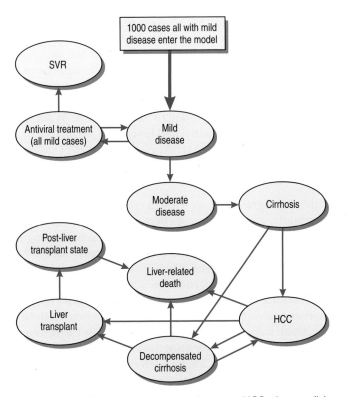

Figure 12.3 Markov model; SVR = sustained virological response; HCC = hepatocellular carcinoma; (reproduced from Wright M, Grieve R, Roberts J et al, 2006, with permission).

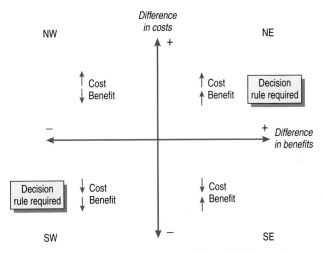

Figure 12.4 Cost-effectiveness plane showing cost and benefit differences between alternative treatments. NE, northeast; NW, northwest; SE, southeast; SW, southwest.

The incremental cost-effectiveness ratio (ICER) is the measure commonly used. It combines costs and benefits as a ratio of the two different mean costs (between the two comparison arms) and the two different mean effectiveness measures (between the two comparison arms). Although an economic

The economics of clinical decision making

evaluation study is not the only information source considered for allocation decisions, proponents of new health technologies tend to compare the ICER value against the (approximate) maximum amount the decision maker is willing to pay for an additional unit of benefit. In the absence of other considerations, a health technology can be considered cost effective only if the decision maker's willingness to pay for an additional QALY (or other effectiveness measure) is greater (or equal) to the ICER. Willingness-to-pay thresholds are not defined explicitly, and how these are arrived at is the subject of much discussion elsewhere (cf Appleby et al 2007, Culyer et al 2007).

Assessing uncertainty

It is important to recognise that, as with all estimates derived from a sample, there is uncertainty around the cost-effectiveness/utility estimates, i.e. the ICER. In clinical research, uncertainty is usually presented using confidence intervals. In economic evaluation, the cost-effectiveness acceptability curve (CEAC) is commonly used instead. The CEAC expresses the likelihood that the cost-effectiveness estimate reflects a cost-effective health technology, based on the existing evidence (Fenwick & Byford 2005). The CEAC summarises, for every value of the willingness-to-pay threshold, the evidence in favour of the health technology being cost effective. The CEAC is usually built by simulating several potential scenarios (based on the data we have), and then producing an estimate of the ICER for each of these scenarios. We can then evaluate the proportion of scenarios that identify the health technology as cost effective in relation to the comparator, over a range of willingness-to-pay values. Two published trial-based CEA examples (Iglesias et al 2006, Manca et al 2007) are given to illustrate cost-effectiveness and cost-utility analysis.

Example 1: cost-effectiveness study

Preventing pressure ulcers is often the responsibility of nursing staff, who must make decisions about what pressure-relieving surfaces to use. Such decisions should be informed by clinical and cost-effectiveness information where possible. In terms of cost effectiveness, a recent RCT compared alternating pressure mattresses with alternating pressure overlays from the perspective of the NHS (Iglesias et al 2006). Trial participants were people aged over 55 years admitted to hospital without a pressure ulcer. Participants were randomised to receive either a mattress or overlay and assessed to see whether a pressure ulcer (grade 2 or more) developed. Patients were followed for a maximum of 60 days. Clinically, there was no difference in the proportion of people who developed a pressure ulcer between the trial arms (Nixon et al 2006). In terms of cost effectiveness, the main resource use of interest was length of hospital stay and the cost of the surfaces themselves; all measured during the trial. Benefit was assessed in the natural unit of time taken to develop a pressure ulcer. Mean cost and mean number of ulcer-free days was calculated for each group (Table 12.2).

In this case, the mean cost of treating a patient in the mattress trial arm was £283.60 less than the overlay. Also, patients receiving the mattress had on average 10.6 more ulcer-free days than those receiving the overlay. The point estimate of the relative cost effectiveness of the mattress falls into the southeastern

Table 12.2 Example 1: cost and benefit data			
	Mattress (n = 982)	Overlay (n = 989)	Difference
Mean cost (£)	6509.73	6793.33	−283.60
Ulcer-free days (95% CI)	–	–	10.64 (favouring mattress)

CI, confidence interval.
Adapted from Iglesias et al (2006).

corner of Figure 12.4. The mattress dominates the overlay, which appears to be more expensive and less effective. In this case, making a decision based on the point estimate is easy, calculating the ICER is superfluous – go with the mattress.

Figure 12.5 is a CEAC for this analysis. Although the point estimate suggests that the use of mattress is cost effective, the uncertainty around its use suggests that we can be 80–90% sure that mattresses are cost effective, for any willingness-to-pay value between 0 and £30,000 per pressure-ulcer-free day. Assuming that the decision maker would be willing to pay £30,000 per pressure-ulcer-free day then the economic evaluation study based on the PRESSURE trial suggests the adoption of mattresses rather than overlays as a cost-effective health technology for preventing pressure ulcers.

Example 2: cost-utility analysis

Musculoskeletal back and neck pain are common conditions that cost health services a great deal to treat. Physiotherapy is a common treatment for these musculoskeletal conditions, although a number of different approaches can be used. A recent RCT compared the clinical and cost effectiveness of a new brief physiotherapy pain-management approach using cognitive-behavioural principles (the solution-finding approach) with a commonly used traditional method of physical therapy (the McKenzie approach) for participants with back or neck pain (Moffett et al 2006). The cost-utility analysis (Manca et al 2007) was conducted from an NHS perspective. Costs were

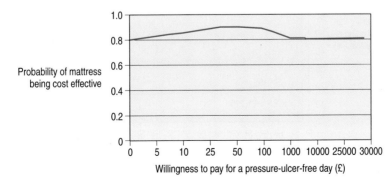

Figure 12.5 Cost-effectiveness acceptability curve (CEAC): pressure mattresses vs. overlays for prevention of pressure ulcers (from Iglesias et al 2006 © BMJ Publishing Group, reproduced with permission).

measured in UK pounds sterling. The main resource use of interest was number of physiotherapy sessions, and GP and nurse visits; these were measured during the trial. Benefit was measured as health-related quality of life using the EQ-5D, which allows the estimation of patient-specific QALYs. Patients were followed up for 12 months.

We can see that patients using the solution-finding approach incurred, on average, fewer costs than those assigned to receive the McKenzie approach. Nevertheless, the solution-finding approach also led to reduced benefit for patients. This then falls into the southwestern corner of Figure 12.4 and a decision rule is required. In the absence of other data, decision makers need to decide whether to save healthcare resources by adopting the less expensive treatment (the solution-finding approach), with the disadvantage of losing health benefits. Relating the incremental mean costs and incremental mean QALYs gives an ICER of £1220 QALY (−£24.4/−0.020) (Table 12.3).

We can investigate the uncertainty around this decision as before. Figure 12.6 shows the CEAC for this analysis. We can see that if the willingness to pay (threshold value) per QALY was 0 (i.e. the decision maker has no budget to pay for health), the solution-finding approach would be cost effective because it offers a cost-saving treatment. However, as soon as willingness to pay per QALY increases, the probability that the solution-finding

Table 12.3 Example 2: cost and benefit data

	Solution finding	MacKenzie	Difference (95% CI)
Mean cost (£)	105.0	129.4	−24.4 (−49.6 to 0.79)
QALYs	0.679	0.699	−0.020 (−0.057 to 0.017)

CI, confidence interval.
Adapted from Manca et al (2007).

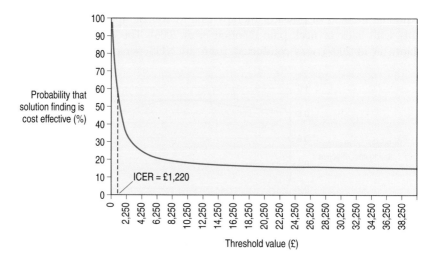

Figure 12.6 CEAC for example 2 (Solution finding vs MacKenzie physiotherapy approaches for patients with neck or back pain); ICER = Incremental cost-effectiveness ratio; (reproduced from Manca A, Dumville J C, Torgerson D J et al. 2007, *Rheumatology*, with permission).

approach is cost effective drops markedly; because although MacKenzie is the more expensive treatment, the cost is deemed worthwhile in terms of the benefit obtained.

CRITICAL APPRAISAL OF COST-EFFECTIVENESS AND COST-UTILITY STUDIES IN HEALTHCARE

Like all forms of research evidence, economic evaluations need critically appraising for validity, clinical importance and applicability before they are given a 'weight' in our decision-making processes. The aim of this section is to guide the reader through the stages of evaluating published CEA. Elsewhere in the book, we have largely steered clear of questions of critical appraisal; due mainly to the preponderance of high quality critical appraisal guides that already exist (see, for example, Cullum et al 2007). But few such tools exist to guide nurses around an economic analysis, hence the inclusion of this section of the chapter.

As with other research designs, CEA appraisal is facilitated by directing a series of tailored questions at the research study. The seminal guide to critical appraisal of economic evaluations was developed by Drummond et al (1997) Here, we will draw on the Drummond checklist as well as the UK requirements for economic evaluation (NICE 2008).

Appraisal questions can be grouped under four main headings: defining and presenting the decision problem, measurement and data, analysis, and discussion. Broadly, these questions can be applied to CEA conducted as part of primary research or DAM studies. For more information, readers are directed to in-depth work by Philips et al (2004) and Ramsey et al (2005).

Defining and presenting the decision problem

Is there a clearly-phrased, answerable research question?

A CEA study should clearly outline its aim(s). Although this information is often contained in other sections of the study, presenting an overview allows the reader to assess quickly how relevant the research is and how well the design addresses the question posed. A well-phrased research question can answer the next four questions.

Does the study compare the cost and consequences of alternative health technologies?

By definition, a CEA must compare two or more health technologies, evaluating their costs and consequences. Included health technologies should be clear from the outset.

Is the patient population(s) clear?

Study findings are only useful when it is clear who they apply to. The reader should be provided with a clear description of the disease(s) or condition(s) being evaluated, along with a clear description of the patient population.

Which clinical settings (policies) were explored in the study?

There may be varying clinical policies or settings influencing the use of a new technology. For example, in their recent CEA, Gillies et al (2008) modelled different policies regarding the screening and prevention of type 2 diabetes. One policy involved a one-off screening at age 45; the second involved up to two additional screenings at ages 50 and 60.

In all CEA, the reader should assess how the policies evaluated relate to practice. Important details may include how, when, and where the health technologies were delivered and at what frequency. This information tells us how the health technologies evaluated relate to current standard practice(s). Importantly, when a single clinical policy is evaluated internal validity (concerning the quality of the data) is often high but external validity (concerning the generalisability of the evidence) can be limited.

Whose perspective is the study being conducted from?

A good CEA will be explicit about the perspective the evaluation is being conducted from. The perspective establishes the relevance of the study for specific decision makers because it dictates which costs and consequences should be measured (see appraisal questions for 'measurement and data').

Are relevant alternatives assessed and clearly described?

A CEA should evaluate health technologies relevant to current practice. Comparing a new technology with an out-dated or unsuitable comparator limits the conclusions that can be related to current practice. Ideally, for comprehensive decision making the CEA must compare the use of the new technology with *all* the relevant strategies (NICE 2001). When appraising a study, the reader must assess whether there are important comparators excluded from the study. Finally, it has been argued that a CEA should only be conducted on effective health technologies (Drummond et al 1997). This means that evidence of clinical effectiveness should be cited within the CEA.

Measurement and data

What type of study has been conducted, and why?

In any CEA, the choice of study design must be appropriate for the underlying research question. If comprehensive and adequate information is available from one RCT, the reader must assess if the objectives of the CEA can be answered using this single data source as the results will depend on the trial characteristics.

Have all important and relevant costs and consequences been identified?

It is important to verify this.

Are all important costs included?

Important costs are those incurred when applying the health technology and those associated with its impact. Thus, decisions about which costs to include require a clear understanding of the health technologies being delivered as well as the epidemiology of the relevant condition. As highlighted above, a full description of the health technologies and the perspective taken will help you make a judgement regarding the completeness of included costs.

It is unlikely that a CEA will have measured all costs associated with alternative technologies: it is not the same as a burden of illness (or cost of illness) study (Akobundu et al 2006). As CEA evaluates the differences in costs and consequences between health technologies, some cost categories can legitimately be excluded. A CEA need not consider costs incurred due to future, unrelated illness occurring in years of life unaffected by the current technologies of interest (Gold et al 1996).

Do the costs included reflect the relevant perspective?

The study perspective will dictate the relevant costs to assess. We have discussed that if the cost perspective is that of the healthcare provider, resources may include staff time, drugs prescribed, and/or length of hospital stay. When a societal perspective is taken, the measurement of all costs, regardless of who bears them, is required. To ensure a comprehensive and useful assessment of cost effectiveness, when a study does not take a societal perspective for its main analysis, relevant societal data can be presented for reference. For example, in the cost-utility analysis described previously, which investigated physiotherapy treatments for back and neck pain, the perspective for the main analysis was that of the NHS. However, the study also looked at private treatment costs incurred by trial participants, and the costs of usual activity missed by patients.

Do the outcomes measured relate to the research question?

A CEA should clearly state the consequences assessed and how these were measured. If natural units were used (e.g. life years, time disease free) these need to be relevant to the decision maker, and fully justified. Moreover, effectiveness outcomes must capture all the health gains and losses associated with use of the technology (e.g. adverse events). From a policy perspective, a cost-utility approach is arguably the most valuable because it allows comparison of value for money across multiple diseases and health technologies. This is useful when considering the adoption of the new technology since comparisons can be made with benefits from the technologies being superseded.

Over what time period are costs and consequences being assessed?

Cost and consequences must be considered over an appropriate and clearly stated time period. The defined time period should be capable of capturing the differential costs and consequences of the health technology. If the time horizon is smaller than the potential timeframe of costs incurred and/or benefits gained from the health technologies being evaluated, the conclusions of the study are limited. Where data for the required time period are not available, extrapolation from the data over longer time periods can be undertaken.

How were the cost and consequences measured?

After evaluating whether relevant costs and consequences have been identified, the reader must appraise how well they were measured. This includes assessment of *what* data have been collected, *how* the data were collected, *when* they were collected, and *how they were synthesised.*

Identifying all important costs and consequences should help dictate *what* data should be collected. *How* and *when* data were collected relates to the study type. In studies such as RCTs, resource use and effectiveness data can be collected prospectively from health professionals and participants at the appropriate times.

When appraising a DAM, one should evaluate whether systematic searches were used to capture all relevant research (Sutton et al 1998). Included data should be *synthesised* systematically using recognised evidence synthesis techniques, such as meta-analysis and indirect treatment comparisons (Glenny 2005, Nixon et al 2007).

In DAM studies, relative treatment effects should be estimated from at least one relevant and robust RCT, if not from multiple RCTs. As RCT data may not be available, or the data limited, supplemental good-quality observational studies will often be required. For example, for long-term outcomes data (including mortality, adverse events, or unanticipated benefits) other data sources might include cohort studies for parameters relating to the natural history of the condition, and cross-sectional surveys for resource use and costs. When there is no evidence to inform aspects of the CEA then expert opinion might be used – with caution. All sources of included data should be provided.

Modelling studies should be explicit about the limitations of included data (e.g. the use of observational data for effectiveness parameter estimation). Any attempts to overcome these limitations (e.g. by using quasi-experimental studies; Manning & Claxton 1997) should be described and the impact of these quantified.

Were the costs and consequences valued credibly?

A common method used to estimate costs in CEA is to measure units of resource use associated with the health technologies. Prices are then assigned to each unit (known as the 'unit cost'). Unit costs can be obtained directly from source, i.e. a hospital finance department. If this is the case, the mechanism by which the costs used in the study were calculated should be explained. In practice, limited time and data mean that unit costs are often taken from publicly available sources (Table 12.4). Such sources should

Table 12.4 Possible sources of UK unit costs	
Direct costs	*Source of unit costs (UK)*
Staff time	Personal Social Services Research Unit (PSSRU): unit costs of health and social care (Curtis & Netten 2006)
Hotel cost of night in hospitals	Chartered Institute of Public Finance and Accountancy (CIPFA 2003) NHS reference costs (DoH 2004)
Cost of medication	British National Formulary (BNF)
Cost of overheads and equipment	Manufacturers; NHS Trusts

be clearly referenced. These unit costs are useful tools for CEA; they are widely used and increase the comparability of results across studies. However, it is acknowledged that these unit costs can be imperfect tools because market prices and real values differ in many circumstances (Gold et al 1996). Unit costs should be reported separately from the volume of resource use. Finally, in any CEA it is important the reader knows the monetary unit used (euros, pounds sterling, US dollars) and the year to which the unit costs relate.

When conducting a cost-utility analysis, one must value 'life lived' through a utility index. NICE recommends the use of validated generic health state descriptors (i.e. EQ-5D) and utilities from preference elicitation conducted with a population sample, such as in Dolan et al (1995). Where patient preferences have been measured directly in a study, clear details regarding the methods should be described.

Were costs and consequences discounted where required?

In economic terms, we generally prefer to spend money in the future but obtain benefits in the present. CEAs must adjust their values to reflect this preference – a process called 'discounting'. Discounting costs accounts for the fact that there is an opportunity cost to spending money now rather than in the future. Benefits should also be discounted. Again there is a time preference to obtaining health benefits, this preference being inverse to costs: we prefer to have benefits now rather than in the future (Torgerson & Raferty 1999, Weinstein & Stason 1977). The values used for discounting in a CEA should be clearly stated.

Analysis

Was the analysis appropriate?

CEA is a young and rapidly developing methodology. Important analytic developments take place regularly and can be complex. Below we outline some of the main issues in assessing how trial-based costs and consequences are calculated. These are (where relevant): whether the analysis accounted for censored (incompletely observed) and missing data, if any distributional assumptions were made, if correlation between costs and effects was accounted for and the methodology for dealing with data from different countries.

- Not accounting for censored and missing data can lead to biased mean estimates. In such cases the imputation of missing values can be conducted (Burton et al 2007) or other analytical methodologies used, i.e. the restricted mean approach and the inverse probability weighting approach (Lin 2000, Willan et al 2005).
- Costs and consequences are often assumed to be normally distributed; however, care must be taken as this assumption is often not true. Recently, both frequentist and Bayesian methods have applied non-normal distributions (such as the gamma distribution) to cost-effectiveness estimation.
- It is important to consider the correlation between costs and consequences for accurate estimates. Bootstrapping (a resampling technique used to obtain estimates of summary statistics) has been the most generalised methodology but both frequentist and Bayesian bivariate regression are valid methodologies.
- Models with interaction-terms or hierarchical models can be applied to explore between-country variations in multinational trials (Manca & Willan 2006).

Additionally, there is increasing recognition in CEA about the importance of adjusting statistical analysis for important prognostic and baseline variables (Nixon & Thompson 2005). This is particularly important if there is evidence of imbalance at baseline in the trial.

As the purpose of models is to represent complex situations as simply as possible, selecting the appropriate design and structure is vital. When appraising a DAM, the reader must assess if the model structure and design describes the problem of interest as well as if the maths add up and are correct. The structure of the model must include all important stages of the condition of interest. However, the model must also be practical and parsimonious. All models will require assumptions to be made and these must be documented as the internal and external validity of the model relies on the reasonableness of its assumptions. Additional detail on appraising DAMs can be found in Philips et al (2004).

Was subgroup analysis conducted, if relevant?

Heterogeneity is as relevant to CEA as it is to RCTs and systematic reviews: that is the cost-effectiveness outcomes might differ between patient subgroups. Not considering heterogeneity can bias cost-effectiveness results and/or lead to imprecise estimates. The identification of patient subgroups for whom the technology might potentially be cost effective is one of NICE's goals for CEA (NICE 2004). For, example, teriparatide (a drug aimed at reducing risk of osteoporotic fracture) was found to be cost effective, but only in patients with a very high fracture risk (Stevenson et al 2005).

This finding contributed to national guidance on bisphosphonates (used in the treatment and prevention of osteoporosis) use (NICE 2005). You should use your knowledge of patient groups and disease to decide whether any subgroup analyses would potentially be important (e.g. younger versus older patients with a stroke and therapy regimens).

Was an incremental analysis conducted?

A CEA aims to evaluate the incremental difference in costs and consequences between health technologies (see Figures 12.2 and 12.3). Where required, an ICER should be calculated.

Was uncertainty adequately assessed?

When evaluating health technologies based on sampled data, there is uncertainty regarding how well the estimate reflects the 'true' value in a population. Evaluating uncertainty in parameters should be done through probabilistic sensitivity analysis with all parameters considered jointly (Briggs et al 2006). Where probability distributions are used to compute the sensitivity analysis, these should be spelled out. Uncertainty should be expressed using CEACs (see Figures 12.5 and 12.6), alongside cost-effectiveness planes or frontier curves. Uncertainty evaluation can be complemented using sensitivity analysis, where characteristics of the main analysis are varied to assess their impact on the results. For example, the VenUS I trial investigated the cost effectiveness of two compression bandaging systems (four-layer bandaging versus short stretch) in the treatment of venous leg ulcers (Iglesias et al 2004). A sensitivity analysis was conducted to assess whether costing the four-layer bandaging as commercially available kits rather than using their consistent parts (base case) impacted on the cost effectiveness. It did not.

Discussion of results

Finally, a good study should present its findings in light of research that has gone before it; outlining how this new piece of works adds to the current evidence based. No piece of research is perfect and authors should be open about the limitations of their work. Limitations include issues already discussed such as assumptions made, limited generalisability and analytical issues such as how missing data were managed. Finally the authors should suggest how cost-effective health technologies may be implemented in current practice.

NHS ECONOMIC EVALUATION DATABASE

This chapter has described how to assess whether a high-quality CEA has been conducted and reported. There is an important, publicly available resource that aids the appraisal process. The NHS Economic Evaluation Database (NHS EED; see www.crd.york.ac.uk/crdweb/) is funded by the

UK Department of Health's NHS Research and Development Programme and housed at the Centre for Reviews and Dissemination (University of York, UK). At the end of December 2007 the database contained 6768 abstracts of economic evaluations. Each abstract is a detailed and structured record describing the economic evaluation. This is also supplemented by a critical commentary that provides a summary of the reliability and the generalisability of the evaluation and a discussion of the implications for the NHS.

RESOURCES

For those keen to learn more about health economic ways of thinking, a great start can be found at www.nlm.nih.gov/nichsr/edu/healthecon/index. html. This is a self-study series of modules on key concepts and techniques in the discipline.

EXERCISES

Part of the challenge in using evidence from economic analysis in your decision making is 'thinking economically'. As an exercise, consider establishing a nurse-led clinic for the management of a chronic condition you might meet in practice (diabetes, asthma, peripheral vascular disease).

1. What are the likely costs involved in the innovation (a nurse-led clinic counts as an innovation)?
2. How could you ensure that the outcomes you consider are those that matter to patients and not just you – as a provider?
3. What are the potential benefits?
4. What decision alternatives are you considering?

REFERENCES

Akobundu E, Ju J, Blatt L et al 2006 Cost-of-illness studies: a review of current methods. Pharmacoeconomics 24:869–890

Appleby J, Devlin N, Parkin D 2007 NICE's cost effectiveness threshold. British Medical Journal 335:358–359

Brazier J E, Roberts J 2004 The estimation of a preference-based measure of health from the SF-12. Medical Care 42:851–859

Brennan A, Chick S E, Davies R. 2006 A taxonomy of model structures for economic evaluation of health technologies. Health Economics 15:1295–1310

Briggs A, Sculpher M, Claxton K. 2006 Decision modelling for health economic evaluation. Oxford University Press, Oxford

Burls A, Clark, W, Stewart, T et al 2002 Zanamivir for the treatment of influenza in adults: a systematic review and economic evaluation. Health Technology Assessment (Winchester, England) 6(9):1–87

Burton A, Billingham L J, Bryan S 2007 Cost-effectiveness in clinical trials: using multiple imputation to deal with incomplete cost data. Clinical Trials 4:154–161

Cullum N, Ciliska D, Haynes B et al 2007 Evidence-based nursing: an introduction. Wiley/Blackwell, London

Culyer A, McCabe C, Briggs A, et al 2007 Searching for a threshold, not setting one: the role of the National Institute for Health and Clinical Excellence. Journal of Health Services Research and Policy 12:56–58

Department of Health 2004 NHS Reference costs 2004. Department of Health, London

Dolan P, Gudex C, Kind P et al 1995 A social tariff for EuroQol: results from a UK general population survey. University of York Centre for Health Economics Discussion Paper Series (no. 138), Centre for Health Economics, York

Drummond M F, O'Brien B, Stoddart G L et al 1997 Methods for the economic evaluation of healthcare programmes, 2nd edn. Oxford University Press, Oxford

Fenwick E, Byford S 2005 A guide to cost-effectiveness acceptability curves. British Journal of Psychiatry 187:106–108

Gillies C, Lambert, P C, Abrams, K R et al 2008 Different strategies for screening and prevention of type 2 diabetes in adults: cost effectiveness analysis. British Medical Journal 336:1180–1185

Glenny A M, Altman D G, Song F et al 2005 Indirect comparisons of competing interventions. Health Technology Assessment (Winchester, England) 9:1–134

Gold M R, Siegel J E, Russell L B et al 1996 Cost-effectiveness in health and medicine. Oxford University Press, Oxford

Iglesias C, Nelson E A, Cullum N A et al on behalf of the VenUS Team 2004 VenUS I: a randomised controlled trial of two types of bandage for treating venous leg ulcers. Health Technology Assessment (Winchester, England) 8(29):iii, 1–105

Iglesias C, Nixon J, Cranny G, et al 2006 Pressure relieving support surfaces (PRESSURE) trial: cost effectiveness analysis. British Medical Journal 332:1416

Kind P 1996 The EuroQol instrument: an index of health-related quality of life. In: Spilker B (ed) Quality of life and pharmacoeconomics in clinical trials, 2nd edn. Lippincott-Raven, Philadelphia

Lin D Y 2000 Linear regression analysis of censored medical costs. Statistical Medicine 1:35–47

Manca A, Dumville J C, Torgerson D J et al 2007 Randomized trial of two physiotherapy interventions for primary care back and neck pain patients: cost effectiveness analysis. Rheumatology 46:1495–1501, British Society for Rheumatology, Oxford University Press

Manca A, Willan A R 2006 'Lost in translation': accounting for between-country differences in the analysis of multinational cost-effectiveness data. Pharmacoeconomics 24:1101–1119

Manning R, Claxton K. 1997 Experimental and econometric solutions to selection bias. Paper presented at the Health Economists Study Group

McCabe C, Stevens K, Roberts J et al 2005 Health state values for the HUI 2 descriptive system: results from a UK survey. Health Economics 14:231–244

Moffett J K, Jackson D A, Gardiner E D, et al 2006 Randomized trial of two physiotherapy interventions for primary care neck and back pain patients: 'McKenzie' vs brief physiotherapy pain management. Rheumatology 45:1514–1521

National Institute of Health and Clinical Excellence (NICE) 2001 NICE technical guidance for manufacturers and sponsors on making a submission to a technology appraisal. NICE, London

National Institute of Health and Clinical Excellence (NICE) 2005 The clinical effectiveness and cost effectiveness of technologies for the secondary prevention of osteoporotic fractures in postmenopausal women. Technology Appraisal (TA87). NICE, London

National Institute of Clinical and Health Excellence (NICE) May 2008 Guide to the methods of technology appraisal. Online. Available: www.nice.org.uk/media/B52/A7/TAMethodsGuide updated June 2008.pdf [Feb 2009]

Neumann P J, Goldie S J, Weinstein M C 2000 Preference-based measures in economic evaluation in healthcare. Annual Review of Public Health 21:587–611

Nixon J, Cranny G, Iglesias C et al 2006 Randomised, controlled trial of alternating pressure mattresses compared with alternating pressure overlays for the prevention of pressure ulcers: PRESSURE (pressure relieving support surfaces) trial. British Medical Journal 332:1413

Nixon R M, Thompson S G 2005 Methods for incorporating covariate adjustment, subgroup analysis and between-centre differences into cost-effectiveness evaluations. Health Economics 14:1217–1229

Nixon R M, Bansback N, Brennan A 2007 Using mixed treatment comparisons and meta-regression to perform indirect comparisons to estimate the efficacy of biologic treatments in rheumatoid arthritis. Statistical Medicine 26:1237–1254

Philips Z, Ginnelly L, Sculpher M et al 2004 Review of guidelines for good practice in decision-analytic modelling in health technology assessment. Health Technology Assessment (Winchester, England) 8:iii–iv

Ramsey S, Willke R, Briggs A et al 2005 Good research practices for cost-effectiveness analysis alongside clinical trials: the ISPOR RCT-CEA Task Force report. Value Health 8:521–533

Sculpher M J, Claxton K, Drummond M et al 2006 Whither trial-based economic evaluation for healthcare decision making? Health Economics 15:677–687

Shiell A, Donaldson C, Mitton C et al 2002 Health economic evaluation. Journal of Epidemiology and Community Health 56:85–88

Siebert U. 2003 When should decision-analytic modelling be used in the economic evaluation of healthcare? European Journal of Health Economics 4:143–150

Sonnenberg F A, Beck J R 1993 Markov models in medical decision making: a practical guide. Medical Decision Making 13:322–338

Stevenson M, Jones M L, De Nigris E et al 2005 A systematic review and economic evaluation of alendronate, etidronate, risedronate, raloxifene and teriparatide for the prevention and treatment of postmenopausal osteoporosis. Health Technology Assessment (Winchester, England) 9:1–160

Sutton A J, Abrams K R, Jones D R et al 1998 Systematic reviews of trials and other studies. Health Technology Assessment (Winchester, England) 2(19):1–276

Torgerson D J, Raftery J 1999 Economic notes. Discounting. British Medical Journal 319:914–915

Weinstein M C, Stason W B 1977 Foundations of cost-effectiveness analysis for health and medical practices. New England Journal of Medicine 296:716–721

Willan A R, Briggs A H, Hoch J S 2004 Regression methods for covariate adjustment and subgroup analysis for non-censored cost-effectiveness data. Health Economics 13:461–475

Wright M, Grieve R, Roberts J et al 2006 on behalf of the UK Mild Hepatitis C Trial Investigators. Health benefits of antiviral therapy for mild chronic hepatitis C: randomised controlled trial and economic evaluation. Health Technology Assessment (Winchester, England) 10(21):iii, 1–113

Involving patients in decision making

Vikki Entwistle and Ian Watt

13

CHAPTER CONTENTS

KEY ISSUES

- The key concepts relating to patient involvement in decision making
- The most influential models for shared decision making and their limitations
- How nurses can facilitate patient involvement in practice

INTRODUCTION

Nurses today face and make an increasing range of decisions about patient care. Some are predominantly technical and are made by drawing on specialised knowledge and research-based information about the effects of different interventions, whereas others also need to draw on the values of individual patients. Table 2.1 (see p. 15), highlights the range of decision types faced by nurses (McCaughan et al 2005).

Nurses have always taken responsibility for important decisions about patient care but as the scope of nursing roles increases, nurses face and have responsibility for a broadening range of decisions. Indeed, some nurses are now employed in roles in which a major part of their job is to provide decision support to patients (e.g. in call centres such as NHS Direct, offering health-related information and advice).

It is increasingly expected that nurses, like other health professionals, will involve patients in decisions about their care as part of the provision of good quality healthcare. Many professional and patient organisations also advocate that patients should be involved in some way in decisions about their healthcare. For example, the Canadian Association of Nurses in Oncology (CANO) requires nurses to, 'collaborate with patients in developing a plan that fits the individual's preferences, beliefs and needs' (CANO 2001). The Long Term Conditions Alliance (LTCA – an 'umbrella' organisation for patient groups in the UK) aims to, 'promote participation by individuals in their own care and treatment and greater control over their own lives' (LTCA 2007). The US Preventive Services Task Force regards, patient–clinician partnership, as 'central to decision making' (Sheridan et al 2004).

This emphasis on patient involvement represents a major shift in the norms within which most healthcare professionals were expected to practise up until comparatively recently. This shift reflects a number of factors, including changes in social values as well as developments in healthcare and shifts in patient expectations. People in many countries are now generally less deferential to authority. Patients have thus become less willing to put up with paternalistic models of healthcare in which it is assumed that the professional knows best and makes decisions on behalf of patients without involving them. Developments in healthcare mean that most problems now have more than one reasonable management option. As different people prefer different options, it is important that individuals are involved in the decision-making process. There is also a growing – albeit imperfect – evidence base that supports the belief that involving patients in decision making can improve their healthcare outcomes (Coulter & Ellins 2007).

This has important implications for nurses. Consider, for example, a nurse working in a diabetes clinic. A single consultation in this clinic might require consideration of a range of health issues; as the following scenario illustrates:

" Mr A is a 57-year-old man with type 2 diabetes mellitus and is attending the clinic for annual review. He is on maximum dose of oral hypoglycaemics and yet his latest blood tests indicate his diabetes is poorly controlled. He has raised serum cholesterol. During the course of the review he mentions that over the last few months he has experienced episodes of chest pain when he has exerted himself. He has also developed a diabetic foot ulcer since he was last seen. "

The health issues identified in this routine (and simplified) scenario give rise to a number of possible management decisions including:

- Should Mr A continue with oral hypoglycaemic medication alone or should he be started on insulin?
- Should Mr A do nothing about his raised cholesterol, start a low-cholesterol diet, or start on cholesterol-lowering medication?
- Should Mr A be referred for a further opinion about his chest pain, be referred for further investigation, or simply monitored for a few more months?
- How should Mr A's diabetic foot ulcer be managed?

In the past, it might not have been within nurses' remit to make these decisions, but this is changing as the scope of nursing is extended. The various options for each health issue have different advantages and disadvantages for Mr A's health and quality of life. In the past, clinicians might simply have considered these in their own minds and made decisions without sharing their reasoning with Mr A or asking for his opinion. Mr A would simply have been presented with a course of action with which he was expected to comply. In the current environment, however, clinicians are encouraged to help patients to participate in decisions about their care and simply dictating a course of action to a patient without giving them an explanation or a hint of a say in the matter would be interpreted as poor quality care. The nurse working in the diabetic clinic would be expected to involve Mr A in the decisions.

KEY CONCEPTS

There are various ways in which patients might be said to be involved in healthcare decision making, and various criteria that might be used for assessing their involvement. In this section, we review basic models of professional–patient interaction during decision making, key considerations relating to the involvement of patients in decision processes, and the evaluation of different approaches to patient involvement.

Basic models of professional–patient interaction

There are three basic models of interaction between patients and healthcare professionals for treatment decision making in routine care: the paternalistic, shared decision making and informed patient models (Charles et al 1997, 1999). These models all assume that a patient has a health problem for which there are several relevant treatment options. They differ primarily in terms of the ways they envisage combining a healthcare professional's knowledge of the treatment options with the patient's personal preferences regarding those options and their attributes. They highlight three main activities: information transfer, deliberation and the selection of a treatment option to implement. The key features of these models are summarised in Table 13.1.

Involving patients in decision making

Table 13.1 Models of treatment decision making			
	Paternalistic model	*Shared decision-making model*	*Informed (patient) model*
Information transfer	Healthcare professionals transfer to patients the minimum information about healthcare options necessary for informed consent	Healthcare professionals give patients all the information about the options that is deemed necessary for decision making. Patients give healthcare professionals information about their personal preferences	Healthcare professionals transfer to patients all the information about the options that is deemed necessary for decision making
Deliberation	Healthcare professionals consider what would be best for each patient	Healthcare professionals and patients both consider what would be best	The patient considers what would be best for him or her
Decision about implementing treatment	Healthcare professionals decide which option will be implemented in each case	Healthcare professionals and patients agree together which option will be implemented	Patients decide which option will be implemented in their case

Based on Charles et al (1997, 1999).

Patients are quite obviously involved in the decision-making process in the shared decision-making model and the informed-patient model. Some patients might also *feel* involved in decision making that conforms to the paternalistic model if healthcare professionals explain their deliberations and decisions to them and leave them scope to discuss and decline a recommended option (Entwistle & Watt 2006, Entwistle et al 2008).

The models were developed on the basis of research into the roles played by doctors and patients in decision making about the treatment of breast cancer. It is thus not surprising that they seem most readily applicable to situations involving patients with acute health problems for which there is a well-defined set of treatment options. In other situations, a broader range of considerations may be important, including:

What happens before healthcare options are discussed?

We might consider several phases of decision making prior to the appraisal of a set of healthcare options (Box 13.1), and there are several reasons for thinking that it might be important to involve patients in these phases (Entwistle & Watt 2006). In primary care, for example, healthcare professionals might need to work with patients to decide an agenda for a consultation before they focus on one problem and consider the options associated with that (Murray et al 2006). In many situations, important work will need to be done to define or clarify the nature of the patient's health problem before potential solutions can be identified and appraised. Healthcare professionals and patients will need to share their thoughts and reach some kind of shared understanding about the nature of the problem if they are to be able to work together effectively to consider the options for dealing with it (Bugge et al 2006).

What happens after an option has been selected?

In the context of the management of long-term conditions in particular, patients are often required to administer their own treatment regimes. Their experiences may need to be reviewed and regimes adjusted on numerous occasions.

Box 13.1 Aspects of decision making

Decision making can be characterised and analysed in a range of ways. We might, for example, distinguish between a series of activities associated with decision making in healthcare contexts:

- Recognition and clarification of a problem (e.g. symptoms, concerns, diagnosis)
- Identification of potential solutions (e.g. tests, possible treatments)
- Appraisal of potential solutions
- Selection of one potential solution as the course of action to be followed
- Implementation of the chosen course of action (e.g. prescribing and taking of medication)
- Evaluation of the chosen course of action (e.g. monitoring of symptom resolution, side effects)

This might be better viewed as a continuation of patient involvement in a sequence or cycle of decision-making activity rather than something that happens separately after a particular healthcare option has been selected (Entwistle & Watt 2006).

What about the relationship between nurses and patients?

The management of long-term conditions also highlights that involvement in decision making is often more than the exchange of information and opinions about treatment options. In this and other contexts, the nature of the relationship between patients and their healthcare professionals may be a particularly significant feature in treatment decision making. Montori et al (2006) have suggested that a phase of 'establishing partnership' should be added to the shared decision-making model for the care of people with conditions such as diabetes, and we have suggested that patients' and clinicians' thoughts and feelings about their relationship with each other might be important domains of involvement (Entwistle & Watt 2006).

Although the models are helpful in distinguishing the key features of three basic patterns of interaction between healthcare professionals and patients during decision making, they don't explain *how*, for example, healthcare professionals and patients can deliberate together and reach agreement as outlined in the shared decision-making model (Wirtz et al 2006). This is considered further in the section, How do you involve patients?

Reasons for involving patients and criteria for evaluating decision making

As noted in the introduction, there are various reasons for sharing decisions for patients. These suggest different approaches to sharing decisions, and also different criteria for evaluating decision-making processes and outcomes (Entwistle et al 1998a).

One important reason for the increased interest in sharing decision making with patients is the recognition that for many health problems or issues there are several treatment or management options, and different people may have good reasons for favouring different solutions. This led to an interest in involving patients in decision making with a view to ensuring that the option selected in any particular case was the one that was most consistent with the individual patient's (informed) preferences relating to the different options and their attributes. The congruence between the healthcare a person receives and their personal values and preferences is now recognised as an important indicator of decision quality, an important goal of efforts to share decisions with patients, and a key criterion for evaluating efforts to support patient involvement in decision making (Box 13.2).

Another, related, reason for the increased interest in sharing decision making with patients has been a concern to respect patients' autonomy. The importance of informing patients about the potential consequences of different healthcare options and enabling them to make their own uncoerced decisions about the interventions they will receive has been a major theme in bioethics in recent years. This has led to a focus on the roles patients and

> **Box 13.2 International Patient Decision Aids Standards (IPDAS) criteria for assessing the effectiveness of decision aids**
>
> - Does the patient decision aid ensure that decision making is informed and values based?
>
> **DECISION PROCESSES LEADING TO DECISION QUALITY**
>
> Does the decision aid help patients to:
>
> - Recognise a decision needs to be made?
> - Know options and their features?
> - Understand that values affect decision?
> - Be clear about option features that matter most?
> - Discuss values with their practitioner?
> - Become involved in preferred ways?
>
> **DECISION QUALITY**
>
> Does the patient decision aid:
>
> - Improve the match between the chosen option and the features that matter most to the informed patient?
>
> ---
>
> Source: International Patient Decision Aids Standards Collaboration (2005) Criteria for judging the quality of patient decision aids. Online. Available: www.ipdas.ohri.ca/IPDAS_checklist.pdf [accessed 29 August 2007]

healthcare professionals play in decision-making processes, and a tendency to view the quality of decisions as somehow dependent on the question of who made them. In some situations, efforts to enable patients to make their own decisions might be appropriate, but a number of concerns have been raised recently about the narrowness of the dominant understanding of respect for autonomy in bioethics. In particular, it has been suggested that this overemphasises the importance of patients as independent choosers, especially when people are sick (Joffe et al 2003, Kukla 2005, Manson and O'Neill 2007). Also, it is increasingly recognised that unless they are very well supported, patients may make poor decisions about their healthcare. This may be because they have not adequately understood the nature and implications of the different options, because they struggle to recognise what matters most to them in relation to these, or because they succumb to errors in information processing (to which we are all prone, but which can be particularly problematic when we are ill and/or upset; Schwartz 2004, Ubel 2002).

Interest in sharing decision making with patients has also emerged from considerations of how to optimise the benefits that patients derive from healthcare. For decisions about lifestyle changes or medications that patients will take for themselves, for example, it seems plausible that patients who have been involved in the process of making the decision will better understand the rationale for the change or medication, be more committed to making or taking it, and thus be more likely to derive the intended health benefits (Collins et al 2007). Patients who are involved in treatment decisions may also benefit from an increased sense of understanding, control, and perhaps of being cared for and respected by the healthcare professionals with whom they engage.

While there are numerous good reasons for involving patients in decision making, the health consequences of different forms of patient involvement in different decision-making contexts are still largely unknown; it is possible that there may be disadvantages as well as benefits (Entwistle et al 1998b, McAffery et al 2007). Patients may experience 'decisional conflict' as they consider decisions for themselves, and may experience 'decision regret' as they reflect back on choices they have made – especially if the outcomes of the chosen intervention turn out to be poor (Brehaut et al 2003, O'Connor 1995). The health consequences of these experiences are poorly understood, but the experiences themselves are arguably important considerations in evaluations of different forms of patient involvement in decision making and efforts to promote these.

Questions of which rationales for involving patients are most important and which criteria should be given most weight in evaluations of different approaches to patient involvement, and different interventions to promote these, are the subject of significant debate; debate that we will not attempt to resolve in this chapter. It is important to note, however, that the answers to these questions may depend in part on the specific features of decision situations themselves. This is considered further in the section Issues and implications, below.

HOW DO YOU INVOLVE PATIENTS?

Some healthcare practitioners routinely practise in a way that facilitates the sharing of decisions with their patients. However, research that involves observing consultations often identifies deficiencies in the extent to which health professionals tell patients about healthcare options and elicit their views about these (Elwyn et al 2005, van den Brink-Muinen et al 2006). Surveys also continue to show that many patients report not being as involved as they would like to be in decisions about their care (Healthcare Commission 2005). In view of this, there is a growing interest in the skills needed by professionals to share decisions with patients, and in the development of training and support for health professionals that might help them to meet patient demand for greater involvement in decisions about their care.

Competencies for the practice of shared decision making have been proposed for both health professionals and patients (Elwyn et al 2000, Towle & Godolphin 1999). We focus here on those required of health professionals. Towle & Godolphin (1999) suggest that health professionals who seek to share decision making with patients need to:

1. Develop a partnership with the patient.
2. Establish or review the patient's preferences for information (such as amount or format).
3. Establish or review the patient's preferences for a role in decision making (such as risk taking and degree of involvement of self and others) and the existence and nature of any uncertainty about the course of action to take.
4. Ascertain and respond to patient's ideas, concerns and expectations (such as about disease management options).

5. Identify choices (including ideas and information that the patient may have) and evaluate the research evidence in relation to the individual patient.
6. Present (or direct patient to) evidence, taking into account competencies 2 and 3, framing effects (how presentation of the information may influence decision making), etc. Help patient to reflect on and assess the impact of alternative decisions with regard to his or her values and lifestyle.
7. Make or negotiate a decision in partnership with the patient and resolve conflict.
8. Agree an action plan and complete arrangements for follow up.

This list suggests a framework not just for practice but also for teaching, learning, and research. However, the competencies within it are not simple to define or to master. Each refers to at least one complex concept capable of several interpretations. If we consider the seventh competency, for example, we might ask just what it means to make a decision 'in partnership' with a patient, or just how conflict should be resolved when it occurs. Most people will require preparation and practice before they can demonstrate the competencies effectively.

Some rules of thumb might be helpful. If we consider the task of ascertaining a patient's ideas, concerns, and expectations, for example (the first part of the fourth competency), you might find the mnemonic ICE (ideas, concerns, expectations) useful and, in recognition of the fact that patients do not necessarily offer their ideas, concerns, and expectations spontaneously (or even be confident about communicating them to health professionals when asked), specific questions such as those listed in Box 13.3

Box 13.3 Possible questions for eliciting patients' ideas, concerns and expectations

IDEAS

- What do you think the treatment options are?
- Have you had any thoughts about how we might best deal with your problems?
- Have you read anything about how we might deal with your problem?

CONCERNS

- What concerns you most about the possibility of an operation?
- You seem anxious about starting on the tablets, do you think they might cause a problem?
- Is there something particularly concerning you about the immunisation?

EXPECTATIONS

- What had you hoped we might do to help your problem?
- If we go down this treatment path – what do you hope the result will be?
- What do you think would reassure you?

might be useful props. However, learning and using such phrases is unlikely to be sufficient to facilitate appropriate forms of involvement.

A well-nuanced application of a range of communication skills is likely to be needed, including:

- listening skills (e.g. encouraging, paraphrasing, reflecting feeling)
- questioning skills (e.g. open and closed questions)
- sending messages skills (e.g. providing feedback and providing information).

In addition, health professionals will need to tailor the approach they use to facilitate patient involvement to the attributes of each individual patient, their communication skills, ability to access and understand information in different languages and formats, and readiness to engage in decision making and discussions with health professionals.

The competencies for shared decision making should not be viewed in isolation and ideally need to be applied within a patient-centred approach (Stewart et al 1995). Although shared decision making is an important aspect of care, it is not the only thing that is important. The starting point for most healthcare interactions is the formation of a positive relationship between professional and patient, which requires compassion, empathy, and caring on the part of the professional. Without a positive relationship it is unlikely that patients will feel fully supported and involved in decision-making processes. The words of customer service staff who are taught to say 'have a nice day' to customers can sound hollow because they are often delivered in an unthinking and automatic way, lacking in any emotional engagement. In a similar way, if clinicians simply learn and rely on stock phrases for shared decision making, but lack a positive motivation to provide patient-centred care, patients may be left feeling inadequately involved in their care. For people with diabetes, for example, the ethos and feel of healthcare interactions has been found to be particularly important for a sense of involvement (Entwistle et al 2008).

Decision aids

The effective communication skills that are essential for supporting shared decision making might in some cases be complemented by resources designed specifically to help patients and health professionals who are facing difficult treatment or management option decisions. Decision aids are interventions designed to help people make specific and deliberative choices among options (including the status quo) by providing (at the minimum) information on the options and outcomes relevant to a patient's health. Aids may also include information on the disease or condition, probabilities of outcomes tailored to personal health-risk factors, an explicit exercise to clarify values, information on others' opinions, and guidance or coaching in the steps of decision making and communicating with others (O'Connor et al 1999).

Decision aids have been variously designed to be used within, or as adjuncts to, consultations between patients and clinicians. They come in a variety of formats including pamphlets, videos, and internet resources. They have been found to improve people's knowledge of management options, promote realistic expectations of their benefits and harms, reduce difficulty with decision making, increase patient participation in the decision-making process, and promote congruence between the treatment options that individuals receive and their informed preferences. However, their effects on health status and quality of life remain uncertain. (O'Connor et al 1999, 2007).

Decision aids vary in their quality; a feature that influences their impact and effectiveness. The standards developed by the International Patient Decision Aid Standards (IPDAS) Collaboration, might help health professionals and others to appraise decision aids before using them in practice. (Elwyn et al 2006, www.ipdas.ohri.ca).

Decision support

The competencies required for decision support in the context of healthcare consultations are important, but nurses sometimes find themselves in situations in which they are required to support patients who are facing decisions made by, and whilst under the care of, other health professionals. They may, for example, be asked questions by patients for whom they are providing supportive nursing care, or be asked for advice while working in health-related advisory or decision counselling roles. In such situations, a more focused framework for thinking about decision support might be helpful.

The Ottawa Decision Support Framework was developed to guide decision support interventions in a variety of settings in which no single healthcare option is clearly best, outcomes may be value laden, and deliberation challenging. It encourages healthcare providers to: (1) assess decision-support needs; (2) provide support tailored to those needs; and (3) evaluate clients' satisfaction with decision-making processes and outcomes. Assessments of decision-support needs involve exploring clients' perceptions of the decision that they face and the difficulties they are experiencing, their views about others involved in the decision, and the personal and external resources that are available to help them make the decision. Once the main sources of decisional conflict have been identified, particular forms of decision support, such as information (e.g. about health situation, options, and their outcomes, or others' experiences with particular outcomes), assistance with clarifying personal preferences, or guidance/coaching (e.g. in the processes of decision-making, communication with others, or access to resources and support) can be provided as appropriate (Murray et al 2004, O'Connor et al 1998).

ISSUES AND IMPLICATIONS

Attempts to involve patients in decisions about their care raise a number of practical and ethical questions. We introduce three key issues here.

1. Do patients want to participate?

Patients express varied preferences relating to their involvement in treatment and other healthcare decisions. A number of studies have used techniques that ask people to consider a set of short descriptions of different ways in which healthcare professionals and patients reach decisions and to say which of these they would prefer (Beaver et al 1999, Degner et al 1997, Strull et al 1984). An illustrative example of the type of question and descriptions used is shown in Box 13.4.

In most studies conducted in Anglophone counties, the majority of patients report that they prefer one of the roles in which both patient and doctor explicitly contribute to the decision-making process (roles like B, C, or D in Box 13.4) (Say et al 2006). Some aggregate differences can be discerned between people from different social and cultural groups (e.g. younger people, better-educated people, and women are less likely than older people, people with less education, and men to say they would like doctors to make treatment decisions for them). Even with these differences, the assumption in practice that, for example, any *particular* older man with limited education would prefer not to be involved is unwarranted.

People's views about the ways in which they should or would like to be involved in treatment decisions also vary according to their health condition and the types of decision they are facing (Say et al 2006). Studies that have asked patients to indicate *who* they think should undertake different decision-making tasks (e.g. problem clarification, option identification, option appraisal and selection) have found that their views differ across these tasks (Deber et al 2007).

The appropriateness of different forms of involvement is probably, at least in part, dependent on patients' preferences relating to these. However, it is important to remember that the basis of patients' expressed preferences for involvement might be unclear. If people have not previously experienced being given clear information and supported in contributing to or making healthcare decisions, they might not imagine themselves capable of understanding the options and making good decisions.

Box 13.4   The kind of question that is typically used to investigate patients' preferences for involvement in decision-making

Thinking about (decisions about your healthcare), which of the following do you prefer?

A. The doctor/nurse makes the decision
B. The doctor/nurse makes the decision after considering my opinion
C. The doctor/nurse and I make the decision together
D. I make the decision after considering the doctor's/nurse's opinions
E. I make the decision

2. In what situations should decisions be shared with patients?

If we think of the vast array of possible options that might be identified in the course of a person's healthcare, it seems impossible that patients could have whatever influence they wanted over decisions about them all. Some limits seem required on the grounds of practicality. Health services would become very much less efficient if there were no constraints on what patients could choose (imagine what might happen if, for example, patients thought they could demand a poorly evaluated and expensive alternative to a well-established and effective drug; to have their surgery in the operating theatre with their lucky number; or to have a particular brand of wound dressing that the hospital doesn't usually stock because it makes bulk purchases of another brand's equivalents).

Many constraints on individual choice are set by healthcare policies and by the protocols and purchasing decisions of service providers. Service users are increasingly represented on the groups that set the policies and protocols and make or monitor the purchasing decisions, and most of the constraints are reasonable and widely accepted. For example, most people are apparently happy for decisions to be made (carefully and) collectively about the types and brands of suture material and dressing that will be used to close and protect the different kinds of wounds that are routinely incurred during elective surgery.

It is important to think, however, about when to offer patients options, which constraints on choice should be explained to them, in what circumstances, and how (Entwistle et al 2006). There are no easy answers, and a number of considerations and values may come into play. Among the features of decision situations that may be pertinent to considerations of how patients can and should be involved in decision-making processes are those relating to:

1. The *people* whose healthcare is being considered. These may vary in terms of:
   a. How well or ill they are
   b. How familiar they are with, and how knowledgeable they are about, their health condition and healthcare options
   c. Their ability to take in and process information
   d. How confident they are discussing their situation and options with healthcare professionals
   e. Their inclination to be engaged in different ways in the decision-making process.
2. The *health issues or problems* to be addressed. These may vary in terms of:
   a. How serious or severe they are
   b. How urgently they need to be addressed
   c. How many healthcare interventions might be used to address them
   d. How similar or diverse the potential healthcare interventions are.
3. The *healthcare interventions* that might reasonably be considered. These may vary in terms of:
   a. How well they have been evaluated
   b. The short- and long-term benefits and harms that might be associated with them

c. The level of certainty attached to their possible outcomes

d. The extent to which their appropriateness or availability might vary with changes in the patient's condition, decisional delay, the adoption of other options

e. The reversibility of any poor outcomes that may result from them.

4. The *healthcare system* in which the decision is to be made may include:

a. Policies or regulations relating to the management of particular conditions and/or the use of particular interventions. These may restrict the availability of certain options to certain patients

b. Financing arrangements that require individual patients to make direct payments for particular interventions. These may bring cost considerations into treatment decision making at the individual level.

Opportunities to involve patients at the time of decision making can be limited. For example, in emergency situations when decisions need to be made quickly, treatment options may be highly complex, and patients are – if not unconscious – unlikely to feel or to be judged fit to process unfamiliar information and make their own well-reasoned decisions about irreversible courses of action that may have serious consequences. In such situations, there is a widespread consensus that health professionals should act quickly, making decisions with a view to preserving life and optimising the patient's chances of a good functional recovery.

By contrast, there may be significantly more opportunities to involve patients in decisions about the ongoing management of their long-term conditions such as diabetes or chronic obstructive pulmonary disease. Many people with such conditions will, especially if they have been well supported by health professionals in the past, have a good understanding of their problems and at least a reasonable appreciation of the different types of treatment that might be appropriate. Decisions about options to change long-term prescription medication regimes can usually be deliberated and deferred in the short term without adverse consequences, and some new medications can be tried out on a short-term basis to see how a particular patient gets on with them before committing to taking them over a longer term. Patients might also be involved in decisions about whether and when to undergo tests to monitor disease progression or the development of complications, although for some conditions in some healthcare systems a standardised schedule will strongly encourage particular choices (or remove choice altogether).

One widely discussed consideration is that of whether there is more than one healthcare option that might be considered reasonable for the healthcare situation, and the extent to which informed individuals would differ in their preferences for these. Some decisions are more sensitive to the different values or preferences of individual patients than others are, and it is widely accepted that it is particularly important to involve patients in the more value-sensitive (or preference-sensitive) decisions.

For example, it may be more important to inform a patient and family members about their options and encourage them to consider what would suit them best if they have: (1) terminal cancer (and the decision is about where to die); compared with (2) septicaemia (and the decision is about whether to receive antibiotic treatment or not). For people with septicaemia, treatment with antibiotics dramatically increases the chances of survival. The vast majority of people place a high value on survival, so the decision is not sensitive to individual preferences and there seems little need to ask patients to consider the statistics and weigh-up for themselves whether they would prefer to receive antibiotics. Indeed, the cognitive and emotional burden that would be placed on the patient by such a request would probably outweigh any benefit to be derived by making the decision in this context. This does not mean that there is no need to explain that antibiotic treatment is recommended and why, or that the patient's consent shouldn't be politely requested rather than roughly assumed.

By contrast, in a situation in which a person with terminal cancer is discussing with his or her palliative care nurse whether to die at home, in the hospice, or in the hospital, there is no clear evidence that one option is vastly better than the others in all significant respects. The decision is much more sensitive to individual patients' (and family members') circumstances, values, and preferences, and their input is much more obviously required for a good decision.

However, the distinction between values-sensitive and other decisions may be less clear cut than it first appears. Given the diversity of people's views, a case could be made for saying that most healthcare decisions are values-sensitive to some degree (there may always be at least a tiny minority of people who would reject an intervention that most people would overwhelmingly prefer). This consideration, combined with a concern not to impose unwanted interventions on individuals promotes a tendency to offer information and choice to everyone about everything – which we started by suggesting would be impractical!

That there is a difficult balance to be struck here is further highlighted when we consider the question of how individuals should be involved in decisions about healthcare interventions that are promoted – or even mandated – for public health purposes. Health visitors and practice nurses who are required to provide vaccinations for young children on standard schedules can sometimes find themselves 'pulled' between a concern to respect the preferences of parents who would prefer not to have their children vaccinated and a concern to promote widespread uptake of vaccinations to eliminate the risk of serious disease outbreaks within populations. These situations raise some interesting ethical tensions that have not been clearly resolved.

3. To what extent are nurses able to share decisions with patients?

As the previous section suggested, the options that nurses are able to offer to patients can be variously constrained by, among other things, national policies, local clinical protocols, and the procurement arrangements of the organisations for which they work. Nurses may feel more or less willing to support patients who are inclined to make choices that in the nurses' professional opinion may be detrimental to the patient's health. The implications of sharing decisions with patients for professional accountability have been largely neglected in this literature (Wirtz et al 2006) but fear of allegations of professional misconduct may tend to militate against the facilitation of patient involvement (or at least of support for certain patient preferences) in some situations. This issue needs further investigation and debate.

Nurses' capacity and inclination to involve patients and family members in healthcare decisions can be strongly influenced by the policies and cultural norms of their particular practice environments. For example, one study found that nurses and doctors working in wards used for the assessment and provision of respite care for older people with dementia did not involve family members to the extent that both they and the family members would have found helpful. In part, this was because there were no guidelines or requirements for such involvement, time and staffing pressures militated against it, and staff were not aware of the extent to which carers felt unable to participate in hospital systems that they experienced as oppressive (Walker & Dewar 2001).

Even in situations in which nurses have a specific remit to support patients facing treatment decisions, they may be constrained by the circumstances in which they work. An investigation of the decision support provided by nurses who worked in a call centre that aims, among other things, to enable callers to make 'sound health decisions' found that there was no clear, structured process for handling calls in which people sought help relating to decisions they were facing. Nurses working on the service lacked the knowledge, skills, and confidence to help callers to clarify their own values or preferences. When the service stocked patient-oriented decision aids for people facing particular decisions, these were difficult to use over the phone and organisational pressure to minimise the length of individual calls was a significant barrier to the provision of adequate support for people facing values-sensitive decisions (Stacey et al 2005).

SUMMARY

It is increasingly expected that nurses will involve patients in decisions about their care, and there are several good reasons for this. There are a number of ways in which patients might be said to be involved in decisions about their care, and different forms of involvement might be appropriate in different situations. The shared decision-making model, which emphasises the importance of an exchange of information about treatment options, mutual deliberation of these and the reaching of agreement about a course of action to implement, is a useful starting point but may need modification.

For some decision situations, nurses might find decision aids and structured approaches to the provision of decision support to be useful. Well-nuanced approaches to involving patients in decision making are likely to require a broad range of interpersonal competencies and a motivation to deliver patient centred care.

The formal rules and cultures of working environments may tend either to constrain or to promote the efforts of individual nurses to involve patients in their care.

Involving patients in decision making

RESOURCES

A great portal to a plethora of information, tools, and sites to help with steering patients through the complexities of choice in healthcare us: www. decisionaid.ohri.ca/index.html

Involve is part of the UK NHS dedicated to promoting public participation in healthcare decision making at a variety of levels (including policy making and research and development: www.involve.org.uk/home

Nothing beats a decent narrative when it comes to communicating some of the challenges of healthcare decision making. Healthtalkonline is a searchable multimedia database of patient experiences of heath states and care. Not only can it help show patients that other patients face similar challenges, but it can also help you better understand what your patients might be going through: www.healthtalkonline.org

---

EXERCISES

The list of competencies for shared decision making in the section How do you involve patients? provides a useful framework for communication skills training. It breaks the process of involving patients in decision making down into a manageable series of steps for discussion, role play, and reflection.

A number of key practical and ethical issues relating to the involvement of patients in decision making are as yet unresolved. Students and experienced nurses alike might find it helpful to discuss these with reference to specific examples. You could encourage individuals to present examples from their experiences in different placement or practice environments (or even from their experiences as patients or family carers) and then to discuss:

- Situations in which it might be more or less appropriate to follow a shared-treatment decision making or an informed-choice model (to encourage participants to share their reasons and their views).
- Challenges and concerns about involving patients in decisions.
- Suggestions about changes or interventions that might make it easier for nurses to involve patients in appropriate ways in decisions about their care.

REFERENCES

Beaver K, Bogg J, Luker K A 1999 Decision making role preferences and information needs: a comparison of colorectal and breast cancer. Health Expectations 2:266–276

Brehaut J A, O'Connor A M, Wood T J et al 2003 Validation of a decision regret scale. Medical Decision Making 23: 281–292

Bugge C, Entwistle V A, Watt I S 2006 Information that is not exchanged during consultations: significance for decision-making. Social Science and Medicine 63: 2065–2078

Canadian Association of Nurses in Oncology (CANO) 2001 Standards of care. Online. Available: www.cano-acio. org [accessed 28 August 2007]

Charles C, Gafni A, Whelan T 1997 Shared decision making in the medical encounter: what does it mean? (Or: it takes at least two to tango). Social Science and Medicine 44:681–692

Charles C, Gafni A, Whelan T 1999 Decision-making in the physician–patient encounter: revisiting the shared treatment decision making model. Social Science and Medicine 49:651–661

Collins S, Britten N, Ruusuvuori J et al 2007 Patient participation in healthcare consultations – qualitative perspectives. Oxford University Press, Maidenhead

Coulter A, Ellins J 2007 Effectiveness of strategies for informing, educating, and involving patients. British Medical Journal 335:2427

Deber R B, Kraetschmer N, Urowitz S et al 2007 Do people want to be autonomous patients? Preferred roles in treatment decision making in several patient populations. Health Expectations 10:248–258

Degner L F, Sloan J A, Venkatesh P 1997 The control preferences scale. Canadian Journal of Nursing Research 29:21–43

Elwyn G, Edwards A, Kinnersley P et al 2000 Shared decision making and the concept of equipoise: the competencies of involving patients in healthcare choices. British Journal of General Practice 50: 892–899

Elwyn G, Hutchings H, Edwards A et al 2005 The OPTION scale: measuring the extent that clinicians involve patients in decision-making tasks. Health Expectations 8:34–42

Elwyn G, O'Connor A, Stacey D et al 2006 Developing a quality criteria framework for patient decision aids: online international Delphi consensus process. British Medical Journal 333: 417 [online 22 August 2006]

Entwistle V A, Watt I S 2006 Patient involvement in treatment decision making: the case for a broader conceptual framework. Patient Education and Counselling 63(3): 268–278

Entwistle V, Sowden A, Watt I 1998a Evaluating interventions to promote patient involvement in decision-making: by what criteria should effectiveness be judged? Journal of Health Services Research and Policy 3:100–107

Entwistle V A, Sheldon T A, Sowden A J et al 1998b Evidence informed patient choice: practical issues of involving patients in decisions about healthcare technologies. International Journal of Technology Assessment in Healthcare 14: 212–225

Entwistle V A, Williams B, Skea Z et al 2006 Which surgical decisions should patients participate in? Reflections on women's recollections of discussions about different types of hysterectomy. Social Science and Medicine 62: 499–509

Entwistle V A, Prior M, Skea Z C et al 2008 Involvement in decision-making: a qualitative investigation of its meaning for people with diabetes. Social Science and Medicine 66: 362–375

Healthcare Commission 2005 Primary care trust survey: key findings report, appendices. Online. Available: www.healthcarecommission.org.uk/_db/_documents/04019374.pdf [accessed 7 November 2006]

Joffe S, Manocchia M, Weeks J C et al 2003 What do patients value in their hospital care? An empirical perspective on autonomy centred bioethics. Journal of Medical Ethics 29:103–108

Kukla R 2005 Conscientious autonomy: displacing decisions in healthcare. Hastings Center Report 35:34–44

Long Term Conditions Alliance (LTCA) 2007 About LTCA. Online. Available: www.ltca.org.uk [accessed 28 May 2008]

McAffery K, Shepherd H L, Trevena L et al 2007 Shared decision-making in Australia. Zeitschrift für ärztliche Fortbildung und Qualitätssicherung 101(4):205–211

McCaughan D, Thompson C, Cullum N et al 2005 Nurse practitioner and practice nurses' use of research information in clinical decision making: findings from an exploratory study. Family Practice 22: 490–497

Manson N C, O'Neill O 2007 Rethinking informed consent in bioethics. Cambridge University Press, Cambridge

Montori V, Gafni A, Charles C 2006 A shared treatment decision-making approach between patients with chronic conditions and their clinicians: the case of diabetes. Health Expectations 9:25–36

Murray M A, Miller T, Fiset et al 2004 Decision support: helping patients and their families to find a balance at the end of life. International Journal of Palliative Nursing 10: 270–277

Murray E, Charles C, Gafni A 2006 Shared decision-making in primary care:

tailoring the Charles et al. model to fit the context of general practice. Patient Education and Counselling 62:205–211

O'Connor A M 1995 Validation of a decisional conflict scale. Medical Decision Making 15:25–30

O'Connor A M, Tugwell P, Wells G A et al 1998 A decision aid for women considering hormone replacement therapy after menopause: decision support framework and evaluation. Patient Education and Counseling, 33:267–279

O'Connor A M, Rostom A, Fiset V et al 1999 Decision aids for patients facing health treatment or screening decision: a systematic review. British Medical Journal 319:731–734

O'Connor A M, Bennett C, Stacey D et al 2007 Do patient decision aids meet effectiveness criteria of the international patient decision aids standards collaboration? Medical Decision Making 27(5):554–574

Say R, Murtagh M, Thomson R 2006 Patients' preference for involvement in medical decision-making: a narrative review. Patient Education and Counseling 60:102–114

Schwartz B 2004 The paradox of choice: why more is less. Harper Collins, New York

Sheridan S L, Harris R P, Woolf S H 2004 Shared decision making about screening and chemoprevention. American Journal of Preventive Medicine 26:56–66

Stacey D, Graham I D, O'Connor A M et al 2005 Barriers and facilitators influencing

call center nurses' decision support for callers facing values-sensitive decisions: a mixed methods study. Worldviews on Evidence-Based Nursing 2(4):184–195

Stewart M M, Brown J B, Weston W W et al (eds) 1995 Patient-centered medicine: transforming the clinical method. Sage, Thousand Oaks, CA

Strull W M, Lo B, Charles G 1984 Do patients want to participate in medical decision making? Journal of the American Medical Association, 252: 2990–2994

Towle A, Godolphin W 1999 Framework for teaching and learning informed shared decision making. British Medical Journal 319:766–771

Ubel PA 2002 Is information always a good thing? Helping patients make 'good' decisions. Medical Care 40 (9, supplement): v39–v44

van den Brink-Muinen A, van Dulmen S M, de Haes H C J M et al 2006 Has patients' involvement in the decision-making process changed over time? Health Expectations 9:333–342

Walker E, Dewar B 2001 How do we facilitate carers' involvement in decision making? Journal of Advanced Nursing 34(3): 329–337

Wirtz V, Cribb A, Barber N 2006 Patient–doctor decision-making about treatment within the consultation: a critical analysis of models. Social Science and Medicine 62: 116–124

Communicating risks and benefits

Dawn Dowding and Carl Thompson

14

KEY ISSUES

- What is risk communication?
- Why risk communication is important
- Verbal descriptions of risk
- Numerical presentations of risk
- Graphical presentations of risk

WHAT IS RISK COMMUNICATION?

In Chapter 3, we outlined how to express uncertainty using numbers and the language of probability. In healthcare, we often have to communicate our uncertainties to other healthcare professionals or more commonly, to patients. We communicate the risks, benefits, and uncertainties of our actions to:

- Encourage a person to change their behaviour to reduce their risk of a 'bad' thing happening to them in the future. By, for example, encouraging a patient to stop smoking and by providing them with information about their risk of developing heart disease if they do not.
- Ensure that a person is fully informed about the risks and benefits associated with a medical or nursing intervention as part of securing informed consent.
- Avoid over-reactions to potential but rare hazards. For example, reassuring an adolescent in primary care about the lack of evidence to link using his or her mobile phone to developing cancer (Lipkus 2007).

In this chapter, we explore the different ways in which this type of information can be communicated. We also provide some insights into what may be the best way of communicating risk for different types of decision problem.

WHY IS RISK COMMUNICATION IMPORTANT?

As should already be apparent from other chapters in this book, health professionals and patients have to make decisions in conditions of uncertainty. We need to communicate this uncertainty to ensure that patients and colleagues can contextualise the choices they face. To make *informed* decisions, we need to have some idea of what the chances are of different outcomes occurring (based on research evidence where possible). If patients have a good understanding of the decisions they are faced with, then the chances of them adhering to treatment are also raised (Epstein et al 2004).

How we communicate information to patients will affect the decisions they take. Look at the two scenarios in Box 14.1 It should be apparent that despite being phrased in two different ways, the two scenarios are providing the same information. In scenario 1, the information about the potential outcomes of surgery and radiation therapy are provided in terms of how many people are likely to survive, and in scenario 2 they are provided in terms of how many people are likely to die. A number of experiments have been carried out giving people either scenario 1 or scenario 2 and asking them which treatment they would choose. What is typically found is that the proportion of individuals who would choose to have radiation therapy is around 18% for scenario 1 and around 44% for scenario 2 (Tversky & Kahneman 1988). In other words, people are more likely to find radiation therapy 'less risky' when its outcomes are phrased in terms of a *reduction* in the risk of immediate death (0% for radiation therapy vs. 10% for surgery) rather than an *increase* in the likelihood of immediate survival (100% for radiation therapy vs. 90% for surgery). The choice depends on how it is 'framed'.

This framing effect happens in a number of different types of healthcare decision. Moxey et al (2003) carried out a systematic review evaluating the

---

Box 14.1   The framing of decisions

SCENARIO 1

Surgery: of 100 people having surgery, 90 live through the postoperative period, 68 are alive at the end of the first year, and 34 are alive at the end of 5 years.
   Radiation therapy: of 100 people having radiation therapy, all live through the treatment, 77 are alive at the end of 1 year, and 22 are alive at the end of 5 years.

SCENARIO 2

Surgery: of 100 people having surgery, 10 die during surgery or the postoperative period, 32 die by the end of the first year, and 66 die by the end of 5 years.
   Radiation therapy: of 100 people having radiation therapy, none die during treatment, 23 die by the end of 1 year, and 78 die by the end of 5 years.

effect of framing outcomes in different ways on decisions taken by patients. They looked at studies that examined decisions on surgical treatment, medical treatment, immunisation, and health behaviour change. When probabilities were expressed in terms of survival (positive framing), more people chose a surgical option or increased their preference for invasive or toxic treatments. In studies that looked at immunisation decisions, a positive frame increased participants' expectations of benefits and reduced their expectation of side effects. Similarly, in studies examining the impact of framing on health behaviour, choices framed in terms of gains to health rather than losses meant that individuals were more likely to exhibit the desired health behaviour.

So the way that information about risks are described (framed) affects the decisions that individuals take. As nurses not only do we have a duty to ensure that patients are informed about the decisions they are faced with, we also need to ensure that we do not unduly influence those decisions. Therefore, ensuring that we communicate information about risks and benefits of medical and nursing interventions in a way that individuals can understand, but that is as objective as possible, is important. Individuals are all different, communicating information to patients involves being able to talk about risk in more than one way (Moxey et al 2003).

VERBAL DESCRIPTIONS OF RISK

One of the most common ways in which we can communicate the risk of an event occurring is by using verbal descriptions such as 'rarely' or 'frequently'. The number of different phrases we can use to talk about risk is considerable. Sutherland and colleagues (1991) examined the variety of ways of communicating risks to cancer patients. They counted the different words used to describe risk on 15 different consent forms for clinical trials being undertaken in their unit. They found 13 different phrases for describing the probability of a risk or benefit of different treatments. In another study, Timmermans and colleagues (2004) used 18 different phrases to describe risk. The full list of all the different phrases used in these two studies is given in Table 14.1.

Intuitively, we think that these qualitative expressions are easy to understand. But what they *mean* to different individuals varies greatly. In the same study, Sutherland et al (1991) asked cancer patients to give a numerical estimate for each word. The estimate was the frequency with which they thought an event would occur from 0% through to 100%. What they found was a wide variation between patients about the likelihood induced by the word. Doctors at different levels of experience were also asked to give numerical estimates of the qualitative terms used in the study (Timmermans et al 2004). As with the Sutherland study, Timmermans found large differences in doctors' interpretations of verbal expressions. 'Extremely rare' ranged from 0% to 15% and the value of 'very likely' ranged from 40% to 99%.

So what does this mean in practice? Box 14.2 contains an example of patient information about non-steroidal anti-inflammatory drugs (NSAIDs). We have put all the descriptive phrases used to describe the risks associated with taking NSAIDs in bold. The patient information suggests that *sometimes* using NSAID will cause bleeding and ulcer development. Think for a minute

Table 14.1   Different verbal descriptions of probability

From Sutherland et al (1991)	From Timmermans (1994)
May occur	Extremely rarely
Occasionally	A very low percent
Possible	A very small percent
Very rarely	Rather unlikely
Rarely	A low chance
Less common	A modest chance
Small chance	Sometimes
Common	Cannot be excluded
Frequently	Possibly
Unlikely	Not always
Likely	A reasonably large
Unusual	Quite possible
Usually	Quite high
	Often
	A large chance
	Quite likely
	Usually
	Very likely

Box 14.2   Verbal descriptions of probability used in patient information

FROM CLINICAL KNOWLEDGE SUMMARIES

www.cks.library.nhs.uk/patient_information_leaflet/anti_inflammatories_non_steroidal

Most people who take NSAIDs do not experience any major side effects. However, you should always read the leaflet that comes with the tablets as it will list all the cautions and possible side effects. The **most commonly** reported side effect of long-term use of NSAIDs is stomach irritation. If taken over long periods of time, NSAIDs can irritate your stomach lining and may cause it to bleed. **Sometimes**, this can lead to an ulcer developing. If you have to take NSAIDs for a persistent or recurring problem, your doctor may also prescribe anti-ulcer medication, to prevent ulcers. If you are taking NSAIDs and you develop upper abdominal pains, pass blood or black stools, or vomit blood, you should stop taking the medication immediately. Also, you should see your doctor as soon as possible or go to the nearest casualty department. NSAIDs can worsen the effects of kidney disorders, so are not advised for people with this condition. **In rare cases**, NSAIDs may cause an allergic reaction, usually resulting in a painless skin rash.

---

about what you think this means. Does it mean that 5% of people will develop an ulcer? 10%? More than 10%? In fact, the evidence from research studies suggests that around 20–30% of patients will probably develop an ulcer if they take NSAIDs (North of England Dyspepsia Guideline Development Group 2004). Do you think that the phrase *sometimes* reflects the frequency with which this side effect occurs? Would it make a difference to your choice if faced with having to take NSAIDs or an alternative? Using verbal descriptions of risk or probability in our communications may lead to misinterpretations of the actual risks associated with particular interventions.

NUMERICAL PRESENTATIONS OF RISK

One way of overcoming the problems of communicating risk using qualitative descriptions is to increase the precision of information by using numbers. This can be done in a number of ways. Table 14.2 gives an overview of some common presentations of risk and benefit. All of the figures used in the example in Table14.2 refer to the same set of research results but it is clear that the numbers used to present the risks or benefits vary greatly. Depending on the numerical presentation you use, you could be suggesting that using nicotine replacement therapy (NRT) increases the chances of stopping smoking by 70% (relative risk) or by 7% (absolute risk). Like framing,

Table 14.2	Numerical presentations of risk	
Risk presentation	Definition	Example
Frequency	Raw observations of the frequency with which an event occurs in the population*	3840 patients out of 22,732 gave up smoking for more than 6 months with nicotine replacement therapy, compared to 2122 patients out of 20,308 who received placebo. Alternatively, you could say that 17 in 100 people give up smoking using nicotine replacement therapy, compared to 10 in 100 people who received a placebo
Probability	A measure that quantifies the uncertainty associated with an event*	The probability of a person giving up smoking if they take nicotine replacement therapy is 17%, compared to 10% without nicotine replacement therapy
Absolute risk	The absolute arithmetic difference in rates of bad/good outcomes between experimental and control participants in a trial**	Taking nicotine replacement therapy increases the chance that you will give up smoking by 7%
Relative risk reduction/ benefit increase	The proportional reduction in rates of bad outcomes/increase in rates of good outcomes between experimental and control participants in a trial**	Taking nicotine replacement therapy increases the chances of you stopping smoking by 70%
Number needed to treat	The number of patients who need to be treated to achieve one additional favourable outcome**	You would need to treat 14 patients with nicotine replacement therapy for one person to stop smoking

*Moore and McQuay (2006).
**Sackett DL et al (2000).

the ways in which risk is presented numerically also affects the types of decisions that patients take.

In relation to Table 14.2, a recent Cochrane review has evaluated the evidence for using NRT to help individuals stop smoking (Stead et al 2008). The results from the 132 trials, for any type of nicotine therapy compared to placebo are given in Table 14.2 in different formats. Actual rates: 3840 out of 22,732 on NRT gave up after 6 months vs. 2122 out of 20,308 in control.

In a systematic review of studies examining the effects of presenting different numerical formats of risk to physicians and patients Covey (2007) identified three distinct ways of presenting relative risk:

- Explicitly using the term 'relative' in the description of risk (e.g. 'Using NRT results in a relative increase in the chance of stopping smoking of 70%').
- Using the term 'reduced/increased' or 'reduced by/increased by' (e.g. NRT increases the likelihood of stopping smoking by 70%).
- Stating the risk as a percentage (e.g. for NRT a 70% increase in smoking cessation was demonstrated).

Just as with relative risks, Covey (2007) also highlights variability in the way that absolute risk in studies may be presented: clinicians often use a mixture of percentages and frequencies.

When individuals are given risk information in the format of relative rather than absolute risk (or its reciprocal, the number needed to treat; NNT), they are more likely to rate a treatment more favourably or choose it as their favoured option (Covey 2007). The formats in which relative or absolute risks are presented also influence choice. Individuals are more likely to favour a treatment when relative risk is phrased as a percentage, and less likely to favour it if they are also given information on the baseline risk (absolute risk in a group with no treatment), or given absolute risks in the format of frequency rather than percentages (Covey 2007). A separate systematic review (Trevena et al 2006) suggests that patients understand risk information better if it is communicated in the form of natural frequencies rather than probabilities – a finding also seen in the non-clinical world (Gigerenzer 2002). Trevena and colleagues (2006) point out that patients understand changes in risk if they are first given baseline figures with which to compare the difference.

So what is the most effective way for you to communicate numerically the risks and/or benefits associated with specific treatments to your patients? In general, you should probably use natural frequencies (such as, 'in 100 people just like you, 17 people will give up smoking using NRT') rather than probabilities ('the probability of a person giving up smoking if they take NRT is 17%'). You should probably also use absolute rather than relative risks, and provide some idea of the baseline measure of risk (if appropriate). For example, a woman's lifetime absolute risk of breast cancer is one in nine. That is to say, one woman in every nine will develop breast cancer at some point in their lives. It is also good practice to ensure that the denominator that you use to express frequencies is common across all of the information you provide (e.g. always give numbers as X out of 100, or X out of 1000 rather than a mixture of the two).

Another area where communication of risks using numbers is common is the clinical discussion that accompanies the results of diagnostic tests or the potential risks and benefits associated with health or illness screening. This often involves explaining *conditional probabilities* to patients (or other healthcare professionals; this is discussed in Chapters 3 and 9). In this instance, you need to take into account the chance or probability of someone with a positive test/screening result having a disease *given* the prevalence of the condition in the population, and the diagnostic accuracy of the diagnostic/screening test. Gigerenzer (2002) argues that it is intuitively quite difficult for healthcare professionals (and patients) to understand this type of information, even if you understand how to make sense of it using techniques such as 2 × 2 tables that were outlined in Chapter 11. However, if you present the same information in the form of natural frequencies, individuals have much less difficulty working out what the chances are of an individual having the disease (Gigerenzer 2002). As an example, Box 14.3 gives an example of a decision problem in both probability and natural frequency formats.

For decisions associated with screening or diagnostic tests, where you need to work out and communicate the likelihood of an individual with a particular test result actually having (or not having) the disease in question, you may be better considering the decision problem in the form of natural frequencies.

GRAPHICAL PRESENTATIONS OF RISK

A key issue when considering how the communication of risk to patients (and other healthcare professionals) is our inability to understand numeric information at all; sometimes referred to as 'collective innumeracy' (Sedrakyan & Shih 2007). An alternative that is more precise than using verbal descriptors,

---

Box 14.3   Conditional probabilities vs. natural frequencies

CONDITIONAL PROBABILITIES

Take a woman aged 40–50 in a particular region of the country:

"The probability that one of these women has breast cancer is 0.8%. If a woman has breast cancer, the probability is 90% that she will have a positive mammogram. If a woman does not have breast cancer, the probability is 7% that she will still have a positive mammogram. Imagine a woman who has a positive mammogram. What is the probability that she actually has breast cancer?"

NATURAL FREQUENCIES

Take a woman aged 40–50 in a particular region of the country:

"Eight out of every 1000 women have breast cancer. Of these eight women with breast cancer, seven will have a positive mammogram. Of the remaining 992 women who don't have cancer, some 70 will still have a positive mammogram. Imagine a sample of women who have positive mammograms in screening. How many of these women actually have breast cancer?"

and possibly easier to understand than numbers, is to use graphics. Graphs may be easier to understand because they provide information in a format that is more easily processed (Ancker et al 2006).

Formats for graphically presenting risk information include bar graphs (histograms), pie charts, icon arrays (stick or facial displays), line graphs, risk ladders, risk tables, and risk scales (see the examples in Figure 14.1). Lipkus & Hollands (1999) suggest that using graphics to present risks should:

- show how large or small the risk is
- compare the size of two risks (relative risk)
- indicate risk over time (cumulative risk)
- highlight the variability in risk (uncertainty)
- show interactions between risk factors.

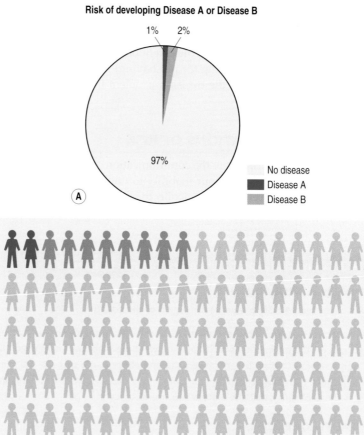

Figure 14.1 Examples of different ways of graphically presenting risk. (A) pie chart; (B) icon displays;

Continued

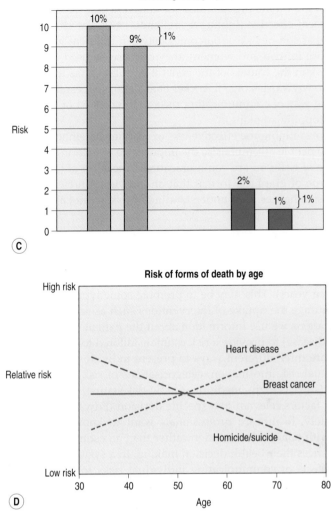

Figure 14.1 – cont'd (C) bar graphs; (D) line graph.

The type of risk you are trying to communicate should be matched to the most appropriate type of graph for displaying that risk. For instance, risk ladders are useful for helping people to identify the risks associated with different types of behaviour, anchored against high and low reference points (Lipkus & Hollands 1999). Stick figures or faces (icon displays) are commonly used to provide individuals with information about their risk of developing a condition (such as breast cancer) over a period of time, and how that risk changes with different interventions (e.g. taking hormone replacement therapy). However, this form of risk presentation might not always be popular with individuals (Lipkus & Hollands 1999). When used to present small probabilities, they can encourage people to be risk averse.

Line graphs are useful and effective for giving people risk information on an event over time (Lipkus & Hollands 1999). Pie charts are often used to communicate the proportion of individuals at risk of developing illnesses and, so long as joint probabilities for different risk factors are presented together, seem effective (Lipkus & Hollands 1999). Bar charts or histograms allow comparison of risk of outcomes between different groups (e.g. risk of heart disease in men and women), they can also be used to look at an individual's risk in the context of the general population (as in the 'QRisk' scoring system: www.qrisk.org/). Ancker et al (2006) suggest that bar graphs are an effective way of communicating risks in the context of behaviour change (such as stopping smoking).

Studies examining the effectiveness of graphical methods of communicating risks to people all emphasise the importance of tailoring the method used to the type of risk you are communicating. Ancker et al (2006) also suggest that the type of graphical format that an individual prefers and the format which most enhances their understanding of risk are not always the same.

THE BENEFITS OF INDIVIDUAL RISK COMMUNICATION

In healthcare, we are often trying to communicate a patient's *individual* risk of an event occurring (e.g. such as their risk of developing heart disease in the next ten years). This may be to promote some type of behaviour change or to encourage the uptake of interventions such as screening. In individual risk estimations we use information about the patient (such as their risk factors for a disease) to provide a risk estimate tailored to them (as with QRisk).

There are three different ways to present individual risk: individual risk scores/actual risk information, categorisations of risk status based on these estimates (such as high-, medium-, or low-risk status), or a discussion of personal risk factors relevant to a specific decision (Edwards et al 2003).

Ultimately, healthcare professionals want to know whether providing patients with tailored information rather than an estimate based on populations enhances their health decision making. In a systematic review examining the effects of communicating individual risks for screening decisions, Edwards et al (2003) found that providing individualised risk profiles was associated with higher uptake of screening tests (such as mammography, breast cancer risk, gene testing, and screening for high cholesterol). They also identified a trend suggesting that individuals at higher risk of a disease were more likely to choose to be screened if they were given individual risk information. Of course, this will not help if screening itself is ineffective and fails to prevent deaths or promote health.

SUMMARY

The way in which you communicate the risks and benefits associated with different healthcare interventions to patients can affect the decisions that patients subsequently make. It is important, therefore, that you understand what you are trying to achieve when communicating such information, and choose the most appropriate format for communicating the information to patients in ways that they can understand. Despite qualitative expressions of risk being open to misinterpretation, this type of communication is very common. This could be because clinicians are reluctant to give numerical estimates, and so imply a level of precision that does not exist (Timmermans et al 2004) or that the precise risk for an individual patient is unknown (Timmermans et al 2004). However, if you want to ensure that patients understand what the risks are associated with either a healthcare intervention, or their own behaviour, then using verbal descriptors of risk are probably ineffective.

Numerical ways of presenting risk information can provide a more accurate evaluation of risk (Lipkus 2007). When giving risk information numerically ensure that you use the same denominator, avoid decimal places, try to use frequencies rather than probabilities, where possible use absolute rather than relative risks, and if you do have to use relative risks make sure that you have a baseline value for individuals to compare to (Lipkus 2007).

If you are using graphs to provide risk information, then try to choose a format that suits the type of decision that a person is being faced with. Bar graphs are useful to help individuals make comparisons between different interventions, line graphs are useful for showing trends over time, pie charts for judging proportions, and icons for displaying the number of individuals affected by a disease within a population (Lipkus 2007). If you do use graphs, then make sure that you provide clear explanations of what they show to the person looking at them.

EXERCISES

Using the QRisk (www.qrisk.org/) calculator, imagine you are running a health-promotion clinic in primary care. Your population has a Jarman score of 42 (higher than average indicating a higher demand for primary care). How might you use the QRisk tool to communicate the need for lifestyle changes in the community members that you are working with?

REFERENCES

Ancker J, Senathirajah Y, Kukafka R et al 2006 Design features of graphs in health risk communication: A systematic review. Journal of the American Medical Informatics Association 13:608–618

Covey J 2007 A meta-analysis of the effects of presenting treatment benefits in different formats. Medical Decision Making 27:638–654

Edwards A, Unigwe S, Elwyn G et al 2003 Effects of communicating individual risks in screening programmes: Cochrane systematic review. British Medical Journal 327:703–709.

Epstein R, Alper B Quill T 2004 Communicating evidence for participatory decision making. Journal of the American Medical Association 291:2359–2366

Gigerenzer G 2002 Reckoning with risk. Learning to live with uncertainty. Penguin, London

Lipkus I 2007 Numeric, verbal, and visual formats of conveying health risks: suggested best practices and future recommendations. Medical Decision Making 27:696–713

Lipkus I, Hollands J 1999 The visual communication of risk. Journal of the National Cancer Institute Monographs 25:149–163

Moore A, McQuay H 2006 Bandolier's little book of making sense of the medical evidence. Oxford University Press, Oxford, 390–409

Moxey A, O'Connell D, McGettigan P 2003 Describing treatment effects to patients. How they are expressed makes a difference. Journal of General Internal Medicine 18:959

North of England Dyspepsia Guideline Development Group 2004 Dyspepsia: managing dyspepsia in adults in primary care (report no. 112). Centre for Health Services Research Report, University of Newcastle upon Tyne

Sackett D L, Straus S E, Richardson W S et al 2000 Evidence-based medicine. How to practice and teach EBM. Churchill Livingstone. Edinburgh, p 251–252

Sedrakyan A, Shih C 2007 Improving depiction of benefits and harms. Analyses of studies of well-known therapeutics and review of high-impact medical journals. Medical Care 45:S23–S28

Stead L F, Perera R, Bullen C et al 2008 Nicotine replacement therapy for smoking cessation. Cochrane Database of Systematic Reviews Issue 1. Art. No. CD000146. DOI: 10.1002/14651858. CD000146.pub3

Sutherland H, Lockwood G, Tritchler D et al 1991 Communicating probabilistic information to cancer patients: is there 'noise' on the line? Social Science and Medicine 32 725–731

Timmermans D, Molewijk B, Stigglebout A et al 2004 Different formats for communicating surgical risks to patients and the effect on choice of treatment. Patient Education and Counseling 54:255–263

Trevena L, Davey H, Baratt A et al 2006 A systematic review on communicating with patients about evidence. Journal of Evaluation in Clinical Practice 12:13–23

Tversky A, Kahneman D 1988 Rational choice and the framing of decisions. In: Bell D, Raiffa H, Tversky A (eds) Decision making. Descriptive, normative and prescriptive interactions. Cambridge University Press, Cambridge, UK 167–192

Teaching clinical decision making and judgement

Carl Thompson and Dawn Dowding

KEY ISSUES

- Key issues in teaching clinical decision making and judgement in nursing
- Teaching strategies
- Resources of helping with teaching clinical decision making and judgement in nursing

KEY ISSUES IN TEACHING CLINICAL DECISION MAKING AND JUDGEMENT IN NURSING

The content of this chapter is based predominantly on our experience of teaching clinical decision making and judgement to nurses and doctors with a range of clinical experience. Teaching decision making is challenging; it is predominantly a cognitive (thought) process, which makes it difficult to explain, demonstrate, and assess (Christie et al 2000). As should be apparent to you from reading the rest of this book, there is no simple explanation for how we make clinical decisions and judgements, and no one 'right' way of reaching a specific clinical decision or judgement. Therefore, in this chapter we outline approaches to teaching decision making that we have adopted, based on our understanding of the research literature examining how clinicians make clinical judgements and decisions, and our belief that we should be providing nurses (and other healthcare professionals) with a 'toolkit' that they can use to ensure that their decisions are based (where possible) on good-quality research evidence. This toolkit includes ways of identifying research evidence, and strategies for combining the results of research studies that are appropriate for different types of decision problem. Our overall aim is to encourage nurses to question their approach to decision making in practice, and hopefully adopt some of the techniques we teach them (where appropriate) to help with their decision making.

What follows are suggestions that cover some of the areas of clinical decision making and judgement discussed in this book. For each section, we have provided an outline set of learning outcomes, which reflect the types of learning we would anticipate students achieving at different levels of experience.

SOME THEORETICAL UNDERPINNINGS

Both the authors came to teaching first as practising nurses (teaching other nurses), then as students (undertaking PhDs and teaching to earn some extra cash), and finally as researchers (eager to get the results of their research into the hands and heads of practitioners). It is only comparatively recently that any educational theories of how to learn and teach have helped us make sense of what we have been doing for over ten years. More importantly, it is only in the last 5 years that we have realised that having a theoretical basis to the teaching we do makes planning sessions and courses easier, and our efforts more valuable.

We have found five approaches to learning and teaching to be particularly useful: adult learning theory (Knowles et al 1984); self-directed learning (Candy 1991); problem-based learning (Wood 2003); self-efficacy (Bandura 1986); and reflective practice (Schön 1987). It would be great if we could honestly state that we organise these individual theories into a coherent framework. The truth is that our approach is somewhat more pragmatic. The deployment of each as the basis for planned learning is primarily a function of the educational levels, clinical experience, and 'raw materials' that we have to work with (e.g. sessions based around appraising research papers verses discussions of ethics). So, problem-based learning works well with degree students who are faced with a treatment or diagnostic decision situation and some research evidence to critically appraise and incorporate into their judgements and choices. A discussion of the ethics of screening choices as continuing professional development with experienced nurses lends itself more to reflective approaches and promotion of self-efficacy.

It is beyond the scope of this book to examine these theories in detail. It is helpful, however, to sketch out the main elements of the theories as they apply to learning and teaching in the context of promoting clinical decision-making skills.

ADULT LEARNING THEORY

The aim of adult learning theory (Knowles et al 1984) is to produce learners who have a degree of independence and self-direction; clearly, traits that are required for informed decision makers. The approach makes five assumptions about the learners:

1. Adults are independent and self-directing.

2. Learners accumulate rich banks of experience; this is a rich resource for learning.
3. Students value learning that integrates with the demands of their everyday life.
4. Adult learners are more interested in immediate, problem-centred approaches than in subject-centred ones.
5. It is internal drivers that provide the motivation to learn rather than external ones.

With these assumptions in mind, we try to weave six principles into our lesson planning:

1. We stress the need to make learners feel comfortable and safe expressing themselves. This sounds like 'motherhood and apple pie' but the truth is that clinical decision making is a professional skill and as professionals ('in action' or 'in waiting') nurses often feel dubious about making choices, and providing a rationale for those choices in the presence of others.
2. We try to involve learners in planning the curriculum for a course, module, or session. Clearly, we are teachers and it would be a poor show if we imparted no new knowledge to students by the end of a session. However, breaking down their clinical practice and involving the students in identifying and explaining their own knowledge needs is a great starting point for delivery. Involving students in identifying their own needs also helps foster internal motivation.
3. We ask learners to draft their own learning objectives. The aim is to foster a sense of control over their learning. It also helps us know when milestones (or at least the student's milestones) have been achieved – or not.
4. We steer students towards identifying resources for learning and to work out strategies for using these that fit with their objectives and ours. An example would be the use of websites to search for synopses of research, such as the journal *Evidence-Based Nursing* (www.ebn.bmj.com). Students often worry that simply searching for a key word (such as 'leg ulcers') is not sufficient – some of them might have experienced PubMed or Medline searching in the past. By getting them to reflect on the information *source* (a collection of pre-appraised research) it usually becomes clear that using the resource in ways that would be woefully inadequate in PubMed is acceptable in this particular context.
5. We try to support students in the execution of their learning plans. With the advent of computerised virtual learning environments, this means that we can encourage students to 'blog' their problems and the 'work rounds' they devise. Doing this provides us with a window into the variations in the performance in the group and enables us to point students in the direction of other students who can help. The teaching function helps the more able student learn as well. This kind of coordination was far more difficult when we simply relied on face-to-face teaching, which makes it easier for less able students to 'hide' in a class.
6. Finally, we ask students to appraise and evaluate their own learning. This is usually a useful exercise in critical reflection but also acts as a means of stopping the group defaulting to the level of the 'average'.

SELF-DIRECTED LEARNING

Again, like 'adult learning', this is more of an approach than a full-blown theory. The overall aim is to produce decision makers that feel able to take responsibility for their learning, autonomy (and the responsibilities that come with it) and choices. Candy (1991) developed a series of composite traits that he felt were associated with being self-directed: being methodical and disciplined, logical and analytical, collaborative, curious and motivated, persistent and responsible, being a confident learner, and being self-aware or reflective.

For us, the typical evidence-based process of formulating a clinical question, searching for research, critically appraising it, and planning for implementation (Cullum et al 2008) is the perfect vehicle for fostering these skills. The sequential and reflective nature of each stage (e.g. Is this question likely to be answerable? Is this an effective search strategy? How valid is this evidence? What do the results mean? Is this statistically significant, clinically significant, both or neither?) mean that progress is stepped, has checks and balances, involves personal thresholds before taking action and is linked to meaningful choices and context (the questions and planned actions arise from clinical uncertainties).

PROBLEM-BASED LEARNING

Building on theories of adult learning and self-direction is the more formalised process (and associated theoretical framework) of problem-based learning (PBL), which can be thought of as a means of learning in which:

" Students use 'triggers' from a problem case or scenario to define their own learning objectives. Subsequently they do independent, self-directed study before returning to the group to discuss and refine their acquired knowledge. (Wood 2003) "

We find PBL useful for developing skills particularly suited to team or collective decision making – a characteristic of many nursing care environments. Skills such as teamwork; chairing a group; self-directed learning and use of resources; listening; presentation skills; cooperation and respect for colleagues' views based on the evidence presented in support of planned choices are all well served by the PBL approach.

We build PBL sessions around a key clinical scenario and seven key steps (Wood 2003; Box 15.1).

A key component of any PBL session is the clinical scenario to be used as the 'problem trigger'. We compare our scenarios against a seven-point checklist (Wood 2003; Box 15.2).

SELF-EFFICACY

As you will have gathered, many of the approaches we use (developing scenarios 'backwards' from evidence; the stepwise exposure to key stages in evidence-based practice; use of appraisal for thinking critically rather than

Box 15.1 Seven steps in a PBL session (adapted from Wood 2003)

Step 1: identifying and clarifying unfamiliar material in the scenario; one of the learners (the 'scribe') writes down or records any issues that remain unexplained after discussion

Step 2: defining the problem or problems to be discussed; there is usually a variety of views expressed by students and all need to be considered by the group. Again, the scribe records the group's list of agreed problems

Step 3: 'brainstorming' the problem(s); encourage students to suggest possible rationales based on their pre-existing knowledge. Students 'feed off each other' by drawing on each other's knowledge and identifying areas of incomplete knowledge; again, the scribe records all of the debate

Step 4: reviewing steps 2 and 3; arrange explanations into tentative solutions. Scribe organises the explanations and restructures if necessary

Step 5: formulating learning objectives and then encouraging the group to reach consensus on the learning objectives; the PBL tutor ensures learning objectives are focused, achievable, comprehensive, and appropriate

Step 6: private study. In this stage, all the students gather their own information related to each learning objective

Step 7: sharing of the group results of private study; this is our opportunity to check learning against the goals we have as tutors. Any assessment we do of the group we do at this stage

Box 15.2 Checklist for clinical scenarios

1. Are the learning objectives defined by the students after studying the scenario likely to be consistent with *our* learning objectives?
2. Are the problem(s) in the scenario appropriate given the stage of the curriculum and the level of the students' understanding and experiential knowledge base?
3. Are the scenarios interesting enough for the students (given where they are now) and will they have relevance to their future practice?
4. Have we paid enough attention to presenting conceptual or abstract concepts (risk, number needed to treat (NNT), likelihood ratios, sensitivity, etc.) in the context of a clinical scenario? Our aim is to encourage integration of knowledge into decision making and this is nigh on impossible if key concepts remain divorced from context and choices.
5. Do the scenarios contain sufficient cues to stimulate discussion and encourage students to seek explanations for the issues presented?
6. Is the problem sufficiently open? If a problem is too narrow then discussion is curtailed too early in the process and any benefits negated.
7. Do the scenarios promote participation by the students by allowing them to seek useful information from various learning resources? A tip for teachers here is to 'reverse engineer' evidence-based synopses (e.g. www.ebn.bmj.com) and syntheses (e.g. Cochrane Library) and base a question on the (evidence-based) answers. Whilst this is categorically *not* how to use evidence in practice – it is handy for teaching and generating some positive learning feedback for students.

purely for assessing the validity, results and applicability of research; group work and cooperative learning) are designed to build students' confidence in their ability to deal with differing decision situations (self-efficacy).

The four key weapons in our armoury are:

1. Students' sense of achieving desired performance (theirs and ours).
2. Watching others 'walking the walk' and learning by doing.
3. Providing a sound scientific, epidemiological, logical or just relevant persuasive argument for why we are doing what we are doing.
4. Making students aware that being nervous or anxious is an aid to successful performance and not a hindrance – even evidence-based practice can be exciting.

Bandura (1969) suggests that if we get it right we can heighten students' sense of self-efficacy. The flip-side of course is that if we fail then our efforts are detrimental. We see our role as five-fold in relation to developing self-efficacy in our learners:

1. Demonstrating decision-making skills.
2. Clearly and unambiguously specifying the outcomes and goals we want to see in students.
3. Giving students the basic 'building block' knowledge and skills to enable skills such as integration of research evidence into decision making.
4. Allowing students access to guided practice with corrective feedback – sometime using simulations (Thompson et al 2005).
5. Providing students with the chance to reflect on their development during and after their training.

REFLECTION AND DECISION MAKING

The 'swampy lowlands' (Schön 1987) of professional practice often bear little resemblance to the classroom. The high noise-to-signal ratio of a ward or clinic; a lack of feedback on judgements and choices; social pressures and structures that interfere with our sense of self-efficacy; and the pressure to perform, with sanctions for those who are perceived to fail, all serve to increase the gap between 'theory' and 'practice'. Reflection is an overworked expression in nurse education (on a single day in 2007, during breaks in teaching, one of us walked past a lecture theatre at an unnamed university. Of the four available sessions in the day, 3 were remarkable for having PowerPoint slides up with the heading 'reflection' on). Despite its ubiquitous presence, Donald Schön's ideas are still of relevance to teaching decision making.

We strive to expose nurses to two kinds of reflection on our courses. The first, 'reflection in action', is fostered by giving nurses new and unfamiliar tasks and asking them to use the knowledge and experience they already have. A simple example of this kind of reflection is to ask nurses who are parents whether they would be willing to let their child take a drug that had been tested on only 10 people and for which the evidence for its effect were the anectdotes provided by those who took it, or would they prefer the drug that had been tested on 10,000 randomly selected people who were followed up for 3 years and compared with a different, randomly selected group of 10,000 people given a sugar pill. Very little scientific knowledge is required to provide an intuitive answer. However, going on to build an explanation as to *why* you prefer the second option is the trigger for motivation and self-directed learning.

The second approach, 'reflection on action', usually takes place after a session or spell in clinical practice. We have already seen that the negative effects of heuristics can be combated by asking ourselves questions such as, 'are there other contributory factors that might have led to the outcome?' and how might the situation have turned out differently?' The same is true of gleaning the benefits from experience.

All of these approaches offer a broad theoretical foundation for the specific areas of clinical decision making and judgement we will outline now.

TEACHING STRATEGIES

Understanding the difference between judgements and decisions

Learning outcomes

- Define the terms 'judgement' and decision.
- Give examples of judgements and decisions.
- Identify judgements and decisions in clinical situations.

Rationale

As was highlighted in Chapter 5, the process of clinical reasoning involves both judgements (assessments of alternatives) and decisions (choosing between alternatives). The two processes involve different types of cognitive process, and the analysis and integration of different types of information. We therefore find it useful at the beginning of a module to ensure that students understand the difference between clinical judgements and clinical decisions. This separation of the two concepts enables students to analyse (later on) how they use information for the two different types of task.

Suggested exercises

We use two approaches to explore the concept of judgements and decisions, depending on the level of clinical experience of the students we are teaching. Nursing and medical students at undergraduate level, with limited clinical experience, often find it difficult to identify and explain a clinical scenario in enough detail to fully explore the concepts of judgements and decisions. We provide this group of students with predefined clinical scenarios. For more experienced students with more clinical experience (normally postgraduate students), we would construct clinical scenarios using examples from their practice. We often do this in groups, asking each individual to identify one scenario where they think the outcome was good, and another where the outcome was bad, and describe it to their fellow group members. As a group they are then asked to choose one example of each type of scenario to describe fully to the rest of the class. In groups, we ask students to identify:

- What actions they would take/have taken and why.
- What information they have based these actions on.

What normally happens is that students can identify actions (decisions) and often justify them using their assessment of a patient (judgements). They will often also give you a list of information on which their assessments (judgements) were based. We use the feedback from the groups to explore the concepts of judgements and decisions, giving formal definitions of each. We also explore the way in which judgements often feed into decision making, and the role of information in making assessments/judgements and informing decision choices.

Exploring the process of clinical decision making and judgement

Learning outcomes

- Define different approaches to the study of judgement and decision making (descriptive, normative, prescriptive).
- Outline the process of clinical reasoning.
- Define the terms 'expert' and 'expertise'.
- Compare the process of clinical reasoning (as above) to the description of judgement outlined by cognitive continuum theory (CCT).

Rationale

As we saw in Chapter 5, there are various different approaches to the study of clinical decision making and judgement, and a number of different descriptive theories that have been developed to describe how clinicians reach clinical judgements. In this set of exercises we are trying to illustrate to students how there are a number of different possible explanations for the same phenomena (and therefore no right answer!). We also try to identify that although there are these different explanations, there are also some commonalities across the different theories (e.g. intuitive reasoning, analytical reasoning, the role of experience and knowledge in decision making).

Exercises

Again, the way that we approach this topic varies depending on the experience level of the nurses we are teaching. With less experienced students, you will probably have to use a predefined case scenario/study. With more experienced students, you could either use a more sophisticated case study or ask them to describe in detail a clinical scenario from their own practice, which you can use as the basis for the exercises.

There are a number of ways in which the case study/scenario can be used to help students explore different approaches to clinical judgement and decision making. These include:

- On the basis of a full description of a patient case, write down the processes that they think they have used to reach certain judgements and decisions (either individually or in groups).
- Give the students a brief outline of a patient case and encourage them to ask for further information or describe what their next actions would be. Write down what questions they ask, and what decisions they make. You can then have a discussion with students about how they have reached their conclusions and factors that influenced their decisions.
- Ask students to 'think aloud' as they try to make judgements and decisions about a patient case scenario (see Lee & Ryan-Wegner 1997 for a full description of this approach). In this type of approach students would ask for further information or state a decision action, providing a rationale at the time for why they are doing so. This approach requires a detailed scenario where you can release information incrementally, and someone to scribe what a student is discussing in detail.
- Play students a video of an interaction between a nurse and patient, and ask them to write down all the judgements and decisions they can identify during the encounter and any obvious reasoning processes they can identify that the nurse has used.

The purpose of all of the above is to encourage students to move beyond identifying judgements and decisions and the information they use, to examine *how* such information is combined and integrated into judgements and decisions. It also encourages students to begin to think through the reasoning processes they may use, and the basis for their judgement and decision making. Depending on the level of expertise of the students, they will probably describe the hypothetico-deductive reasoning approach, and may possibly also refer to intuition or similar. We often split students into groups and ask them to define what they consider an expert to be, and also how they would define expertise, which we then include within wider discussions stimulated by the case study. Finally, we put a slide up illustrating the cognitive continuum and explain its premises, before asking them (in groups) to list what they think the similarities and differences are between the reasoning processes they have identified they use, and the tenets of CCT.

The concept of error

Learning outcomes

- To be able to distinguish between errors, slips and lapses and to explain the role of planning in decision errors.
- Outline the main causes of errors in the individual.
- Outline the main systemic causes of errors.
- Plan a strategy to reduce errors in their own clinical practice.

Rationale

The potential for errors will always be a feature of clinical decision making. Nurses are at the forefront of efforts to improve governance, quality, and patient safety, and their judgements and choices matter. We link errors (patient safety) and decision making because it is decisions and judgements that often act as the crucible in which latent and active conditions for failure (Reason 2000) come together.

The main obstacle to teaching the prevention of errors is the same as in clinical practice: how to provide sufficient feedback to make errors 'visible' to the decision maker. If feedback is not presented then learning from, or training for, errors and error reduction will always be an abstract process.

Exercises

The most powerful exercises are the most interactive. When you have a large group to teach (> 100) you can utilise the power of large samples and conduct some of the classic 'experiments' of Kahneman and Tversky (Tversky & Kahneman 1974). Plous' (1993) text on the psychology of decision making is a rich source of such experiments in a more accessible form than the originals. Some of the most popular (actually, not popular, but effective) exercises we do with students include variations of the overconfidence test in Box 7.3 (p. 113). Sometimes we let students choose a colleague to help them 'guesstimate' the answers. They still get less than 90% correct. The other 'serious' interactive exercise we often find useful is a derivation of the classic 'confusion of the inverse' probability of Eddy's mammogram question:

> " A says she feels unnaturally tired and listless after her first child. In your experience, this means there's a 1 in 100 chance that she may be depressed. She fills in the Edinburgh Postnatal Depression Scale. This accurately classifies roughly 80% of depressed women and 90% of non-depressed women.
> Q1. (for one half of the group) What would you say the woman's chances of being depressed are?
> Q2. (for second half of group) Given your prior belief that she had a 1% chance and test results that are only 80–90% reliable what would you say the chances of depression are? "

What you hope for is that: (1) both groups get it wrong; and (2) the first group provides higher estimates than the second. In our experience, the first group will suggest around 75% and the second around 60% (the correct answer is *circa* 7 or 8%). Both groups usually get it wrong and this gives you an opening to discuss diagnostic reasoning.

These are fairly serious and advanced exercises but sometimes we just want to achieve the task of making everyone feel comfortable and safe talking about errors, and human propensities to use information in certain ways. This next task is CCT's 'killer' crowd stopper; however, after 10 years of using it in teaching it is time to pass on the secret!

1. Think of a number between 10 and 20.
2. Add the two digits together.
3. Subtract the new number away from the first number (between 10 and 20) you thought of.
4. Subtract 5 from this.

5. Convert the number you are thinking of to a letter... so if you are thinking of 1 it's A, 2 is B, 3 is C, etc.
6. Now, think of a country that begins with the letter you are thinking of.
7. Now, the second letter of that country - think of an animal that begins with that letter.

So long as you have a few people in the class, the effect is dramatic. Most people give the 'right' answers (see Answers on page 265 at the end of this chapter). If you do this in Australia however, be aware that many people will say emu rather than elephant. Why? Because the trick relies on simple maths and the availability heuristic; for most Europeans the knowledge that is easiest to recall for a task in which the country must begin with D is Denmark. Again, this is lots of fun, but gives you a window through which to begin to talk about heuristics and bias and availability in particular. I often then go on to explore with learners those examples of knowledge that are easy to recall but which prove to be erroneous when examined systematically: concentrated oxygen administration for neonates for example.

These exercises tend to focus on the individual and of course are devoid of much clinical context (although of course you can pull context into the discussions that follow them). To introduce the notion of errors in systems into the group, one exercise that we have found very useful is to provide a clinical scenario. If you want an exemplar that is designed for this job then reports such as 'To err is human' (Institute of Medicine 2000) or 'Organisation with a memory' (Department of Health 2000) have plenty that can be adapted for the classroom. Depending on the experience of the group and the time available we will ask them to first – as individuals – classify errors, slips, lapses, and mistakes. Then we will get them as a group to share their classifications. If we are talking about agreement or variability between clinicians, we may (following a 'mini lecture') get them to calculate kappa (a measure of agreement beyond chance) and talk about what this means at this point. We will, however, also have discussions about the causes of the errors and mistakes identified. If time allows or we have a couple of sessions, we will introduce some tools to help the group identify the causative factors in the system. Short sessions can utilise tools such as the '5 whys' (www.sdo.nihr.ac.uk/files/adhoc/change-management-booklet.pdf) and longer sessions will allow students to learn about and begin to make use of more detailed approaches such as root cause analysis (www.msnpsa.nhs.uk/rcatoolkit/course/iindex.htm).

All of these avoid asking people to 'talk about mistakes that they have made'. In our experience, this rarely works and only succeeds in making people feel really uncomfortable. The exercise – with enough clinical context injected – is close enough to clinical practice to have some meaning and encourage personal reflection on their own practices and errors.

Clinical decision analysis

Learning outcomes

- Give examples of decision situations that would be suitable for a clinical decision analysis.

- Construct a decision tree for a clinical decision.
- Identify probabilities from appropriate research literature or subjective estimations.
- Describe methods for eliciting patient utilities.
- Populate a decision tree with probabilities and utilities.
- Calculate a simple decision analysis and identify the most appropriate course of action.
- Carry out a simple sensitivity analysis on a decision tree.
- Summarise the advantages and disadvantages of using clinical decision analysis as a way of assisting clinical decision making in nursing.

Rationale

As discussed in Chapter 11, clinical decision analysis is one approach that can be used as a way of assisting nurses to make decisions for specific types of clinical problem. As an approach, it has a number of benefits, including encouraging nurses to think through different decision options, encouraging them to identify appropriate research evidence to help inform their decisions, and explicitly encouraging them to think about the implications of specific decisions for patients. We have found that teaching nurses the techniques of clinical decision analysis encourages them to think about their decision making in a different way, giving them an entirely different outlook on their clinical practice. We encourage them to think about decision analysis as one technique they can use (for some types of decision) to help them talk through decision options with patients. Often, just the process of structuring a decision in the form of a decision tree helps both nurses and patients clarify their thinking about a specific decision task.

Exercises

We have taught decision analysis using a combination of lectures and group work and more recently as an interactive module using our university's virtual learning environment. In both approaches most of the teaching is focused on students working either individually or in groups to construct their own clinical decision analysis. We give them a decision problem which should: be detailed enough for them to identify appropriate decision options; reflect a decision scenario with genuine uncertainty (i.e. it isn't clear what the optimum decision should be) and where there are potential risk/benefit trade-offs that patients need to be aware of for different decision options. We then get students to complete the following tasks:

1. Construct a decision tree (identifying different decision options and the potential outcomes that could result from each option).
2. Identify the probability or likelihood of each outcome occurring, using published evidence where available or subjective assessments (where it isn't). We often use this process as a way of reflecting on the potential problems of using subjective assessments (such as overconfidence and the influence of heuristics). Students often find the identification of probabilities from research evidence problematic; sometimes this is

because they need to think through what information they actually need, and sometimes it is because of the difficulties of translating the results of studies (which may be given in the form of odds ratios or mean differences) into probability estimates. Where possible, we encourage students to look for raw data tables of the occurrence of events, and get them to calculate their own probabilities. They also need to identify the range of possible values (for sensitivity analysis), which requires an understanding of confidence intervals.

3. Populate the decision tree with appropriate probability estimates.
4. Elicit utilities for the different outcomes in their tree using an established method (such as a standard gamble). We give them a worksheet to use as a guide for this, and ask them to elicit utilities from a friend or family member (not patients!). This exercise will often stimulate a lot of discussion about how we measure utility and what it is that the different methods are measuring. If carried out in a group, it often becomes clear that different group members have different utilities for the same outcome, which we use as the basis for a discussion about the importance of recognising the variation in patient utility.
5. Populate the decision tree with appropriate utility estimates.
6. Calculate the decision tree and identify the 'best' option (should be the branch with the highest value).
7. Carry out a sensitivity analysis, in which students vary the figures in their decision tree and see what effect it has on the optimum decision.

Students normally need a lot of support to carry out these tasks. However, by the end of the process they are normally able to discuss what they see as the potential benefits and limitations of such an approach to clinical decision making.

The process of diagnosis

We should state at the outset that we don't teach 'diagnosis', as in history taking, physical examination, forming differentials, and offering a diagnostic label. Partly, this is because we are not clinically skilled or medical doctors, nor do we have enough knowledge of particular health conditions. We teach diagnostic *reasoning*, which is about knowing the value of information and using that information alongside our own experience and research evidence to make diagnostic judgements. We do, however, work alongside skilled clinicians to develop educational programmes designed to help clinical staff in particular disciplines: heart failure, palliative care, and critical care outreach.

Learning outcomes

• Be able to integrate the concepts of prevalence (and prior probability), sensitivity, specificity, positive, and negative predictive value into diagnostic reasoning.

- Be able to demonstrate Bayesian probability revision 'on the fly' for some simulated clinical problems, e.g. prior x likelihood ratio = posterior.
- Successfully develop and use 2 × 2 tables and likelihood ratio nomograms.

Rationale

One author (CT) wrote an article for a nursing journal in which the prevalence of urinary tract infections was altered in an attempt to illustrate how test performance (post-test probability) alters in different clinical settings even though sensitivity and specificity stays the same. The reviewer scrutinising the paper refused point blank to believe that a test could produce differing values in differing clinical contexts ('Otherwise how could they get it licensed?'). Nurses need to know about the clinical epidemiology behind the process of being confronted with disparate information (signs, symptoms) and having to classify patients into groups as a basis for action appropriate for the group they are in: the process of diagnosis.

With the advent of nurse practitioners and nurse prescribing, nurses are beginning to 'diagnose' in the legal and medical sense of classifying people into disease groups. However, even those nurses without the medical responsibility of diagnosing use diagnostic reasoning. At the formalised end of diagnostic activity there are the various approaches to nursing diagnosis www.nanda.org/ and www.acendio.net/. At the informal end, however, nurses classify patients into groups in practice based on the information they see, hear, and feel every day.

Although we are beginning to teach nurses procedures such as physical examination and the clinical necessity of tests for 'assessment' (e.g. Doppler readings in leg ulcer assessment or the MMSE in elder assessment in A&E), we have a much weaker history of teaching nurses about the clinical *value* of such tests. The MMSE in primary care settings, using standardized diagnostic instruments (e.g. the DSM-IV) as a 'gold standard' has a sensitivity of between 71 and 92%, and specificity from 56 to 96%. The predictive value of a positive test, in a population with 10% prevalence of dementia, might range from 15 to 72%. Moreover, its accuracy depends on the age, education, and ethnicity of the individual; it is most accurate for white individuals who have at least a high-school education (www.ahrq.gov/clinic/3rduspstf/dementia/dementrr.htm).

GENERAL POINTS

The focus of our teaching is not to teach students *how* to reason, but more to help them understand the different *ways* that they might reason, and to provide them with a variety of different strategies for using information more systematically or appropriately to inform their judgement and decision making. We feel it is important to emphasise the variety of different ways that judgement and decision making can be described and analysed. However, just as important is the need to highlight that for specific judgement and decision tasks taking a more analytical approach may be beneficial; both for their patients *and* for them. If nothing else, using techniques such as decision analysis or calculating the potential benefits or a diagnostic test will enable nurses to *explain* and *justify* how they have reached their decisions in a more coherent and evidence based way.

Exercises

Let us separate out diagnostic reasoning from the background knowledge or 'building blocks' (sensitivity, positive predictive value, likelihood ratios) required for making 'foreground' (Sackett et al 2000) diagnostic decisions.

Table 15.1 illustrates some of the strategies we use with clinical teachers (expert nurse practitioners or doctors training nurses) and learners to foster the skills needed to manage diagnostic uncertainty. You will note that there are few (if any) 'evidence-based' concepts involved. This framework is about breaking down the initial 'startled bunny' reaction of learners when confronted with the sheer amounts of information and uncertainty in a diagnostic decision situation into something altogether more manageable. When learners are comfortable with the stepwise approach to diagnosis, you can begin to introduce concepts that will help them attach appropriate weights to the information (test results, signs, symptoms, prevalence, and priors) they are faced with. We based the framework on the similar needs of novice doctors to acquire diagnostic reasoning skills (Bowen 2006). This is designed around a group-learning environment (e.g. a simulation with a patient-actor or a clinical teaching 'round' or clinic.

The final question of Table 15.1 ('how did you rule it out?') introduces the idea of the 'value' of information in diagnostic decision problems.

The only real way we have found to get students to grasp the relationship between patient characteristics, prior beliefs, the properties of 'tests', and the 'performance' of those tests (i.e. post-test probability) is to guide students through the five techniques for diagnostic reasoning in Chapter 9. Although some students are more attuned to specific techniques than others, in our experience almost all students prefer the nomogram approach. The crucial thing here is to make sure that the techniques are all applied to the same scenario or patient problem. The aim is to get students familiar with the techniques to the point where they become part of their reasoning, rather than to apply them to lots of different conditions; only some of which will have been experienced.

We have found that giving students a hands-on series of 2×2 calculations in which the prevalence is changed (Figure 15.1) and then asking them to report on *how* they revised their ideas to the group and explain *why* is helpful in steering students towards and intuitive approach to handling information on the value of a 'test'.

ANSWERS

You were thinking of 'Denmark' and 'elephant'.

Table 15.1 A framework for fostering diagnostic reasoning in learners

Diagnostic reasoning skill	'Clues' in learners	What's wrong	Educational strategy	Example
Acquiring data and reporting to colleagues	Learner's presentation to the group lacks important information	The learner has failed to spot what is important, to obtain important information, or both.	Use a clinical expert to model the acquisition of clinically important findings to the learner and ask the learner to present the findings again	'Have a look at Nurse Consultant X's history and exam taking. Look at the things he or she does that are particularly good for extracting information. Now let's discuss what you saw'
Problem 'sense making'	Disorganised presentation or discussion of findings (or both) The 'summing up' by the student bears only a loose resemblance to the case	Student has no experience with the clinical problem or lacks a 'conceptual' approach to it (i.e. has not done their homework). The student has not adequately found a way of making sense (representing) of the diagnostic problem, lacks coherence in their understanding of the case, or both	Ask the expert to think aloud when eliciting important findings in order to link important findings to expert problem representation. Having explained the importance of representing diagnostic problems, ask the student to summarise findings in two or three sentences and compare it to an expert's version	'Now we've had a look at the findings you think are important, let's think together about how they point to type II diabetes. I'm thinking about type 2 diabetes because…' 'Concise and accurate problem representation is a critical stage in generating differential diagnoses. Can you give me a couple of sentences summarising this case? Here's how I think it might look'
Generating diagnosis hypotheses; selecting the appropriate 'script' given the case	Lots of provisional diagnoses offered with no sense of likelihood or priority Discussion of differential	Learner has not identified a way of making sense of the problem or an appropriate script (organised set of knowledge) given the data. Either the learner has failed to identify a script for the data they are faced with or	Ask student to: (1) list important findings; (2) create a representation of potential diagnostic problems using selected findings; (3) prioritise diagnostic approaches that are most likely to identify discriminating features for each diagnostic problem being considered.	'What are the main findings? Can you summarise these? What are the diagnostic considerations for type 2 diabetes? Why?' 'What are your primary and secondary diagnoses? What features of this patient help you discriminate between them?'

	diagnoses not linked to the data in the case	they are unable to compare and contrast the scripts they are working with	Ask the learner to support the diagnosis being offered with reference to the findings from the case (the easy bit), now ask for an alternative plausible diagnosis and have the student compare it with other plausible diagnoses. You might also venture your own (or an expert's) analysis of the case	
Cognitive feedback	Diagnoses are far fetched	Learner has poor understanding of the case or has failed to grasp and use notions of relative probability (rare and common cases)	Ask the student to describe a prototypical presentation for the diagnosis ventured and explicitly to compare prototypical findings with data derived from the case. Identify any extra data required to rule in the diagnosis	'What is the classic presentation for type 2 diabetes? What findings in this case fit this typical presentation? Are there enough key features to carry on down this line of reasoning? What other information do you need?'
Developmental stage	Presentation or reasoning below the expected level for a common problem	Learner has not created an appropriate 'anchor' (prototype of likely conditions), lacks experience with kinds of presenting patient or a combination of both	Ascertain true levels of student experience with this kind of patient. Identify patients who fit the typical presentation of a problem and make sure the student cares for them; make sure students always compare their hunches (i.e. initial diagnosis) with at least one plausible alternative and spell out the discriminating information present or required	'Have you looked after other patients with type II diabetes? What do you remember about those patients? I want you to go away and read up on depression (based on the notion that depression is a plausible alternative). Identify key and discriminating features and tomorrow tell me what you have learned'

Continued

Table 15.1 A framework for fostering diagnostic reasoning in learners—Cont'd

Diagnostic reasoning skill	'Clues' in learners	What's wrong	Educational strategy	Example
Contextual awareness	Disorganised presentation of a complex and ill-defined problem. Evidence of varying levels of understanding within the group	The learner might have multiple working diagnoses in their 'problem space' and risks overload or prematurely 'closing' on a diagnosis or both. The ability to reason is a function of experience (with cases) as well as stage in training. Within the group, there is likely to be a broad spread of experience even if stage of training is held constant	Ask student to identify and defend primary and secondary diagnoses with reference to discriminating features; show the student your own (or expert) clinical reasoning for the case and how you made sense of the problem. Show and tell: ask two or three other learners to bring their problem representations to the session. Use questioning to ascertain levels of expertise; get the more 'expert' ones to reason aloud; again, spell out your own (or a true expert's) reasoning	'Tell me how your primary diagnosis is supported by the clinical findings.' 'Choose a reasonable alternative diagnosis and tell me why it does not fit the clinical findings.' (Repeat for each plausible diagnostic representation.) [Then ask the group] 'Does anyone have a different problem representation?' [Ask the most experienced student or staff member: 'Tell us your primary diagnosis and how is it supported by the clinical findings. Did you consider any other diagnosis and if so how did you rule it out?']

Adapted from Bowen (2006).

Prevalence = 10/1000 = 0.01 (PPV 0.06, NPV 0.99, LR+ 7.42, LR– 0.11)

	Truth		
	Yes	No	
Positive test	9	120	Total who test positive
Negative test	1	870	Total who test negative
	Total with condition	Total without condition	Total sample

Prevalence = 300/1000 = 0.30 (PPV 0.76, NPV 0.95, LR= 7.41, LR– 0.11)

	Truth		
	Yes	No	
Positive test	270	85	Total who test positive
Negative test	30	615	Total who test negative
	Total with condition	Total without condition	Total sample

Prevalence = 500/1000 = 0.50 (PPV 0.88, NPV 0.89, LR+ 7.37, LR– 0.11)

	Truth		
	Yes	No	
Positive test	450	61	Total who test positive
Negative test	50	439	Total who test negative
	Total with condition	Total without condition	Total sample

NB: Get the students to work out the maths **AND** tell us what it means for their decision making

Figure 15.1 The effect of changing prevalence.

RESOURCES

We have identified a number of resources that we find useful to assist us with our teaching. As well as this book(!) and the references specifically mentioned in this chapter, these include:

Higgs J, Jones M 2000 Clinical reasoning in the health professions, 2nd edn. Butterworth Heinemann, Oxford UK. *This book has a number of chapters addressing different ways of teaching clinical reasoning.*

Hunink M, Glasziou P, Siegel J et al 2001 Decision making in health and medicine. Integrating evidence and values. Cambridge University Press, Cambridge UK. *An excellent text that outlines the stages of clinical decision analysis that can be used as the basis for teaching the process to students. Has a number of exercises.*

Straus S E, Richardson W S, Glasziou P et al 2005 Evidence based medicine: how to practise and teach EBM, 3rd edn. Elsevier, London. *The excellent teaching methods chapter is a good resource for planning courses and avoiding common pitfalls. The fact that it is written for doctors does not matter for this chapter.*

www.treeage.com/*A decision analysis software package that can be used to construct and calculate decision trees. Has a 30-day trial download that students can use to help them with the process. Students do need to be reasonably computer literate to make full use of the program.*

The excellent 'tips for teachers' series in the Canadian Medical Association Journal (CMAJ) has tips for teaching evidence-based medicine but these are often directly relevant to teaching decision making generally. All the pdfs can be accessed here: www.pgme.utoronto.ca/Resources/CanMEDS/Scholar.htm

A nice resource for cognitive errors is the 'Thinker': http://cat.xula.edu/thinker/ decisions/heuristics/ by Bart Everson & Elliott Hammer. This is a fairly interactive on-line set of tools for understanding common heuristics and bias.

REFERENCES

Bandura A 1969 Social learning of moral judgments. Journal of Personality and Social Psychology 11:275–279

Bandura A 1986 Social foundations of thought and action: a social cognitive theory. Prentice-Hall, Englewood Cliffs, NJ

Bowen J L 2006 Educational strategies to promote clinical diagnostic reasoning. The New England Journal of Medicine 355:2217–2225

Candy P C. 1991 Self-direction for lifelong learning: a comprehensive guide to theory and practice. Jossey-Bass, San Francisco

Christie A, Worley P, Jones M 2000 The Internet and clinical reasoning. In: Higgs J, Jones M (eds) Clinical reasoning in the health professions, 2nd edn. Butterworth Heinemann, Oxford UK, p 148–155

Cullum N, Ciliska D, Marks S et al 2008 An introduction to evidence based nursing. In: Cullum N, Ciliska D, Haynes B et al (eds) Evidence based nursing. Blackwell, London, p 1–8

Department of Health 2000 Organisation with a memory. HMSO, London

Institute of Medicine 2000 To err is human: building a safer health system. National Academy Press, Washington, DC

Knowles M S and associates 1984 Andragogy in action: applying modern principles of adult learning. Jossey-Bass, San Francisco

Lee J, Ryan-Wegner N 1997 The 'think aloud' seminar for teaching clinical reasoning: a case study of a child with pharyngitis. Journal of Pediatric Health Care 11(3):101–110

Plous S 1993 The psychology of judgment and decision making. McGraw Hill, New York

Reason J 2000 Human error: models and management. British Medical Journal 320:768–770

Sackett D, Straus S E, Richardson W S et al 2000 Evidence based medicine – how to practice and teach EBM, 2nd edn. Churchill Livingstone, London

Schön D A 1987 Educating the reflective practitioner: toward a new design for teaching and learning in the professions. Jossey-Bass, San Francisco

Thompson C A, Foster A, Cole I et al 2005 Using social judgement theory to model nurses' use of clinical information in critical care education. Nurse Education Today 25:68–77

Tversky A, Kahneman D 1974 Judgment under uncertainty: heuristics and biases. Science 185:1124–1131

Wood D F 2003 ABC of learning and teaching in medicine: problem based learning. British Medical Journal 326: 328–330

INDEX

Index

INDEX

3